Health and Medicine at Sea, 1700–1900

Maritime medicine, together with its links to the development of empire, is a burgeoning area of historical interest and enquiry. This book, based on extensive original research, explores the history of health and medicine in maritime and imperial contexts in a key period, reflecting the growing professionalization of medicine at sea from the establishment of the Sick and Hurt Board to the end of the Victorian era. The chapters, written by leading experts in the field, are grouped around two central themes: Royal Naval medical policy, administration and practice; and health and mortality relating to the migration of peoples across the globe, including slavery, emigration and indentured migration. The book will be of interest to a wide range of historians, particularly those working in the fields of maritime history, the history of medicine, and the history of colonialism and imperialism.

Health and Medicine at Sea, 1700–1900

Edited by

David Boyd Haycock and Sally Archer

THE BOYDELL PRESS

First published 2009
The Boydell Press, Woodbridge

ISBN 978–1–84383–522–6

The Boydell Press is an imprint of Boydell & Brewer Ltd
PO Box 9, Woodbridge, Suffolk IP12 3DF, UK
and of Boydell & Brewer Inc.
668 Mount Hope Ave, Rochester, NY 14604, USA
website: www.boydellandbrewer.com

The publisher has no responsibility for the continued existence
or accuracy of URLs for external or third-party internet websites
referred to in this book, and does not guarantee that any content
on such websites is, or will remain, accurate or appropriate.

A CIP catalogue record for this book is available
from the British Library

This publication is printed on acid-free paper

Printed in Great Britain by
CPI Antony Rowe, Chippenham and Eastbourne

Contents

Figures and Tables

Preface

The nine essays collected in this volume are based on 'The British Maritime History Seminars, 2007: Health and Medicine at Sea', convened by the National Maritime Museum, Greenwich. The seminars took place at the Institute of Historical Research (IHR), University of London, from January to June 2007.

Supporting and sponsoring new research into maritime history is a core priority for the National Maritime Museum, as is disseminating this research to a wider audience through publications, exhibitions, online work, and the Museum's conference, lecture and wider educational programme. In 1999 the Museum launched an initiative to establish an annual series of seminars on British maritime history, and enlisted the help of the naval historian Professor N.A.M. Rodger of Exeter University (now at All Souls College, Oxford), and Professor David Cannadine, then Director of the IHR. Together with Dr Margarette Lincoln and Dr Nigel Rigby of the National Maritime Museum, Professors Rodger and Cannadine subsequently became convenors of the newly-formed 'British Maritime History Seminars'. The series has been held at the IHR ever since, and the National Maritime Museum is indebted to the Institute for its continued enthusiasm and support.

The seminars aim to be a platform for the many new approaches being taken in maritime history, by new and established scholars, with each annual series embracing a different theme. Alongside the Museum's broader research programme, the seminars have been instrumental in encouraging an interdisciplinary approach to the subject. Over the years a variety of themes have been explored, from 'Geographies: Mapping Maritime Cultures and Trades' and 'Britain and the Atlantic World', to 'Seapower and Empire' and 'Cultures and Commerce'. Most recently, the themes have been 'The Sea as a Stage: Enacting and Re-enacting Maritime History' (2008) and 'Ship and Shore' (2009).

The 2007 series on 'Health and Medicine at Sea' was particularly successful, due perhaps to the very cohesive nature of its subject matter. It is the first of the British Maritime History Seminar series to be published, but (we hope) not the last. Most of the essays in this volume are based on the actual seminar papers given in the series, although we are indebted to our contributors for their eagerness to seek out and include even newer research.

Finally, I would like to thank Dr John Cardwell for his very helpful advice and assistance when I was programming the original seminar series in 2006.

Sally Archer
March 2009

Contributors

Laurence Brown is Lecturer in Migration History at the University of Manchester. His research has explored how projects for indentured Indian labour were globalized through networks of migration linking the Caribbean, the Indian Ocean and the Pacific. He is currently working on a global history of indenture using GIS to explore the medical regimes and material conditions of the plantation.

M. John Cardwell is Curator of the Royal Commonwealth Society Collection at Cambridge University Library. He is author of *Arts and Arms: Literature, Politics and Patriotism during the Seven Years' War* (2004) and co-author of *Nelson's Surgeon: William Beatty, Naval Medicine and the Battle of Trafalgar* (2005), which received the 2006 prize for best non-clinical medical book from the Royal Society of Medicine and the Society of Authors.

Erica M. Charters is Lecturer in the History of Medicine at the University of Oxford, having previously lectured at the University of Bath Spa and University of Liverpool. Her research examines disease, state power, warfare, and how these intersect in the eighteenth century, especially in colonial contexts. She is currently working on a comparative examination of French warfare, as well as the treatment of prisoners of war during the mid eighteenth century.

Pat Crimmin was Senior Lecturer in History at Royal Holloway, University of London, and Caird Senior Fellow at the National Maritime Museum, 1998–99. She has served on the councils of the Navy Records Society and the Society for Nautical Research, and serves on the editorial board of *The Mariner's Mirror*. She is the author of articles on various aspects of naval administration, as well as biographies in the *Oxford Dictionary of National Biography*. She is currently researching the role of the Sick and Hurt Board, c. 1715–1806, in relation to naval health.

Michael Crumplin is a retired consultant surgeon. He has been a student of medicine in the Republican and Napoleonic Wars for forty years and as a curator and archivist at the College of Surgeons he writes, lectures and advises researchers, authors and the media. He has published three books on early-nineteenth-century military surgery. He is a trustee of the Waterloo Committee and a member of the 2015 commemorative committee.

Robin Haines was formerly Senior Research Fellow at Flinders University of South Australia and is now retired from academic life. She has published widely on migration from the UK to Australia in the nineteenth century, and in recent years has turned her attention to slave, convict, and emigrant health at sea. Her publications include *Emigration and the Labouring Poor* (1997), *Life and Death in the Age of Sail* (2006), *Charles Trevelyan and the Great Irish Famine* (2004), *Doctors at Sea* (2005), and an interactive CD-ROM, *Bound for South Australia* (2004).

Mark Harrison is Professor of the History of Medicine and Director of the Wellcome Unit for the History of Medicine at the University of Oxford. He is the author of numerous books and articles on various aspects of the history of war, commerce, imperialism and medicine. His publications include *Climates and Constitutions: Health, Race, Environment and British Imperialism in India, 1600–1850* (1999) and *Disease and the Modern World: 1500 to the Present Day* (2004).

David Boyd Haycock was Curator of Seventeenth-Century Imperial and Maritime History at the National Maritime Museum between 2007 and 2009. He has held research fellowships at the University of Oxford, the University of California, Los Angeles, and the London School of Economics. He works in the cultural and economic history of science and medicine, and his most recent publication is *Mortal Coil: A Short History of Living Longer* (2008).

Simon J. Hogerzeil is a resident psychiatrist in The Hague, the Netherlands. He is currently working on a PhD thesis in Psychiatric Epidemiology on immigrants' utilization of mental health care. He co-authored the paper on slave mortality featured in this book during his study of medicine at Leiden University, the Netherlands.

Radica Mahase completed an MA in Modern Indian History at Jawaharlal Nehru University, New Delhi, and a PhD in History at the University of the West Indies, St Augustine, Trinidad. She spent one year as a Commonwealth Visiting Scholar at the Centre for the History of Science, Technology and Medicine at the University of Manchester and is currently a part-time lecturer at the Cipriani College of Labour and Co-operative Studies, Trinidad.

Hamish Maxwell-Stewart is an Associate Professor in the School of History and Classics, University of Tasmania. He is the author or co-author of several books on the history of convict transportation to Australia, including *Closing Hell's Gates* (2008), *American Citizens, British Slaves* (2002) and *Chain Letters: Narrating Convict Lives* (2001).

David Richardson is Professor of Economic History and co-founder of the Wilberforce Institute for the study of Slavery and Emancipation, at the University of Hull. He has held visiting positions at Harvard and Yale. The paper published in this volume arises from a project funded by the Wellcome Trust on the relationship between medicine and the Atlantic slave trade.

Ralph Shlomowitz has degrees from the University of Cape Town, the University of the Witwatersrand, the London School of Economics and Political Science, and the University of Chicago where Robert W. Fogel supervised his PhD dissertation on labour arrangements after the Civil War in the USA. He taught at Flinders University in Adelaide, Australia, from 1975 to 2007. In 2004, he was elected a Fellow of the Academy of the Social Sciences in Australia.

Acknowledgements

Simon J. Hogerzeil and David Richardson, 'Slave Purchasing Strategies and Ship-board Mortality: Day-to-Day Evidence from the Dutch African Trade, 1751–1797' was first published in the *Journal of Economic History*, 67, 1 (March 2007), 160–90 © Economic History Association, published by Cambridge University Press.

The editors would like to thank the following for the use of images in the book:

'An amputation performed at St Thomas's Hospital in the mid eighteenth century' and *The Examination of a Young Surgeon* by George Cruickshank appear courtesy of the Royal College of Surgeons.

Wounded after Waterloo by Sir Charles Bell appears courtesy of the Army Medical Services Museum.

'Title and sample pages from Dr Hooper's revision handbook', 'Removal of the arm at the shoulder-joint', 'Above knee amputation and closure of stump after surgery' appear courtesy of Michael Crumplin.

All other images appear courtesy of the National Maritime Museum, Greenwich.

Abbreviations

ADM	Admiralty records, The National Archives and National Maritime Museum
BL	British Library
GCRO	Gloucestershire County Record Office
MCC	Middelburgsche Commercie Compagnie
NMM	National Maritime Museum
ODNB	*The Oxford Dictionary of National Biography* (Oxford, 2004)
SHB	The Sick and Hurt Board
TNA	The National Archives (Kew)

Introduction
Health, Medicine and the Maritime World:
A History of Two Centuries

David Boyd Haycock

The two centuries between 1700 and 1900 witnessed profound changes in Western medicine, and the period covered by this book (which principally focuses on the experience of Britain and its empire) can be chronologically bookmarked by two key moments: the foundation of Greenwich Hospital in 1694, and the foundation of the London School of Tropical Medicine in 1899. Yet despite the recognition of the need for greater palliative care which led to the establishment of a hospital for old and invalid seamen at Greenwich, in terms of medical history, the eighteenth century began with an air of uncertainty, disagreement, doubt and disappointment. The period ended, however, in great optimism.

To briefly review this process of change, by the beginning of the eighteenth century, chemists, empirics and other 'irregular' practitioners had been attacking the traditional, scholarly method of medical practice (founded on the ancient writings of Galen) for almost two centuries. Influenced by the writings and later followers of the sixteenth-century German physician Paracelsus, these laymen (and sometimes women) were highly critical of a medical system which they felt was dominated by university-educated physicians who had done little to improve the art of healing. But some of those very physicians were also dissatisfied with the results of the so-called 'Scientific Revolution' of the seventeenth century. While this had seen great advances in physics, optics, mathematics and astronomy, it had not resulted in any particular improvements in medical practice. In 1704 Dr Richard Mead, one of the wealthiest and most renowned of London's physicians, pondered why, 'notwithstanding the considerable advances made in the study of nature by the moderns ... this useful art [of medicine] has not received those benefits, which might reasonably be expected from a surer method of reasoning'. Indeed, he went so far as fretting that 'medicine still deals so much in conjecture, that it hardly deserves the name of a science'.[1] Sir Richard Blackmore, who like

---

[1] Richard Mead, *A Treatise Concerning the Influence of the Sun and the Moon upon Human Bodies* (London, 1748) pp. v–vi; this work had first been published in Latin in 1704, as *De imperio Solis ac Lunae in Corpora Humana et Morbis inde oriundis*, and first appeared in English in Halley's *Miscellanea Curiosa* in 1708.

Mead was a Fellow of the Royal College of Physicians, reflected similarly two decades later:

> It is wonderful, as well as much to be lamented, that this useful and important Art should be improved so little in so many Centuries, and that its State should still continue so uncertain and imperfect. We have hitherto discovered few Remedies of a peculiar specifical Virtue, for the Cure of any Diseases.[2]

Yet, by the end of the following century, a revolution had occurred in medical knowledge. In the 1790s the physician Edward Jenner discovered what would be the world's first vaccination – using cowpox to confer immunity to smallpox. It was quickly heralded as a major advance in medical science. How it worked, however, was a mystery. But through diligent experimental work, in the mid-nineteenth century the French chemist Louis Pasteur helped rapidly to advance understanding of the role bacteria played in the development of many such diseases. Pasteur showed that fermentation and putrefaction were biological processes dependent on the action of specific micro-organisms. Having realized that bacteria invaded the body and quickly multiplied to cause diseases such as rabies and anthrax, he helped to develop the germ theory of disease. Then in 1880, a French army physician, Charles Laveran, first identified protozoa in the red blood cells of people suffering from malaria, whilst around the same time Carlos Juan Finlay first suggested that mosquitoes might play a role in the transfer of yellow fever, which had proved a major killer in the tropics. This was followed in 1882 by the German physician Robert Koch's announcement that a bacillus that he had isolated and identified caused tuberculosis. Micro-organisms, including bacilli and protozoa, were soon recognized as the origin of a range of other killer diseases, including smallpox, cholera, diphtheria, and typhoid fever. Between 1872 and 1903, the causative organisms of almost every common disease were identified.[3] The sciences of bacteriology, immunology and biochemistry were born.[4]

Many of these aforementioned diseases had wreaked havoc on European mariners since the fifteenth century, when advances in shipbuilding and navigational technology had enabled Spanish, Portuguese and Italian sailors to make ever more distant voyages into the waters of the Atlantic – first heading south down the coast of Africa, and then eastwards in search of a new route to the lucrative Asian spice and silk trade. These voyages of discovery were followed in 1492 by Columbus's famous journey westwards, across open waters, in search of those same Oriental markets. The latter adventure, of course, failed in its stated aim, but it did result in the discovery of the 'New World'. By 1522, the first circumnavigation of the Earth had been successfully completed, and the 'terraqueous globe'

---

[2]   Sir Richard Blackmore, *Treatise of Consumptions and other Distempers Belonging to the Breast and Lungs* (London, 2nd edn, 1725), p. xii. But see Roger French and Andrew Cunningham (eds), *The Medical Revolution of the Seventeenth Century* (Cambridge, 1989).
[3]   Thomas Dormandy *The White Death: A History of Tuberculosis* (London, 1999), p. 199n.
[4]   W.F. Bynum *et al.*, *The Western Medical Tradition: 1800 to 2000* (Cambridge, 2006), pp. 123–32.

became a watery stage on which, over the subsequent four centuries, the nations of Western Europe fought for dominance.

This dominance was desirable largely because of the wealth it could bring – at first, in trade and conquest, and then in the establishment of colonial settlements. As John Evelyn (1620–1706) wrote in 1674, 'whoever Commands the Ocean, Commands the Trade of the World, and whoever Commands the Trade of the World, Commands the Riches of the World, and whoever is Master of That, Commands the World itself'.[5] But command of the ocean depended, in part, upon the command of *health* – something that Evelyn recognized. A member of the Council for Foreign Plantations, and an investor in the East India Company, Evelyn was also a Commissioner for Sick and Wounded Seamen during the Anglo-Dutch wars of the mid seventeenth century. He became a strong advocate for the establishment of a permanent naval hospital, and eventually was appointed Treasurer of the Commissioners for Erecting Greenwich Hospital.

Voyages of discovery, colonization and even military endeavour could easily flounder in the face of malnutrition or disease. It is a commonplace that the eighteenth-century Royal Navy suffered far higher mortality from disease than it ever did from the more dramatic events of combat or shipwreck: as Mick Crumplin notes in his essay in this collection, the proportion of deaths from battle strikes during the French Revolutionary and Napoleonic Wars was as low as 6 or 7 per cent.[6] Yet the role that maritime medicine played in the processes of medical improvement over the course of the eighteenth and nineteenth centuries (be it in surgery, sanitation, or mass migration) has still not been fully explored. That maritime medicine *did* play some part in these processes has, however, been acknowledged, and it is aspects of those processes that the nine essays in this book explore.

The volume is divided into two sections. The opening set of five essays examine health and medicine in the Royal Navy in the 150-year period from the permanent establishment of the Sick and Hurt Board early in the eighteenth century to the campaign to improve the position of naval surgeons in the mid nineteenth century. The Royal Navy clearly had an economic as well as a military interest in the health and well-being of its men: for example, it introduced compulsory vaccination of its sailors at a relatively early date.[7] And while the Admiralty might at times have proved slow to recognize the importance of this, or governments tardy to provide the requisite funds to support it, by the end of the Napoleonic Wars it was understood that the better health of its seamen had played an important part in Britain's victory over France. Sir Gilbert Blane, who until 1802 was a Commissioner of the Sick and Hurt Board and the person most responsible for introducing many important changes in naval medical practice during the French

---

5 John Evelyn, *Navigation and Commerce: Their Original and Progress* (London, 1674), p. 15.
6 See Chapter 3 in this collection, p. 64.
7 See N.A.M. Rodger, 'Medicine and Science in the British Navy of the Eighteenth Century', in Christian Buchet (ed.), *L'Homme, La Santé et La Mer: Actes du Colloque international tenu à l'Institut Catholique de Paris les 5 et 6 décember 1995* (Paris, 1997), pp. 333–44, esp. p. 333; and Gilbert Blane, *Elements of Medical Logick* (1819).

Wars, calculated that improvements in health in the Royal Navy between 1779 and 1813 had led to the lives of 6,674 sailors being saved in the latter year alone. Though he acknowledged that the figures were not wholly reliable or comparable, it still appeared certain that '[u]nder such an annual waste of life, the national stock of mariners must have been exhausted in the course of the prolonged warfare from which this country has just emerged.'[8]

However, as Blane pointed out, even though mortality in the Royal Navy by 1814 was much lower when compared with former years, it was still 'very high when compared to that of subjects of the same age, in other situations of life'. A naval mortality rate of 1 in 30.25 in the three last years of the Napoleonic Wars did not compare favourably with a domestic mortality rate of 1 in 57 for men aged 20 to 40 years.[9] Fevers, dysentery and tuberculosis continued to be troublesome problems on board damp, overcrowded naval vessels which often operated for long periods of time away from port, sometimes in insalubrious tropical regions. Lessons would be learnt (usually the hard way) on how to avoid (as best as possible) some of these diseases and disorders; but little could be done to treat them, and even the effective way of using bark (cinchona, the base ingredient of quinine) could be misunderstood, and good practice reversed.[10]

The second set of four essays look at a slightly different, but not unrelated, topic: human migration, both voluntary and involuntary. Britain was increasingly involved in the slave trade following the foundation of the Royal Africa Company in the mid seventeenth century, and it eventually became one of the major carriers of slaves across the Atlantic to the West Indies and North America. But even after an Act of Parliament abolished (at least in theory) the British slave trade in 1807, the forced shipment of enslaved Africans to the Americas continued. And Britain continued another practice of enforced migration, embarking thousands of convicts (male and female) to Australia. At the same time, semi-voluntary migration increased dramatically in the nineteenth century. The Irish famine, the Highland clearances and periodic economic downturns and bad harvests forced hundreds of thousands of men, women and children to leave their homes for new lives in the Americas, Australia, New Zealand, South Africa and elsewhere around the globe. Meanwhile, indentured workers from South Asia travelled in

---

[8]   Gilbert Blane, 'On the Comparative Health of the British Navy, from the Year 1779 to the Year 1814, with Proposals for its Further Improvement' (1815), in Christopher Lloyd (ed.), *The Health of Seamen: Selections from the Works of Dr James Lind, Sir Gilbert Blane and Dr Thomas Trotter* (London, 1965), p. 176. On the possible unreliability of Blane's figures, see Chapter 5 in this volume, p. 112.

[9]   Blane, 'Comparative Health', p. 188: Blane obtained his mortality figures for the general populace from the well known 'Northampton Tables' compiled by the demographer Richard Price in the 1770s.

[10]   On the Navy's acceptance and then rejection of the use of bark (which occurred in favour of venesection in the early nineteenth century), see James Watt, 'Some Forgotten Contributions of Naval Surgeons', *Journal of the Royal Society of Medicine*, 78 (1985), pp. 758–62. A similar error was made in the nineteenth century, when limes replaced lemons and oranges as the Navy's chief antiscorbutic, when in fact limes actually contain less Vitamin C.

ever greater numbers across the seas in search of work, often carried by European ships to work as labourers on European plantations. It has been calculated that in the nineteenth century over one million migrants left India as indentured workers, bound for tropical colonies in the Atlantic, Pacific and Indian Oceans.[11]

As we shall see, all of these voyages – most of them on board sailing ships and some of them lasting many months – involved obvious and sometimes profound dangers to health; but many of the improvements in health and sanitation that helped to improve conditions on board depended upon lessons learnt by the surgeons, physicians, captains and admirals of the Royal Navy.

Medicine in the Royal Navy

The four-volume history *Medicine and the Navy, 1200–1900* (1957–63), written by J.J. Keevil, Jack Coulter and Christopher Lloyd, remains the authoritative account on the subject as it pertains to the Royal Navy. It is an extensive study, based largely on the Admiralty collections that survive at the National Archives and the National Maritime Museum. But its scope remains limited, and it is increasingly out of date. It is unlikely, though, that we will see another study of such scope and range.

In 1997, the eminent naval historian N.A.M. Rodger outlined some of the continuing deficiencies of our knowledge of medicine and science in the eighteenth-century Royal Navy.[12] Many of these still remain little examined, but there have been a number of important recent studies. John Booker, for example, has recently published the first definitive study of the British experience of maritime quarantine, covering the period from the mid seventeenth to the end of the nineteenth century. His book, however, approaches the subject from constitutional (in the political sense) and economic standpoints. As he explains, 'Medical issues are not neglected, but introduced only as far as necessary to explain why quarantine was introduced, altered and finally abandoned.'[13]

Understandably, scurvy is not a subject that has lacked attention from maritime historians, and the literature on the subject is extensive. It is not a theme that is explored directly in this collection, though obviously it was of huge importance to health at sea in the period covered here, and the eventual discovery of an effectual preventative and cure was a major step forward in maritime health. The role played by the surgeon James Lind in this process, and his famous trial on board HMS *Salisbury* in 1747, has tended to be overplayed (as has, potentially, the role of the Royal Navy).[14] Nevertheless, the widespread issuing of fruit juice on board

---

[11] See Chapter 9 in this volume, p. 195.

[12] Rodger, 'Medicine and Science in the British Navy'.

[13] John Booker, *Maritime Quarantine: The British Experience, c.1650–1900* (Aldershot, 2007), p. xiv.

[14] See for example David Harvie, *Limeys: The True Story of One Man's War against Ignorance, the Establishment and the Deadly Scurvy* (Stroud, 2002); Lloyd and Coulter in *Medicine and the*

Royal Naval vessels from the mid 1790s onwards resulted in real improvements in health. As Sir Gilbert Blane observed in 1815, the 'efficacy' of citrus fruits in the treatment of this hitherto deadly malady was 'singular when compared to that of any other remedy in any other disease. It is a certain preventative as well as cure'; nor did it produce 'bad effects on the constitution. … It may therefore be affirmed with truth that it performs not only what no other remedy will perform in this disease, but what no known remedy will effect in any known disease whatever.'[15] When compared with Sir Richard Blackmore's aforementioned remark regarding the lack of discovery of remedies 'of a peculiar specifical Virtue, for the Cure of any Diseases', this was a major step forward.[16]

The work of James Lind, Gilbert Blane and Thomas Trotter in the second half of the eighteenth century made it clear that it was in hygiene, and in the provision of good, fresh food, that real advances could be made in the health of Royal Navy seamen. James Cook's long and relatively healthy voyages appeared to indicate this, even though his conclusions on how his crew largely avoided the scurvy were deeply flawed.[17] Hence, as Vice-Admiral Horatio Nelson observed in 1804: 'The great thing in all military service is health; and you will agree with me that it is easier for an officer to keep men healthy, than for a physician to cure them.'[18] This realization, however, took time: William Cockburn claimed in 1696 that the victuals served to the Royal Navy's sailors were 'a great deal better, and his allowance larger, than in any *Navy* or *Merchant-ships* in the world'.[19] This may have been true; but if so, it said very little for the food and drink being served to foreign sailors, and it is true that much food on board was often unfit for consumption, especially towards the end of long voyages. It is not surprising that scurvy and other vitamin deficiencies were frequent problems – even after the introduction of fruit juice.

Navy, vol. III, also overemphasize Lind's role. For more measured recent assessments, see R.E. Hughes, 'James Lind and the Cure of Scurvy: An Experimental Approach', *Medical History*, 19 (1975), pp. 342–51; William McBride, 'Normal Medical Science and British Treatment of the Sea Scurvy, 1753–75', *Journal of the History of Medicine*, 46 (1990), pp. 158–77; C. Lawrence, 'Disciplining Disease: Scurvy, the Navy, and Imperial Expansion, 1750–1825', in D.P. Miller and P.H. Reill (eds), *Visions of Empire: Voyages, Botany and Representation of Nature* (Cambridge, 1996); and Michael Bartholomew, 'James Lind and Scurvy: A Revaluation', *Journal for Maritime Research* (2002).

[15] Blane, 'Comparative Health', pp. 179–80.

[16] Blackmore, *Treatise of Consumptions*, p. xii; see also Roger French and Andrew Cunningham (eds), *The Medical Revolution of the Seventeenth Century* (Cambridge, 1989).

[17] On Cook's misinterpretation of the supposed effectiveness of malt in assuaging scurvy, as proposed by David MacBride in *An Historical Account of a New Method of Treating the Scurvy at Sea* (London, 1767), see Lloyd and Coulter, *Medicine and the Navy*, vol. 3, pp. 302–15; on the impact of dysentery on this voyage, see David Boyd Haycock, 'Exterminated by the Bloody Flux: Dysentery in Eighteenth-Century Naval and Military Medical Accounts', *Journal of Maritime Research* [www.jmr.nmm.ac.uk] (January 2002).

[18] Horatio Nelson to Dr Mosley, 11 March 1804, quoted in James Watt, 'Surgery at Trafalgar', *The Mariner's Mirror*, 91 (2005), p. 281.

[19] William Cockburn, *An Account of the Nature, Causes, Symptoms and Cure of the Distempers that are Incident to Seafaring People. With Observations on the Diet of the Sea-men in his Majesty's Navy* (London, 1696), pp. 6–7.

N.A.M. Rodger was particularly critical in 1997 that medical administration and naval policy in relation to health remained 'very little studied'.[20] This has started to change, as some of the papers in this collection reveal. Erica Charters shows in her prize-winning essay, which opens this collection, that the ability to feed – and thereby maintain the health – of the sailors in the Western Squadron that blockaded the French Atlantic coast during the Seven Years War played an important (perhaps crucial) part in the overall success of this new maritime strategy. But she also points out that this initiative, which focused on the regular supply of fresh foodstuffs, was both provisional and precarious, and demanded a great deal of organization, administration and expense. Roger Knight's recent project 'Sustaining the Empire: War, the Navy and the Contractor State', funded by the Leverhulme Trust and completed in 2009, provides further insight into the important role that victualling played in the military success of the Royal Navy.[21] The naval hospital – another subject noted by Rodger as under-studied – has also benefited from new research, particularly by Christine Stevenson and Geoffrey Hudson.[22]

Another recent important research project – the fruits of which are to be seen for the first time in this collection – is John Cardwell, Laurence Brockliss and Michael Moss's prosopographical survey into the backgrounds of Royal Navy surgeons. This builds upon a related research project on Army surgeons.[23] The important contribution made by Navy surgeons to the development of maritime medicine during the two centuries covered by this book cannot be overstated, and it is important to have a clearer understanding of who they were, where they originated, and how they learnt their trade. Some surgeons were clearly interested in the improvement of health at sea, and acting or former surgeons helped to develop important new surgical techniques.[24] They also published a number of important British texts on maritime medicine in the eighteenth century; these included James Lind's *Treatise on Scurvy* (1753) and *An Essay on the Most Effectual Means of Preserving the Health of Seamen* (1762), William Northcote's *The Marine*

[20] Rodger, 'Medicine and Science in the British Navy', p. 333.
[21] Focused on the period of the French Revolutionary and Napoleonic Wars, and based at the Greenwich Maritime Institute, University of Greenwich, the project ran in collaboration with the National Maritime Museum from 2006 to 2009. The project website is to be found at: http://www.nmm.ac.uk/researchers/research-areas-and-projects/sustaining-the-empire/
[22] See Christine Stevenson, *Medicine and Magnificence: British Hospital and Asylum Architecture, 1660–1815* (New Haven and London, 2000); and Geoffrey L. Hudson, 'Internal Influences in the Making of the English Military Hospital: The Early-Eighteenth-Century Greenwich', in Geoffrey L. Hudson (ed.), *British Military and Naval Medicine, 1600–1830* (Amsterdam and New York, 2007), pp. 253–72. See also J. Bold, *Greenwich: An Architectural History of the Royal Hospital for Seamen and the Queen's House* (New Haven and London, 2000).
[23] See Marcus Ackroyd, Laurence Brockliss, Michael Moss, Kate Retford and John Stevenson, *Advancing the Army: Medicine, the Professions, and Social Mobility in the British Isles, 1790–1850* (Oxford, 2006).
[24] For an interesting review of these innovations – some of which were, unfortunately, lost before being rediscovered in the later twentieth century, see Watt, 'Some Forgotten Contributions', pp. 753–62.

Practice of Physic and Surgery (1770) and Thomas Trotter's *Medicina Nautica: An Essay on the Diseases of Seamen* (3 volumes, 1797–1803).

Naval surgeons recognized the need to improve maritime health, and also the shortcomings in their own training. In 1742 the surgeon John Atkins proposed the creation of a training facility for surgeons in Portsmouth.[25] Though this appears to have been ignored by the Admiralty, following the disastrous Pacific expedition made under the command of Captain George Anson between 1740 and 1744, when well over a thousand men died from scurvy, a Society of the Navy Surgeons of the Royal Navy of Great Britain was established in 1747. Though short-lived, the Society recognized that sea surgeons could put their particular skills and experiences to use for both naval and public benefit. They published what James Lind described as a 'laudable plan for improving medical knowledge, by the labours of its several members; who have opportunities of inspecting Nature, and examining diseases, under the varied influence of different climates, seasons and soils'. Lind had first intended to publish his now famous book on scurvy 'as a short paper to be published in the memoirs of our medical navy-society'.[26]

Though the Society appears to have folded by 1763, it illustrates the role surgeons could play in the improvement of maritime medicine – a role that often extended well beyond the 'wooden walls' of the ships in which they originally served. Even if – as Margarette Lincoln has suggested – publication by surgeons was sometimes for the purposes of self-interest, promotion or professional advancement, she notes that their works still appear to have been read, with many going into second and further editions.[27] Many surgeons went on to obtain degrees and enjoy medical careers outside the Navy, with some – such as Thomas Trotter – enjoying success as what we would now call general practitioners. There were thus numerous ways in which surgeons were able to transmit their experience beyond the confines of the Navy. As James Watt has observed, over the course of almost four centuries, Royal Navy surgeons 'made important contributions to the understanding of nutritional disorders, to tropical diseases, human metabolism, hygiene, health statistics, medical and surgical audit, health screening, lifesaving and social reform'.[28] Indeed, N.A.M. Rodger has described the eighteenth-century Royal Navy as 'the laboratory' in which many of the social and medical ideas on health and hygiene were worked out, and 'which in time fuelled the nineteenth-century public health movement', and the Navy's suppression of scurvy and smallpox 'can be seen as rehearsals' for the conquest of Asiatic

---

[25] See John Atkins, *The Navy Surgeon, Or, Practical System of Surgery* (2nd edn, London, 1742), preface.

[26] James Lind, *A Treatise of the Scurvy* (Edinburgh, 1753), preface vii–viii; on the history of the Society, see George C. Peachey, *A Memoir of William and John Hunter* (Plymouth, 1924), pp. 79–90.

[27] Margarette Lincoln, 'The Medical Profession and Representation of the Navy, 1750–1815', in Geoffrey L. Hudson (ed.), *British Military and Naval Medicine, 1600–1830* (Amsterdam and New York, 2007), pp. 201–26.

[28] Watt, 'Some Forgotten Contributions', p. 757.

cholera in the 1850s.[29] A recent study by David McLean has in part studied exactly this subject, exploring the key role that surgeons and other Royal Navy personnel in Plymouth played during the second epidemic of Asiatic cholera in Britain, which struck in the late 1840s.[30]What Cardwell's chapter in this book offers is an insight into the hitherto largely unknown backgrounds of those men who chose to join the Royal Navy as surgeons (surgeons were always volunteers: despite the frequent shortage in wartime, they were never pressed into service). Cardwell reveals that many came from relatively humble backgrounds, but through hard work and study they were able to make important contributions to medicine. Cardwell's essay is followed by Michael Crumplin's examination of the education and on-board experiences of the ship's surgeon in the period of the Revolutionary and Napoleonic Wars. A retired surgeon, Crumplin is particularly interested in the medical demands placed upon surgeons. As noted above, combat could be infrequent, but when it occurred, high demands were placed upon the surgeon and his assistants. Skills that had been learnt over the course of an apprenticeship, a brief course of university lectures and some hospital training, together with the everyday accidents that befell a sailing vessel, had to be pressed into immediate service. This training was haphazard: unlike in other European states (and despite the calls of men such as John Atkins), there was no official school for training Army or Navy surgeons until 1806, when John Thomson was appointed to the first professorship of Military Surgery to be founded at a British university. Not surprisingly, given the fact that by the first half of the nineteenth century over 90 per cent of British medical graduates were trained in Scotland, this Regius Chair was established at the University of Edinburgh.[31]

The Sick and Hurt Board, which administered the appointment of surgeons and the running of Navy hospitals over much of this period, is the subject of Pat Crimmin's essay. She has made an exhaustive study of the Sick and Hurt Board Papers in the National Maritime Museum, and her chapter offers further reflections on this under-studied material. In particular, she explores the departmental policies and practices of the Royal Navy's overworked and understaffed medical department during the period of the French Wars. This includes reflections on the inevitable political considerations – both office and departmental politics, and party and service politics. As Crimmin acknowledges, more work needs to be done on this extensive archive; but by exploring how the backdrop of politics influenced the more day-to-day activities of the Sick and Hurt Board, she argues that the problems of naval health in this period, and the difficulties involved in improving it, become more understandable. She thus provides the context in which to examine whether the Board was (to use a phrase popular in politics today) 'fit for purpose'.

---

29 Rodger, 'Medicine and Science in the British Navy', p. 341.
30 See David McLean, *Public Health and Politics in the Age of Reform: Cholera, the State and the Royal Navy in Victorian Britain* (London, 2006).
31 Matthew H. Kaufman, *The Regius Chair of Military Surgery in the University of Edinburgh, 1806–55* (Amsterdam and New York, 2003), p. 18, table 1.1.

Despite its apparent failings and shortcomings, in comparison to France, at least, the system worked surprisingly well. In a recent reassessment of the competence of both French and British naval surgeons at Trafalgar, James Watt concluded that the 'emphasis on cleanliness and antisepsis, practical training, continuing post-graduate education and contributions to specialist journals, coupled with effective surgical techniques developed through wide experience, gave [British] naval surgeons the edge, in the field of trauma, over their civilian counterparts', as well as their counterparts in the French and Spanish navies. 'They had the additional advantage of the support of many naval commanders, whose passion for cleanliness and personal hygiene provided an environment favourable to their efforts.'[32]

However, many of these lessons were lost once the Napoleonic Wars ended in 1815. In the following decades the Royal Navy failed to make the career of a ship's surgeon either an attractive or a lucrative one. By 1840, the situation was so abject that not a single candidate came forward for consideration as a surgeon in the Royal Navy.[33] The mid-nineteenth-century campaign to improve the lot of the naval surgeon and his charges is thus the subject of the final paper in this first section. Mark Harrison begins by discussing the campaign run in The Lancet by its founding editor, Thomas Wakley, to improve pay and conditions for Navy surgeons. This was focused through the lens of the appalling mortality of crews involved in the anti-slavery operations of the West Africa Squadron, and two cases in particular: the ill-fated Niger Expedition of 1841–2, and the steam-sloop Éclair, which allegedly brought yellow fever from West Africa to one of the Cape Verde Islands in 1845. Harrison relates these events to contemporaneous concerns over the health of factory workers in Britain, and concludes that the debate helped create the conditions for what can be seen as a turning point in the history of British naval medicine – for it was then, in the 1840s and (with the Crimean War) the 1850s, that the public mood changed, revealing that it 'was no longer prepared to countenance what it regarded as needless deaths from disease.'[34]

In these years of the mid nineteenth century the first true advances started to be made in the field of treatment of many of the diseases that so ravaged the sailors of the West Africa Squadron. Indeed, the London School of Tropical Medicine, founded in 1899, was a direct outcome of the charitable Seamen's Hospital Society, which had been established following the end of the Napoleonic Wars.[35]

Migration

The surgeon and Physician to the Channel Fleet, Thomas Trotter (c. 1760–1832), provides a clear bridge between the two sets of essays in this collection. The son of

32 Watt, 'Surgery at Trafalgar,' p. 280.
33 Kaufman, The Regius Chair of Military Surgery, p. 20.
34 Chapter 5, p. 127.
35 See Gordon C. Cook's recent extensive study, Disease in the Merchant Navy: A History of the Seamen's Hospital Society (Oxford, 2007).

a Scottish baker from Melrose, Trotter studied medicine at Edinburgh University for two years under Alexander Monro *secundus* before joining the Royal Navy as a surgeon's mate in 1779. Though quickly promoted to the rank of surgeon following his exemplary service at the Battle of Dogger Bank in 1781, he was laid off without the benefit of half pay at the end of the American War of Independence. Trotter was then forced to embrace what he called 'the painful alternative' of employment on board a Liverpool slave ship. Following 'the unpleasant months he spent in the unhallowed trade', in which many slaves died from scurvy, in 1786 he published a book in which he compared the shipboard experiences of sailors and slaves.[36]

Of course, the appalling and inhuman experiences of an enslaved African cannot be too closely compared to those of a press-ganged Briton. But to an eighteenth-century surgeon there were parallels that could be drawn. Pressed men, though robbed of their freedom, were not generally shackled or as ill-treated as slaves; however, they could initially be confined in what were often filthy, over-crowded and disease-ridden holding vessels.[37] As one pressed youth recalled on looking into the steerage of a holding vessel moored off Liverpool in around 1800, 'a hot and pestilential effluvia rose and enveloped me'. Below decks he glimpsed 'a crowded mass of disgusting and fearful heads, with eyes all glaring upwards from that terrible den; and heaps of filthy limbs, trunks, and heads, bundled and scattered, scrambling, laughing, cursing, swearing, and fighting'.[38] He could almost have been describing the scenes on board a slaver: in 1790, Dr Alexander Falconbridge told a Parliamentary Committee that the scenes below decks aboard a slave ship struck by flux and fever 'approached nearer to the resemblance of a slaughter-house than any thing I can compare it to, [and] the stench and foul air were likewise intolerable'.[39] Slaves could spend up to six months in such conditions even before the Atlantic crossing was made, and the potential for the outbreak of disease was clear. Likewise, pressed men – who may also have spent time in gaol before reaching holding vessels – were frequently seen as sources of disease when they were transferred to join the ships in which they would serve. Many surgeons and physicians, including Trotter, were thus opposed to the practice of impressment.[40]

---

[36] Thomas Trotter, *Observations on the Scurvy: With a Review of the Opinions Lately Advanced on that Disease, and a New Theory Defended* (2nd edn, London, 1792), p. xxix; Marcus Rediker, *The Slave Ship: A Human History* (London, 2007), p. 410, note 39.

[37] For an interesting recent social, cultural and literary analysis of the press, see Daniel James Ennis, *Enter the Press-Gang: Naval Impressment in Eighteenth-Century British Literature* (London, 2002). Ennis points out that 'Britons viewed impressment with as much distaste as they viewed chattel slavery, but impressment was so integral to British naval policy that it was legal – and practiced – long after Parliament abolished the slave trade'. Ennis, *Enter the Press-Gang*, p. 16. And a naval captain could sometimes be as sadistic as the master of a slave vessel – though the fate of Captain Hugh Pigot of HMS *Hermione*, murdered in 1797 by his crew on account of his love of the lash, was a rare extreme: see Dudley Pope, *The Black Ship* (London, 1963).

[38] January Searle (ed.), *The History of Pel Verjuice, The Wanderer* (London, 1853), pp. 81–2.

[39] Quoted in Rediker, *The Slave Ship*, p. 274.

[40] See Trotter, *Observations on the Scurvy*, pp. 153–8, and his *A Practicable Plan for Manning the Royal Navy, and Preserving our Maritime Ascendancy, without Impressment* (Newcastle, 1819).

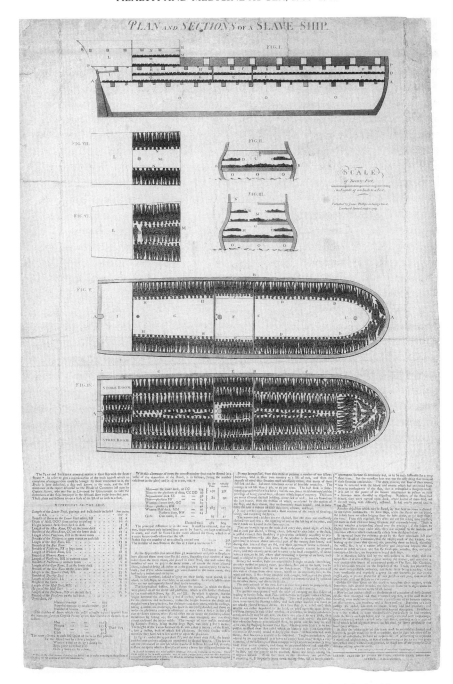

Figure 1. 'Plan and Sections of a Slave Ship' (The *Brooks*) (published by James Phillips, 1789). National Maritime Museum, Greenwich.

The diseases that might present themselves on board slave vessels were also similar to those that occurred on Navy ships: in particular dysentery ('bloody flux'), fevers (including what we now know to have been malaria and yellow fever), scurvy and smallpox. Dr T. Aubrey's *The Sea-Surgeon* of 1729 was especially written 'for the Use of young Sea Surgeons' serving on slave vessels off West Africa. Aubrey blamed the 'Inhumanity, Barbarity, and the greatest of Cruelty of their Commander, and his Crew', together with the 'Ignorance of the Surgeon', for any excess mortality that might occur among 'these poor Creatures'.[41] On Trotter's single slave voyage – made between 1783 and 1784 aboard the now infamous slaver the *Brooks* – fifty-eight out of around 650 slaves, and three crewmen, died.[42] In comparative terms, this was relatively low: it has been calculated that slave mortality rates during the Middle Passage in this period fluctuated from a mean minimum of 11.1 per cent to a mean maximum of 21.9 per cent, while between 20 and 24 per cent of crewmen died (largely of mosquito-borne fevers caught on the African coast).[43] But these were averages, and individual voyages could witness horrifying loss of life. For example, of 700 slaves bound to Barbados on board the Royal Africa Company's vessel *Hannibal* in 1693, only 480 arrived alive.[44]

Following his experience on board the *Brooks*, Trotter became an ardent anti-slavery campaigner. In 1790 he would – along with the captain of the ship, Clement Noble – be called before a Select Committee of the House of Commons to give his expert testimony on the slave trade. Overcrowding in a bid to maximize profits, together with inadequate ventilation in the crowded ships, was considered a principal cause of such high mortality: the factors of the Royal Africa Company had written as early as 1681 that 'the covetousness of commanders crowding in their slaves above the proportion for the advantage of freight is the only reason for the great loss to the company'.[45] Trotter had tried to persuade Noble (who took 'no precautions ... to preserve the health of the slaves')[46] of the need to provide decent provisions for his miserable cargo, but had been ignored by Noble – just as the

---

[41] T. Aubrey, *The Sea-Surgeon, or the Guinea Man's Vade Mecum* (London, 1729), pp. 132–3. For further discussion on this subject, see Richard B. Sheridan, 'The Guinea Surgeons on the Middle Passage: The Provision of Medical Service in the British Slave Trade', *International Journal of African Historical Studies*, 14 (1981), pp. 601–25; and Ralph Shlomowitz and Robin Haines, 'Explaining the Mortality Decline in the Eighteenth-century British Slave Trade', *Economic History Review*, 53 (2003), pp. 262–83. Sheridan argues that 'government regulation and certain developments in medical science contributed in some measure to the decline in slave mortality on the Middle Passage': Sheridan, 'The Guinea Surgeons', pp. 601–2.

[42] Rediker, *The Slave Ship*, p. 333; Trotter, *Observations on the Scurvy*, pp. 65, 69.

[43] Philip D. Curtin, *The Atlantic Slave Trade: A Census* (Madison and London, 1969), pp. 283–4; see also Stephen D. Behrendt, 'Crew Mortality in the Transatlantic Slave Trade in the Eighteenth Century', in *Slavery and Abolition*, 18 (1997), pp. 49–71; and David Eltis and David Richardson (eds), *Routes to Slavery: Direction, Ethnicity and Mortality in the Transatlantic Slave Trade* (London, 1997).

[44] Sheridon, 'The Guinea Surgeons', p. 604.

[45] Hugh Thomas, *The Slave Trade: The History of the Atlantic Slave Trade, 1440–1870* (London, 1997), p. 413.

[46] Trotter, *Observations on the Scurvy*, p. 55. Trotter notes that 'a few gallons of lime-juice' and

Royal Africa Company had ignored the advice of its factors a century before. In fact, it increasingly appears to historians that overcrowding (while clearly cruel and uncomfortable) was not actually a principal cause of additional mortality on board slave ships. The greater problem, it has been suggested, was that overcrowding resulted in under- or poor provisioning – the issue that Trotter identified, but was unable to rectify.[47] Filth was also obviously a clear problem, and it has been calculated that gastrointestinal diseases caused over 40 per cent of slave deaths.[48]

The contentious question of mortality in the transatlantic slave trade has been of considerable interest to historians since the publication in 1969 of Philip D. Curtin's seminal study, *The Atlantic Slave Trade: A Census*. Curtin identified a discernible general tendency of decreasing mortality rate of slaves over the eighteenth and nineteenth centuries. This contrasted with his discovery that the death rate of the crew on board those vessels remained nearly at the same level over the period. 'Apparently,' he concluded, 'the slave traders discovered ways to improve health conditions for slaves in transit, but they were less successful in meeting the dangers of malaria and yellow fever, the principal killers of strangers to the West African coast.'[49] Curtin was undoubtedly correct in his conclusion that, while the trade was profitable to the merchants involved, and for their West Indian and American customers,

> it may be that the social cost of the trade – the cost to European society as a whole – was far greater than its benefits, again to European society as a whole. European historians have been quick to point out that African slave dealers sold their fellow Africans for private profit, contrary to the true interests of African society. It is at least worth asking whether this might not have been true of European merchants as well.[50]

This proposition echoes remarks made by Trotter in 1797. In the first volume of *Medicina Nautica* – perhaps influenced by the arguments of his colleagues in the abolition movement – he suggested that while the European colonies in the Indies, Africa and America had brought 'riches and commerce', they had also 'brought a train of diseases peculiar to their climate, and fatal to the constitutions of northern nations, and which leave us to doubt whether or not we ought to regard these acquisitions as beneficial to society.'[51] As with the case of improving

---

a small quantity of oranges and guavas was the only stock of 'fresh vegetables' on board the ship when it left Africa. Ibid., p. 66.

[47] Thomas, *The Slave Trade*, p. 414, citing H.S. Klein, *The Middle Passage* (Princeton, 1978). In order to prevent rebellion on board their vessels, slavers tended to carry higher numbers of crew than would be required in other merchantmen – a factor that would have added to the problems of space and victualling. See Emma Christopher, *Slave Ship Sailors and their Captive Cargoes, 1730–1807* (Cambridge, 2006), p. 182.

[48] See Richard H. Steckel and Richard A. Jensen, 'New Evidence of the Causes of Slave and Crew Mortality in the Atlantic Slave Trade', *Journal of Economic History*, 46 (1986), pp. 57–77.

[49] Curtin, *The Atlantic Slave Trade*, pp. 276, 283.

[50] Ibid., p. 286.

[51] Thomas Trotter, *Medicina Nautica: An Essay on the Disease of Seamen*, Volume 1 (London, 1797), p. 7.

health in the Royal Navy, there was a clear economic interest in conserving the well-being of both slaves and the mariners who transported them, even if the moral duty of care that we would implicitly assume today was generally ignored. For as Trotter observed, although he recommended that slaves should be well treated, 'few think that they are trampling on the Rights of a Man and a Brother!'[52]

In the four decades since the publication of Curtin's study, research into this topic has developed considerably as new data have been uncovered and analysed. In the opening essay of this second part of the book, Hamish Maxwell-Stuart and Ralph Shlomowitz survey the most recent literature on the subject, addressing the question of what factors explain excess slave mortality in the Middle Passage, and comparing this with the excess mortality of indentured migrant workers from the Pacific Islands. Their survey is followed by an essay by Simon J. Hogerzeil and David Richardson examining records from the Dutch West African slave trade of the second half of the eighteenth century. These data are used to study the day-to-day purchasing activities of traders; this information is then related to reveal new insights into shipboard mortality according to age and sex of slaves, the geographical location of the trade itself, and the season in which slaves were loaded on board. Interestingly, in contrast to other studies, their cliometric analysis shows that male slaves, though on average loaded on board later, had a higher risk of mortality than women or children. (Interestingly, Trotter himself noted some of these points, and recommended smaller slave ships – not in order to prevent overcrowding, but in order to lessen the time that they lay off the African coast gathering their human cargo.)[53] Hogerzeil and Richardson conclude that it is necessary for historians to adopt a broader definition of the Middle Passage, to embrace the whole time that slaves spent on board ship, and to recognize the fact that this could differ enormously between individuals.

From the mortality of slaves, we turn to the transportation of men, women and children from Britain to Australia in the nineteenth century. As Robin Haines shows in her paper, many of the lessons learnt by the Royal Navy in the decades up to and including the French Wars were implemented on board these sometimes equally crowded vessels. This contribution is most clearly seen in the advice given by Assistant Colonial Surgeon William Redfern (1774/5–1833) in his report to Governor Lachlan Macquarie on 30 September 1814, in response to the calamitous mortality on board three convict ships recently arrived in New South Wales. Redfern had joined the Royal Navy in 1797 as a surgeon's mate, but was transported to New South Wales in 1801 for his part in the mutiny at the Nore. He worked as an assistant surgeon at the Norfolk Island penal settlement, for which he was given a free pardon in 1803. He was therefore well placed to make recommendations for the improvement of medical treatment of convicts.

Of equal importance to the attention paid to the minor requirements of the passengers – be they emigrants or convicts – was legislation in support of those

---

[52] Trottter, *Observations on the Scurvy* (1792), p. 243.
[53] Ibid., p. 240.

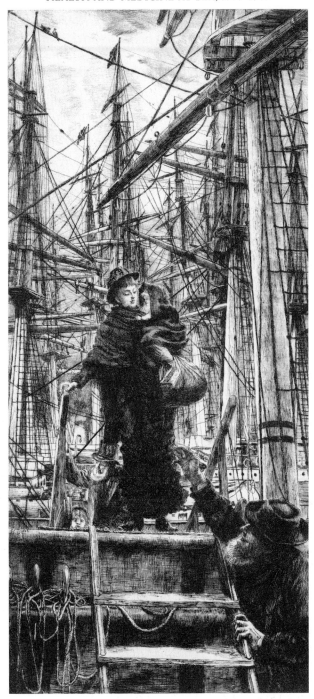

Figure 2. *The Emigrants*, by Jacques-Joseph (James)
Tissot, 1880. National Maritime Museum, Greenwich.

needs, and their strict implementation by surgeons and captains. When the *Lord Wellington*, a ship carrying female convicts from Britain to New South Wales, arrived at the colony in January 1820 after a nine-month voyage, with no deaths on board, and none landed sick, the surgeon attributed this success to a number of causes:

> Firstly, the most excellent care taken of them by Government in providing so amply for all their little wants in so long a voyage ... Secondly, the goodness of their provisions and the liberal supply of various comforts placed at the disposal of the surgeon and superintendent ... Lastly, the constant state of cleanliness, of warmth, and of every general attention to their victualling, to their water and all their minor wants and to keeping them to their religious duties ...[54]

The clear effect of such legislation can be seen in the much lower mortality rates on board government-commissioned ships making the long voyage from Britain to Australia, compared with mortality rates of passengers on the unregulated but shorter voyage to North America.[55] Surgeons thus clearly played an important – and recognized and appreciated – role in the health of a ship's passengers: in 1856, Dr James Harris, surgeon on board the Royal Mail packet ship *Donald Mackay* making the journey from Liverpool to Melbourne, was presented with a testimonial signed by 450 passengers.[56]

The last essay in this collection, by Laurence Brown and Radica Mahase, explores the experiences of a final and equally distinct group of emigrants: those many migrants and their families who left India in the nineteenth century to take up employment as indentured workers for the tropical colonies of the Atlantic, Pacific and Indian Oceans. To many British and colonial abolitionists, such Asian indentureship was merely a 'new system of slavery', and – once more – techniques that had been introduced to improve the lot of slaves (and convicts and other migrants) were explored. But as Brown and Mahase show, this deeply disruptive migrant experience was one in which – in medical terms, if not also in others – two cultures clashed. Clear conflicts and misunderstandings arose between the needs and expectations of migrants, and those of the ship captains and surgeons responsible for transporting them. For Brown and Mahase, these emigrant ships are important sites for reinvestigating what has been termed 'colonial' medicine, and they see them as the location of shifting encounters between British and Indian understandings of medicine.

As the essays in this collection show, maritime medicine in the eighteenth and nineteenth centuries is a rich subject, filled with an array of fascinating and informative archives, events and experiences. Many of these are ripe for further investigation. Individually, these nine essays are interesting and important in their

---

[54] TNA, ADM/101/45/1/2, fol. 17: diary for the *Lord Wellington*, by Edward Foord Bromley, MD, surgeon, Royal Navy and Superintendent of Convicts.
[55] See Chapter 8 in this volume, p. 177.
[56] NMM, MS HSR/N/8.

own right. They highlight some of the recent work that has been undertaken in the history of maritime medicine, and offer results from recent new analysis and projects. Together they offer a broad introduction to the subject, and illustrate some of the exciting new directions that future research will take, or is already taking.

I

'The Intention is Certain Noble': The Western Squadron, Medical Trials, and the Sick and Hurt Board during the Seven Years War (1756–63)

Erica M. Charters

Awarded the Julian Corbett Prize for Research in Modern Naval History, University of London

The Royal Navy's importance to British victories during the Seven Years War, Britain's first global war of empire (1756–63), can hardly be overstated. Triumphs such as Quebec in 1759 and 1760 and Havana in 1762 are best described as amphibious operations. Indeed, as Richard Harding defines amphibious warfare in the eighteenth century as 'a mode of action in which a military force, capable of being fully maintained at sea, is dispatched to accomplish specific objectives on enemy territory', it is difficult to find a military action during the war that was not at least dependent upon naval power.[1] Closer to home, the strategy of the Western Squadron is credited with both protecting colonial military operations and trade, and ending French naval power.

More particularly, as the Western Squadron could operate successfully only by maintaining the health of its men, stationed at sea for long periods, historians have credited the success of British imperial forces during the Seven Years War to the naval administration's procedure of sending out fresh provisions. Here, I re-examine the operation of the Western Squadron in the light of contemporary medical practice and theory. I begin by discussing the health of seamen and the obstacles to maintaining it within the context of the development of Western Squadron operations during the eighteenth century. I then focus on the health

---

[1] R. Harding, *Amphibious Warfare in the Eighteenth-Century: The British Expedition to the West Indies, 1740–1742* (Woodbridge, 1991), qt. p. 2, see also ch. 4; D. Syrett, 'The Methodology of British Amphibious Operations during the Seven Years and American Wars', *Mariner's Mirror*, 58 (1972), pp. 269–80; D. Baugh, 'A War on Water: The Role of the Geographical Extremities in British Success, 1755–63', Plenary Lecture, 'A War for Empire: The Seven Years War in Context' Conference, National Maritime Museum, London (hereafter NMM), 13 July 2006.

of the Squadron during the Seven Years War and especially on the effect fresh victuals had on rates of sickness. This examination demonstrates that the initiative of fresh provisions was provisional and precarious. The Sick and Hurt Board and the Admiralty recognized that the sending out of fresh provisions to the Western Squadron was no long-term solution to the problem of maintaining the health of seamen when at sea for extended periods of time. I conclude by examining the correspondence of the Sick and Hurt Board during the period of the Seven Years War, establishing that their medical research into cures and preventatives for scurvy other than fresh vegetables was not based on ignorance, but rather on the search for a cure achievable within the constraints imposed by ships at sea and the practical demands of naval administration.

The Western Squadron and the Health of Seamen

The Western Squadron was not an innovation of the Seven Years War; the term can be traced back to 1705, even though such a squadron had little practical effect until the wars of the 1740s.[2] Having a fleet of ships constantly cruising to the 'westward' (that is, west of approaches to the English coast, and along the Channel off Brest and Ushant) meant that incoming British merchant vessels could be protected, whilst French fleets and supply ships were prevented from setting out for the colonies or preparing for an invasion of Britain. Both Middleton and Rodger assert that the strategy of the Western Squadron was never comprehensively or clearly elucidated by either Admiral Edward Vernon or George Anson, under whom the practice first developed in the 1740s. Instead, by the mid eighteenth century, what had begun as a practical experiment was now shown to be a viable strategy, albeit one requiring continuing modifications.[3]

Naval historians emphasize the problems inherent in such a stratagem. It was difficult for such a squadron to cruise for extended periods, partly due to the geography of the region near Brest, where wind, rocks and tide combined to threaten its safety.[4] More significantly still, a cruising fleet could not maintain its station for an extended period of time without losing much of its manpower to sickness.[5] As James Lind, the eminent naval physician who was stationed at Haslar hospital during the war, remarked:

---

[2] A.N. Ryan, 'The Royal Navy and the Blockade of Brest, 1689–1805: Theory and Practice', in M. Acerra, J. Merino, J. Meyer (eds), *Les Marines de guerre européennes, XVII–XVIIIe siècles* (Paris, 1985), pp. 176, 181.

[3] Ryan, 'Blockade of Brest', p. 181; M. Duffy, 'The Establishment of the Western Squadron as the Linchpin of British Naval Strategy', in M. Duffy (ed.), *Parameters of British Naval Power, 1650–1850* (Exeter, 1992), pp. 60–81. On the Squadron's role in the Seven Years War, see R. Middleton, 'British Naval Strategy, 1755–1762: The Western Squadron', *Mariner's Mirror*, 75 (1989), pp. 349–67; N.A.M. Rodger, *The Command of the Ocean: A Naval History of Britain, 1649–1815* (2nd edn, London, 2005), ch. 18.

[4] Rodger, *Command*, pp. 279–81.

[5] Ryan, 'Blockade of Brest', p. 182.

> The scurvy is a disease common in the winter and spring, and very fatal to seamen in the Channel cruisers ... when large squadrons of men of war are kept constantly employed in the Channel service, the length of their cruises, generally from ten to thirteen weeks, often occasions a great sickness ...[6]

As significant as Admiral Edward Hawke's defeat of the French navy at the Battle of Quiberon Bay in 1759 may have been for Britain's ultimate victory in the war, his success relied on a fleet that was as large as that under Conflans, fully manned, healthy, and which had been able to maintain a close blockade of Brest for eight months. As N.A.M. Rodger succinctly summarizes the triumph of 1759: 'It had never been possible for a fleet at sea to remain healthy for so long.'[7] This achievement has been attributed to the efficiency of naval administration on shore, and specifically to the sending out of fresh victuals under the direction of Anson and the Victualling Board.[8]

The mid-eighteenth-century naval physician James Lind advocated fresh provisions to prevent scurvy among sailors at sea for extended periods of time. He also proposed a number of measures that would not have had much success in preventing scurvy, such as regular issues of fresh meat, cream of tartar, cider, or the 'rob' (that is, boiled concentrate) of lemons and oranges.[9] As a result, naval historians have concluded that the health of the Western Squadron was maintained not because of contemporary medicine, but rather because of the initiatives of contemporary naval administration. While recognizing that naval officials may have been aware of Lind's medical theories, the historian Stephen Gradish argues that in the case of fresh victuals to the Western Squadron, inspiration came from Anson, organization came from the Victualling Board, and pressure to institute such measures came from both the Admiralty Board and naval officials such as Hawke and Boscawen.[10] Rodger not only concurs that naval administration must be credited but goes as far as asserting that it maintained the health of the fleet *despite* contemporary naval medicine.[11] According to Rodger's analysis, not only

---

[6]   J. Lind, *An Essay on the Most Effectual Means of Preserving the Health of Seamen in the Royal Navy* (3rd edn, London, 1774), pp. 18–19.

[7]   Rodger, *Command*, p. 281.

[8]   See especially S. Gradish, *The Manning of the British Navy During the Seven Years' War* (London, 1980). On naval administration, see D. Baugh, *British Naval Administration in the Age of Walpole* (Princeton, 1965); R. Middleton, 'Naval Administration in the Age of Pitt and Anson, 1755–1763', in J. Black and P. Woodfine (eds), *The British Navy and the Use of Naval Power in the Eighteenth Century* (Leicester, 1988), pp. 109–27; R. Middleton, 'Pitt, Anson and the Admiralty, 1756–1761', *History*, 55:184 (1970), pp. 189–98. For an even broader perspective, see J. Glete, *Navies and Nations: Warships, Navies and State Building in Europe and America, 1500–1800* (Stockholm, 1993).

[9]   Gradish, *Manning*, pp. 129–31; K. Carpenter, *The History of Scurvy and Vitamin C* (Cambridge, 1986), pp. 51–74.

[10]   Gradish, *Manning*, ch. 6.

[11]   N.A.M. Rodger, 'Le scorbut dans la Royal Navy pendant la guerre de Sept Ans, 1756–1763', in A. Lottin, J.-C. Hocquet, S. Lebecq (eds), *Les hommes et la mer dans l'Europe du nord-ouest de l'antiquité à nos jours* (*Revue du Nord*, extra number, 1986), pp. 455–62.

did eighteenth-century medical theory and practice have little to offer the Navy, but the great gains of naval medicine and especially of public health in the nineteenth century should be rightly considered as the offspring of naval administration. Rodger concludes, '[a]ny true history of eighteenth-century naval medicine … must in part be a history of medical knowledge gained by demolishing, or at least circumventing the power of the medical establishment.'[12]

To understand the methods taken by contemporaries to cure and prevent disease we need to understand how contemporaries understood disease. And here, we should also note that it was not simply scurvy that plagued ships' crews. But, as Lind himself recognized, the term 'scurvy' covered a broad swathe of diseases, and so was often used in a general sense. Moreover, eighteenth-century conceptions of the body and disease explained ill health by means of a combination of factors. These emphasized the role of an individual's constitution among various other 'predisposing' and 'occasional' causes. (Modern medical science also finds few diseases that are caused by one factor, and which are not notably influenced by an individual's constitution or exacerbated by environmental circumstances.) Likewise, observation demonstrated to eighteenth-century medical practitioners that one disease often gave rise to another, and that 'scurvy' in itself was not easily distinguished from other diseases.[13] As a consequence, distinguishing between scurvy and fevers in this period is difficult, as well as ahistorical, not only because contemporary observers claimed these diseases were not always distinct, but also because remedies for scurvy and fever were often the same. With miasma and putrefaction as the root causes of ill health, prevention and cure in the form of fresh air, ventilation, fumigation, and a diet of fresh provisions supplemented with acidic foodstuffs (in eighteenth-century terminology): all were recommended to maintain the health of seamen against both fevers and scurvy.

Contemporaries understood that scurvy was the product of a lack of fresh provisions, although the explanation of the disease was not through a lack of a specific vitamin, but rather through the onset of putrefaction. Putrefaction, eighteenth-century medical authorities claimed, was the natural state into which our bodies would descend if we did not continually refresh ourselves with eating, drinking, and constant natural evacuations, including perspiration brought on by exercise.[14] Along with John Pringle, Lind argued that on the basis of their various experiments and years of observations and experience (including Lind's two years as a naval surgeon on Channel service), scurvy was a disease of putrefaction caused by a number of factors. Most important among these was a damp environment, and especially the moist and often unventilated and cold air in which seamen worked and slept, and a diet based on salted meats and unleavened bread. His much-cited

---

[12] N.A.M. Rodger, 'Medicine and Science in the British Navy of the Eighteenth Century', in C. Buchet (ed.), L'Homme, la santé et la mer (Paris, 1997), p. 341.

[13] 'The Water-Dock', The Medical Museum: Or, a Repository of Cases … Home and Abroad, I (London, 1763), pp. 50, 51.

[14] James Lind, A Treatise of the Scurvy … and Cure, of that Disease (Edinburgh, 1753), pp. 272–3.

trial with lemons on board HMS *Salisbury* notwithstanding, Lind did not argue that a lack of fresh fruit and vegetables was the main cause of scurvy.[15] Indeed, his observations as a naval surgeon and physician led him to argue explicitly against such a scenario. He explains that he had had witnessed scurvy on HMS *Salisbury* while cruising in the Channel, despite the fact that the sailors had only recently consumed many vegetables while on shore. Yet, this is not to suggest that Lind did not recognize the benefit of fresh fruit and vegetables to the health of seamen while at sea. He reasons:

> So that although it is a certain and experienced truth, that the use of greens and vegetables is effectual in preventing the disease, and extremely beneficial in the cure; and thus we shall say, that abstinence from them, in certain circumstances, proves the *occasional cause* of the evil: yet there are unquestionably to be found at sea, other strong sources of it; which with respect to the former (or want of vegetables) we shall hereafter distinguish by the name of the *predisposing causes* to it.[16]

Lind thus identified the damp and cramped conditions on board ship as the *'principal and main predisposing cause'* of scurvy, along with a diet lacking in fresh provisions, especially fruit and vegetables, as well as a constitution liable to such a disease.[17]

In sum, disease in general, and scurvy in particular, was best prevented through exercise and a healthy diet, especially one that included fresh provisions, and if that was not possible, one that included what were called 'antiseptics' and 'antiscorbutics': citrus fruits, vinegar, types of grass, ginger, wine, beer made with spruce – all items that had been shown to retard the rotting and putrefaction of meat in various trials.

Lind, and other officials including naval officials, recognized that it was thus the circumstances of a ship at sea that posed the greatest challenge to a crew's health. Regular stops in harbour were therefore the optimal preventative of sickness.[18] This is demonstrated in the terminology used: such stops were called 'refreshments', both for the ships themselves (being scraped and cleaned), and also for the men. Specifically, time on shore provided fresh air (that is, air not as moist as on board ship), exercise, and fresh provisions: all agreed that these were the best cures, as well as the best preventatives, for scurvy. Although the men might be

---

[15] Although most naval historians, such as N.A.M. Rodger, recognize this reading of Lind, there are still a surprising number who credit Lind with observing that lemon juice or fresh vegetables alone would cure scurvy. See, for example, D.I. Harvie, *Limeys: The True Story of One Man's War Against Ignorance, the Establishment and the Deadly Scurvy* (Stroud, 2002).

[16] Lind, *Scurvy*, p. 53.

[17] Ibid., pp. 64, 65, 67; see an excellent summary of Lind's theory of scurvy in W. McBride, '"Normal" Medical Science and British Treatment of the Sea Scurvy, 1753–75', *Journal of the History of Medicine and Allied Sciences*, 46 (1991), pp. 160–63.

[18] Rodger estimates that ships usually spent more than half their time in port during this period. See *The Wooden World: An Anatomy of the Georgian Navy* (London, 1988), pp. 37–9, and appendix II: 'Sea Time', p. 352.

granted a few days' leave once a ship arrived into port after a cruise, what was more certain was that fresh provisions would be served. On so-called 'flesh days', fresh meat was granted to men four days a week, when in port.[19] Logbooks of various ships record the receipt of fresh meat on board when in port, usually in the form of entire bullocks, and they also record the cutting up of this meat to be served to the sick, and if much was left over, to the entire ship's company.[20]

This practice was gradually modified during the summer and autumn of 1759. During this period, the Lords of the Admiralty were explicit about the importance of maintaining a constant blockade of Brest, in the midst of intelligence concerning a French invasion that required supplies to be assembled at Brest. Responding to Hawke's complaint that he had not enough beer and water to remain on station in early October, the Lords assured Hawke that they had already ordered and sent more beer and wine. Such immediate action, the Lords told Hawke, 'will enable you to continue on your station where it is more necessary than ever for you to remain as long as possible at this very critical conjuncture'.[21]

During the same period, officials began to supply the Squadron with vegetables: the procedure which historians have considered as the key to keeping the fleet out for so long.[22] The amount sent, and the regularity with which vegetables were sent, is difficult to ascertain. While regular records of fresh meat received on board exist, and such shipments appear to have been carefully noted, the arrival of vegetables does not appear to have been given the same importance, perhaps because fresh meat was believed to be just as important to maintaining the men's health, and also perhaps because officials were more concerned with keeping careful accounts of the more expensive fresh meat. The practice of sending vegetables out to ships in Quiberon Bay and Belle Isle during the war is noted in the Navy Board's Pay Office books regarding precedents and exceptions for pursers' accounts. It appears that the charge for vegetables was somewhat muddled, as the pursers charged the vegetables as if they were 'a gift to the seamen', and hence not on their accounts, while the Board appears to have charged the cost to each ship's accounts.[23] Also, the records concerning condemned vegetables do not state what was wrong and exactly how much was thrown overboard. This deviation from standard procedure for condemned victuals, where pursers and commanding officers had to follow procedure and keep detailed records of the amount surveyed and condemned,

[19] Duffy, 'Establishment', pp. 67–8.
[20] NMM, ADM L/P.4, Lieutenant's Journal of HMS *Pallas*, 1757–62, and NMM, ADM L/P.3, Journal of HMS *Pallas*, 1757–60.
[21] Admiralty to Hawke, 5 October 1759, The National Archives, London (hereafter TNA), ADM 2/526, ff. 332–3. As beer was widely regarded as an antiscorbutic, see the extensive attempts to remedy bad beer: Gradish, *Manning*, pp. 156–7; on Admiralty efforts to remedy bad beer, see NMM, HWK/11 (Hawke in-letters), August to October 1759, NMM, HWK/14 (Hawke out-letter book), August to October 1759.
[22] TNA, ADM 111/49 (Victualling Board Minutes), 3 August 1759.
[23] TNA, ADM 30/44 (Navy Board Pay Office: Precedents and Exceptions for Pursers' Accounts), f. 170.

again suggests that vegetables were not subject to the same rigorous administrative scrutiny as meat and regular provisions.

As for fresh meat, by early August 1759 officials suggested that, quantities allowing, it could be given to healthy seamen as well as the sick. Admiralty dispatches, Hawke's orders, and lieutenants' logbooks document an evolving practice of providing sick men with fresh meat as a matter of priority, while surplus provisions were occasionally distributed among healthy crew members.[24] The procuring of fresh provisions, including vegetables, was thus an extension of a common practice directed towards curing sick seamen when ships came into port. Lind, Admiralty officials, and commanders all recognized the benefit of fresh provisions. For ships not in port, naval officials searched for alternative means of maintaining the health of crews, such as regular issues of beer. The sending out of fresh meat and vegetables to ships on blockade was clearly first directed only towards the sick seamen, and occurred on an irregular basis. It developed only gradually into a measure applied to the entire squadron sailing under Hawke, just as the Western Squadron initially was a cruising squadron and only under dire necessity, because of a feared French invasion, became a constant blockade of Brest.

The impact and success of this supply of fresh provisions, regardless of Lind's high praise and the victory of Quiberon Bay in November 1759, are somewhat difficult to judge. Hawke and Admiralty officials were obviously pleased when such fresh provisions reached the fleet. Writing to the Admiralty on 28 August 1759, Hawke commented, '[t]he little fresh meat we have had has already showed it self in very salutary effects.'[25] Just three days later, Hawke complained to Pett, the victualling officer at Plymouth, that Pett must ensure fresh provisions would soon be sent again as 'we have been now sixteen weeks within a few days from Spithead, and the men falling down in the scurvey [sic]'.[26] While Hawke noted that most of the seamen were healthy, he repeatedly noted in his correspondence that the crew of HMS Foudroyant were very sickly.[27] As returns for the fleet under Hawke do not appear to survive, the actual rate of sickness among the Squadron cannot be clearly established. Yet comparing muster tables from ships among the Squadron in 1759 with those from 1758 (that is, prior to the regular supply of fresh provisions), there is not a dramatic difference in sick rates for the same time of year and cruise.[28]

This is not to suggest that the Western Squadron's virtually complete blockade of Brest and the Battle of Quiberon Bay could have been achieved without the

---

[24] Admiralty to Hawke, 7 August 1759, TNA, ADM 2/526, ff. 65–6; Admiralty to Victualling Board, 2 August 1759, ADM 2/82, f. 257; Hawke to Captains, 6 August 1759, NMM, HWK/5 (Hawke's Orders).

[25] Hawke to Admiralty, 28 August 1759, TNA, ADM 1/92.

[26] Hawke to Pett, 31 August 1759, NMM, HWK/14.

[27] See, for example, Hawke to Pett, 31 August 1759, NMM, HWK/14.

[28] TNA, ADM 36/6354 (muster book for HMS Pallas, 1758–9); I have followed N.A.M. Rodger and D. Crewe in using muster books to establish sick rates, although there are discrepancies with the few existing monthly and weekly returns.

supplies of fresh provisions. Yet in many ways the blockade was a precarious operation; had circumstances demanded its continuation into the 1760s, success would by no means have been guaranteed. Indeed, with the weather and winds becoming increasingly difficult during the winter of 1759–60, Hawke was then already finding sailing frustrating. By the middle of December, Hawke reported that his ships were short of supplies and some were becoming sickly, while for him, 'I have now been thirty one weeks on board, without setting my foot on shore, and cannot expect that my health will hold out much longer.'[29] He wrote to the Admiralty early in January 1760: '[e]very plan of operation I formed after the 1st of December has proved abortive, through bad weather and want of provisions and necessaries.'[30]

There were constant problems with the small victualling sloops, especially during the rough winter weather. After Hawke's decisive battle in Quiberon Bay, few more were sent out, and Lind reports that scurvy consequently afflicted the crews. Throughout most of his cruise in 1760, Boscawen not only reported sickness among his crew, but also found provision transports damaged by the rocks, and described their supplies as 'so small and uncertain that it will be of very little use.'[31] Likewise, the squadron in the Channel under Keppel during the latter part of 1760 and in 1761 suffered from sickness, including scurvy. When victuallers did reach Keppel, he noted that problems other than bad weather plagued the supply of fresh provisions: many of the sheep had died before they reached his fleet, while vegetables other than potatoes, onions and cabbages 'generally get here in such a condition from being rotten, that the good intent of their Lordships directing such supplys became useless, as well as expensive.'[32]

Supplies of live cattle and good vegetables were surely scarce and expensive, especially during the shortages that prevailed during war years. Vegetables and fruit were not only uncommon fare among the labouring classes in this period, but their supply would have been entirely seasonal.[33] Such regular supplies of live cattle and vegetables for the seven thousand sailors in the squadron, and perhaps double that number during 1759, must also have disrupted local port markets. In June 1760, Boscawen reported to the Admiralty, 'Captain Hughes of the Tamar that convoy'd the Transports with Bullocks and Sheep from Ireland tells me that he is afraid the Populace will not suffer more to be shipp'd at Cork'.[34] Overall,

[29] Hawke to Admiralty, 16 December 1759, NMM, HWK/14.
[30] Hawke to Admiralty, 7 January 1760, TNA, ADM 1/92.
[31] Boscawen to Admiralty, 19 February 1760, and turn-over-note 27 February 1760, TNA, ADM 1/90; Boscawen reported sickness throughout the months February to May 1760. He reports 'remarkable good health' among the squadron on 8 June 1760 after he had sent four ships to Plymouth containing all of the sick crew: Boscawen to Admiralty, 8 June 1760, TNA, ADM 1/90.
[32] Keppel to Admiralty, 6 November 1761, and 26 September 1761 regarding sheep mortality, TNA, ADM 1/91.
[33] Letters by Lind, Grainger, and Huxham in *The Medical Museum*, II (London, 1763–4), pp. 318–418.
[34] Boscawen to Admiralty, 15 June 1760, TNA, ADM 1/90.

such provisioning would have been very expensive, and thus difficult to continue financing over a long period of time, in addition to the various practical problems that plagued supply transports and meant that provisioning at sea was never regular or dependable.[35] While stationed in Quiberon Bay in early 1761, Hawke requested a sufficient number of ships in order to rotate the fleet and send ships to port frequently, 'to preserve their companies, be enabled to perform the duties of the station, and save the exorbitant expence of victuallers, which after all but little answer their intended purpose.'[36] Even after the success and glory of the battle at Quiberon, Hawke described the sailing during the blockade as especially harsh. After his return home early in 1760, he wrote, '[i]ndeed I have had a very long tiresome and fatiguing cruize, and as hard a piece of service to go thro with, as cou'd be put upon any Man; but thank God I waded thro it at last.'[37] Hawke claimed that cruising during the blockade warranted special recognition from the Admiralty, not just because of victory over the French, but because of the difficulty encountered while at sea. He wrote late in 1760 to the Admiralty about the situation of those commanders:

> Being witness last year; while I commanded a Squadron of the King's Ships off Ushant to the great fatigue and pains, which the masters; who conducted squadrons on that dangerous station; I wrote to you on the 23d of Sept 1759 to lay their case before their Lordships.[38]

Even the intrepid Hawke recognized that the conditions of constant blockading were exceptional, and unusually harsh, notwithstanding the supply of fresh meat and vegetables. The supply of fresh provisions that included vegetables, for the four months between July and November 1759, did indeed allow a great naval victory over the French. But because of financial constraints and logistical difficulties it appears that such an operation was not continued for long after Hawke's victory, and nor could it be widely or regularly instituted to ensure dependable operations of a Western Squadron for an extended period of time. While we need to recognize that the Western Squadron's battle and blockade in 1759 were remarkable achievements, it is also apparent that a permanent Western Squadron was not yet possible. The main reason for this was the health of crews. Fresh provisions, regularly provided on shore, were identified by medical officials and naval officials as the key to maintaining health, yet their constant supply to ships at sea stretched naval capabilities during the 1750s and 1760s.

---

[35] Duffy, 'Establishment', pp. 68–9.
[36] Hawke to Admiralty, 13 January 1761, NMM, HWK/15.
[37] Hawke to Lady Kingston, 9 February 1760, NMM, AGC/V/8.
[38] Hawke to Admiralty, 11 October 1760, NMM, HWK/15.

The Sick and Hurt Board and Medical Trials

The body that was widely responsible for medical practice within the Navy was the Sick and Hurt Board, also often called the Sick and Wounded Board. In 1756, the Board comprised four commissioners and four clerks, as well as officials and medical practitioners stationed in various ports upon whom the Board relied for informed correspondence.[39] Its responsibilities during the Seven Years War were the care of sick and wounded seamen, medical practitioners in the Navy, naval hospitals, and all prisoners of war. Given this remit, the Board has been characterized by naval historians more as an administrative committee than a medical authority, and criticized upon this account.[40] Although Gradish notes that by 1756 two of the four commissioners were medical men, James Maxwell being a physician with hospital experience and Henry Tom a former naval ship and hospital surgeon, he concludes that the Sick and Hurt Board is best regarded during this period as an administrative body, without the authority to introduce any medical initiatives.[41] Likewise, Rodger argues not only that contemporary medical knowledge had little to offer the Navy, but also that the Sick and Hurt Board:

> had little to do with ships at sea, and though its members usually included a physician, it too was mainly an administrative rather than a medical or scientific body. Thus the naval administrative system provided no focus outside the Admiralty itself where medical or scientific opinion could be brought to bear on problems of health at sea.[42]

While it is true that, by today's standards, most naval diseases were not curable in the eighteenth century, contemporary medical authorities were optimistic that naval diseases could be treated and even to some extent prevented. Similarly, the correspondence of the Sick and Hurt Board during the Seven Years War, while not demonstrating that they considered themselves authorities beyond the power of the Admiralty, does demonstrate that they believed themselves to be a medical body responsible for evaluating practical cures and preventatives. In this respect, not only were they fully aware of the constraints inherent in shipboard life, but they also combined medical knowledge with bureaucratic practicality, thus challenging Rodger's dichotomy between medicine and naval administration during the period.

The most well known, and in some ways most successful, medical initiative of the Sick and Hurt Board during this period was the introduction of portable soup or broth, the issue of which continued throughout the eighteenth century. Made of beef and mutton left over from the salted naval rations, it was formed into small

---

[39] P.K. Crimmin, 'The Sick and Hurt Board and the Health of Seamen c. 1700–1806', *Journal for Maritime Research* [www.jmr.nmm.ac.uk] (December 1999), p. 4.
[40] C. Lloyd and J.S. Coulter, *Medicine and the Navy 1200–1900. Vol. III: 1714–1815* (Edinburgh, 1961), p. 7; Crimmin, 'Sick and Hurt', pp. 6–7.
[41] Gradish, *Manning*, p. 21.
[42] Rodger, 'Medicine and Science', p. 335.

cakes that were easily stored on board, and then mixed with boiling water and served to the men as soup, often with vegetables or grains. In early August 1757, the Admiralty ordered Hawke to trial some portable soup, with detailed instructions regarding its use. Over the next few weeks, Hawke sent out orders to the captains of various ships under his command, not only detailing where and how to store it as well as how to prepare it, but also notifying the captains that they were 'to direct the Surgeon to make very nice and particular observations on the effects of it, on the Sick more especially those afflicted with the Scurvey and to report to them at the end of every Cruize their opinion of its efficacy and utility'.[43]

As directed, surgeons reported on the efficacy of the broth. The surgeon of HMS *Intrepid* (in Hawke's squadron) wrote in praise of the broth. While he did not claim that the broth cured the sick seamen, he maintained that it was essential in preserving the lives of the sick until they reached the naval hospitals on shore. The surgeon patriotically proclaimed: 'Every British Seafaring Man in His Majesty's Navy ought to be thankful for this great refreshing Benefit ... I hope Success will Crown the design'.[44] Likewise, the surgeon of HMS *Barfleur* reported to the Sick and Hurt Board that the sick seamen he cared for would only eat the broth, which he credited (along with mutton) for 'the loss of so few men afterwards and that none were swept away by the scurvy at sea'.[45]

With such positive reports, the portable broth was more widely instituted and regulated in the Navy. In February 1758, the Sick and Hurt Board distributed prescribed instructions for issuing the broth, including a form to be filled by the surgeons which detailed the length of time and the type of disease from which the patient suffered.[46] In October 1758, the Board still described the portable broth as on trial, although it noted that it was a successful one. In writing to the Admiralty, the Commissioners of the Board also explained that they had hired a new person responsible for making the broth, as the original cook had resigned when the Board had insisted she receive only her stated salary and not any 'irregular Emoluments'.[47] Likewise, the procedure under which the broth was made was also standardized.

The portable soup appears to have been well liked, judging by the requests for it. By February 1759, the Board had to turn down a request for portable soup from Colonel Eyre Coote in India, as they did not have enough with which to supply both the Army and the Navy. They therefore asked the Admiralty for permission to extend production of the soup to Portsmouth and Plymouth.[48] Permission must have been granted, as during the expedition to Belle Isle in 1761, the Board

---

43 Hawke to Young, 12 August 1757, NMM, ADL/M/2; Hawke to Fergussone, 16 November 1757, NMM HWK/5; Hawke to Hobbs, 13 August 1757, NMM HWK/4.
44 SHB to Admiralty, enclosure in 4 January 1758, NMM, ADM F/17 (Sick and Hurt Board out-letters).
45 SHB to Admiralty, enclosure in 24 January 1759, NMM, ADM F/19.
46 SHB to Admiralty, 3 February 1758, NMM, ADM F/17.
47 SHB to Admiralty, 12 October 1758, NMM, ADM F/18.
48 SHB to Admiralty, 24 February 1759, NMM, ADM F/19.

agreed to give its excess portable soup to the Director of the Army Hospitals.[49] By the end of the war, the portable soup had become part of the standard diet at naval hospitals, with greens and grains usually added.[50] With the recipe for the broth itself containing nothing that would have provided vitamin C, it is most likely that it was the common practice of adding vegetables to the broth that made it so healthy.

Dried apples were also tried as a possible cure for scurvy. Early in August 1757, the Sick and Hurt Commissioners advised the Admiralty that eight and a half bushels of dried apples had arrived from North America, 'to make experiments with them on seamen ill of the scurvy'.[51] Hawke was instructed to try this cure carefully on one of his ships, adding, 'we make no question, but you will have the goodness to give orders for the tryal of them to be made under your own Eye'.[52] Hawke's instructions from the Sick and Hurt Commissioners included recipes for apple pudding and apple pie, with sugar, nutmeg, and cinnamon as seasoning. Although apples contain little vitamin C, and once dried and soaked in water contain even less, dried apples and the water in which they were soaked would have had other health benefits – such as fibre and minerals – for men who otherwise ate dried biscuits and salt meat.

Yet, even if the effect of portable broth and dried apples in curing or preventing scurvy is doubtful, the procedures revealed by these initiatives are instructive. Under the authority of the Sick and Hurt Board, suggestions were first instituted as trials or experiments upon the seamen, with surgeons reporting their observations to the Board. If found successful, the Board formally regulated the production and issue of such items. While it appears that portable broth was the only successful initiative during the Seven Years War, the evaluation of various other suggestions reveals the medical theory and workings of the Sick and Hurt Board. In December of 1757, for example, the Board received a request from a Mr Leake to try out his medicine. The Board found that Leake neither would disclose his medicine's contents nor knew anything about sea scurvy, and recommended that no trial should proceed.[53] The Board also turned down a proposal to use oil as a cure and preventative for scurvy, on the theoretical grounds that such a treatment would produce putrid fevers in the conditions of a ship, noting that the individual who proposed the remedy had conducted no experiments that demonstrated anything to the contrary.[54]

While contemporary medical theory was thus used to explicate a proposed cure, the Board repeatedly stressed the need for trials to demonstrate the safety and efficacy of a proposed cure as well. When the Board refused to try Richard

[49] SHB to Admiralty, 5 November 1760 and 28 February 1761, NMM, ADM F/21; see above note 103, p. 250, on provisions to Belle Isle.
[50] Lind, *Health of Seamen*, p. viii; Gradish, *Manning*, p. 160.
[51] SHB to Admiralty, 5 August 1757, NMM, ADM F/16.
[52] SHB to Hawke, 9 August 1757, NMM, HWK/10.
[53] SHB to Admiralty, 5 December 1757, NMM, ADM F/16.
[54] SHB to Admiralty, 27 March 1758, NMM, ADM F/17.

Dunn's medicine to cure fluxes in May 1759, they explained that it was not only because Dunn had not studied medicine, but also because he would not disclose its ingredients. The Board recommended that he 'find proper people who would voluntarily take his medicine and told him we would attend to the effects of it'.[55] Similarly, the Board was wary of the publican William Adams's 'infallible cure for the flux'. Although Adams claimed that the recipe was originally from India, and that he had tried it on himself and others with success in the 1740s, the Board still insisted that Adams produce people or certificates that attested to its more recent success.[56]

If the safety and relative efficacy of a proposed medicine or preventative were established by medical theory and by certificates, the Board then allowed the medicine to be tried on a small number of seamen at a naval hospital. When Edward Hogkin was granted permission to conduct a trial on his cure for the flux, on the Board's direction officials at Haslar hospital selected twelve patients for Hogkin's use. When the Board reported Hogkin's medicine ineffective among these twelve, the Admiralty cancelled the second planned trial at Plymouth hospital.[57] Similarly, Robert Douglas was allowed to try his cure for scurvy on four patients at Haslar, under no less an authority than Lind. Upon further examination, however, the Board concluded that not only was Douglas's cure not original, the main ingredient already having being published in Lind's *Treatise on the Scurvy*, but they also considered it impossible to judge the efficacy of a cure for scurvy among sailors on shore given that their diet contained fresh provisions.[58] As Douglas insisted that his cure could work at sea as well, the Board recommended a sea trial. The orders that accompanied Douglas upon this experiment are especially significant. Vice-Admiral Saunders, as commander-in-chief in the Mediterranean, was instructed:

> to give the said Mr. Douglas all possible assistance for his making the proposed experiment, and that due care be taken that the persons put under his cure are such as are really afflicted with that distemper, and that while under cure they have no other assistance of diet or otherwise than such as the sick of His Majesty's Fleet at sea are generally supplied with; as this is a circumstance particularly to be attended to, to ascertain the real efficacy of the medicine; and as it did not appear upon the experiment made last year in the hospital at Haslar that the patients under his cure and enjoying the benefit of hospital diet etc received the least peculiar Advantage. ...[59]

The Commissioners of the Sick and Hurt Board were thus fully aware that a useful cure for scurvy must be one applicable to the circumstances of a ship at sea. This distinction, and the Commissioners' understanding that a valid cure for scurvy in the Navy had to be effective in the absence of fresh provisions, was again

---

[55] SHB to Admiralty, 24 May 1759, NMM, ADM F/19.
[56] SHB to Admiralty, 11 April 1758, NMM, ADM F/19.
[57] SHB to Admiralty, 14 April 1758, NMM, ADM F/17.
[58] SHB to Admiralty, 21 July 1760, NMM, ADM F/21.
[59] SHB to Admiralty, 22 April 1761, NMM, ADM F/21.

made in the evaluation of wort as a cure for scurvy, as proposed by Dr McBride. The Commissioners stated that they considered wort ineffective on shore, but suggested that it might be useful at sea, where fresh meat and vegetables 'which chiefly contributes to the cure on shore, cannot be had'.[60] Again, in response to a suggestion to carry fresh fruit to sea, the Commissioners noted, 'lemons and oranges and apples would be very useful on a cruize at sea if it was practicable to carry and serve such quantities as would be necessary'.[61] Although fresh provisions had been supplied to ships in the Western Squadron during the preceding years, the Sick and Hurt Board and the Admiralty thus must have been aware that such operations could not be widely instituted in the Navy. The Board's continuing search for a cure for scurvy, rather than denying the advantages of fresh provisions, was simply a search for a practical cure that could be applied throughout the Navy and its operations.

As they had remarked during their evaluation of Douglas's cure for scurvy, the Commissioners were well acquainted with Lind's suggestions in his *Treatise on the Scurvy*.[62] The problem was the logistics and cost of supplying such items to ships during naval operations, a concern that was characteristic of an administrative, as well as a medical, body. The Commissioners, however, did not consider a cure beyond their grasp, especially if one applied contemporary medical theory and demonstrated the efficacy of cures through experiments. According to Lind, contemporary medical theory, and empirical observations, the remedial qualities of oranges and lemons should be found in other so-called 'antiseptics' too, such as wort, vinegar, or apples. The medical challenge for the Commissioners of the Sick and Hurt Board was to find a cure that was affordable and available in sufficient quantities to supply around seventy thousand seamen, but which could also be stored for months at a time in damp and already cramped conditions.

There is nothing to suggest that the medical trials and experiments described here were entirely new to this period. Indeed, a reference to a trial conducted in the 1740s suggests that such procedures had been in use for some years.[63] A standard procedure emerged that allowed assessment of a medicine within different naval contexts: first one trial in one hospital ashore, then a second trial at another hospital, then on board a limited number of ships, and finally widely given to ships while sailing, relying on surgeons' reports to evaluate the efficacy of the medicine at sea. The use of clinical trials and the emphasis on empiricism does not necessarily exclude the Sick and Hurt Board from mainstream medical practice. While physicians were meant to be university-trained, steeped in theory and learning, and lacking in practical experience, the gap between those who actually practised medicine and those who theorized has recently been shown to have been

---

[60] SHB to Admiralty, 1 July 1762, NMM, ADM F/23.
[61] SHB to Admiralty, 27 August 1761, NMM, ADM F/22.
[62] See p. 31 above.
[63] SHB to Admiralty, 30 March 1757, NMM, ADM F/15.

much smaller than traditionally assumed.[64] Within the voluntary hospitals that were established throughout urban areas in Britain during the eighteenth century, clinical observations and clinical trials were made possible; by the 1780s and 1790s they appear to have been common.[65] The detailed research of Andreas-Holger Maehle suggests that the experimental evaluation of drugs, including controlled experiments and individual clinical trials, can be traced back as far as the late seventeenth century. These trials were motivated by therapeutic concerns, as were the trials under the Sick and Hurt Board. Unlike the latter trials, however, for the most part the earlier drug trials were very limited in scope; indeed, often they were confined to the medical practitioner testing on himself. Only in the 1770s and 1780s were they extended to groups of patients in hospital care.[66]

Although the type of medical trial practised by the Sick and Hurt Board was probably not widespread in the mid eighteenth century, there is nothing to suggest that the Commissioners of the Board thought they were inventing a new scientific method. What was different in the case of the Sick and Hurt Board was their ability to institute systematic trials upon a large number of individuals.[67] Having men under their command, and large numbers under their care in hospitals and on board ships, naval medicine was perfectly suited to clinical trials and observations.[68] Not surprisingly, in eighteenth-century France clinical trials also first appeared at military and naval hospitals and then in civilian hospitals.[69]

Conclusion

The Sick and Hurt Board did not seem aware that these medical practices involved a theoretical challenge to standard medicine. As had been the case in

[64] For an examination of the ambiguity and fluidity of medical authority in eighteenth-century England, see Roy Porter, *Health for Sale: Quackery in England* (Manchester, 1989). Military medical historians have noted evidence of practical medicine in the armed forces in early periods: see, for example, H.J. Cook, 'Practical Medicine and the British Armed Forces after the "Glorious Revolution"', *Medical History*, 34 (1990), pp. 1–26. Historians of hospital medicine in the eighteenth century have also noted similar widespread tendencies: see, for example, G. Risse, *Hospital Life in Enlightenment Scotland: Care and Teaching at the Royal Infirmary of Edinburgh* (Cambridge, 1986), chs 4–5; S.C. Lawrence, *Charitable Knowledge: Hospital Pupils and Practitioners in Eighteenth-Century London* (Cambridge, 1996), chs 3–6.

[65] Risse, *Hospital Life*, ch. 4 and epilogue; Lawrence, *Charitable Knowledge*.

[66] For an overview of the nature of clinical trials in this period, see A.-H. Maehle, *Drugs on Trial: Experimental Pharmacology and Therapeutic Innovation in the Eighteenth Century* (Amsterdam, 1999).

[67] For earlier periods and empiricism, see S. Shapin and S. Schaffer, *Leviathan and the Air-Pump: Hobbes, Boyle, and the Experimental Life* (Princeton, 1995); C. Licoppe, *La formation de la pratique scientifique: le discours de l'expérience en France et en Angleterre (1630–1820)* (Paris, 1996) – although these forms of empirical practice are somewhat different from the medical 'trials' of the Navy.

[68] For an earlier period, see Cook, 'Practical Medicine'.

[69] L.W.B. Brockliss and C. Jones, *The Medical World of Early Modern France* (Oxford, 1997), ch. 11.

the development of the Western Squadron, it instead appears that they believed they were simply instituting practical solutions using available resources. With hindsight, such small practices did indeed change the nature of medical enquiry and theory, especially reinforced by the development of hospital medicine during the later eighteenth century. By instituting standardized clinical trials on groups of anonymous men in the Navy, asking for specific observations in order to make judgements regarding the efficacy of the substance on trial, and assuming that these trials could be replicated throughout the Navy in a variety of climates by low-level practitioners, the Board was challenging the usual case-by-case or individual approach to evaluating therapeutic efficacy. Although the medical trials conducted by the Sick and Hurt Board were in many ways simply an extension of an already established practice, this extension had wide-ranging repercussions for the nature of medical practice, and indeed for the relationship it demonstrates between sailors and the Admiralty, and, more broadly, the British state. With thousands of men under their command, the Navy was free to institute these trials upon the bodies of seamen.

By the end of the eighteenth century, such standardized views of the bodies of sailors meant that medical practitioners could statistically evaluate the health and medical care of sailors.[70] The care and money invested in maintaining the health of sailors during the war, whether through fresh provisions or through the search for a practical cure for scurvy, demonstrates that the Royal Navy, like the Army, considered the welfare of these men integral to their responsibilities, and relied on contemporary medical knowledge to do so. By the same token, naval medical care and medical trials during this period also indicate the resources and power available to the British state in the context of naval operations. The administrative resources, manpower, and money expended on providing fresh provisions to the Western Squadron during 1759, and more sporadically in the years after, were remarkable, as were the efforts of the Sick and Hurt Board in trials evaluating medical suggestions and implementing successful innovations, such as portable soup.

In many ways, the supply of fresh provisions to the seamen of the Western Squadron thus parallels the development of the Western Squadron itself. Medical officials had long recognized that fresh provisions would benefit the health of seamen, but due to practical constraints such provisioning was not possible when ships were at sea. When sick seamen were landed on shore, or when ships came into harbour, fresh provisions were supplied. Likewise, a fleet stationed in the westward approaches had long been recognized as an excellent strategy, but the logistical problems of having such a fleet stationed along those coasts for an extended period of time proved almost impossible to solve. Gradually, however, cruises were attempted for longer periods, until in 1759 a fleet sustained a blockade of Brest for eight months. This blockade was recognized not only as unusual, but

[70] U. Tröhler, 'To Improve the Evidence of Medicine': The Eighteenth-Century British Origins of a Critical Approach (Edinburgh, 2000).

also as a drain on the strength of the Royal Navy itself. While in the short term such a long cruise could certainly ensure the security of British coasts and colonies, in the long term such long cruises could wear out the British fleet and her men for years to come, rendering the Royal Navy vulnerable in future campaigns, as was the case in the 1770s and 1780s.

More broadly, this detailed examination of the Sick and Hurt Board's activities demonstrates that naval history and medical history should not be studied as challenges to each other, or indeed in isolation from each other and from wider historical developments. The Sick and Hurt Board in the eighteenth century cannot be accurately characterized as simply a naval administrative body, but neither can it be defined as a body concerned only with medical care. This is clearly demonstrated when medical theories and methods are studied within their contemporary context, including explanations and motivations. As the naval surgeon of HMS *Barfleur* reported in 1758 regarding the introduction of broth for sick sailors at sea, 'the Intention is certain Noble, and I hope Success will Crown the design'.[71]

Comparing the Navy with the Army, it appears at first glance that the Navy was able to maintain a better standard of health among crews, especially because naval officials were able to institute stricter controls to maintain the health of sailors, due to the practice of impressment and the tighter control over men on board ships. Yet this assumption can be challenged on a number of fronts. First, as Rodger's detailed examination of the 'disordered cohesion' of life on board ships during the Seven Years War demonstrates, naval officials commanded not through threats and strict discipline, but rather through persuasion and the recognition of seamen's traditional rights and privileges.[72] Secondly, there was significant overlap between medical services in the Army and Navy, especially as almost all operations were amphibious. As noted, during the expeditions to the coast of France, even provisions for the soldiers were provided by the Navy. James Maxwell, one of the Commissioners of the Sick and Hurt Board during the war, had previously served as a medical official with the British Army, and corresponded with Viscount Barrington (the Secretary at War) regarding the medical services of the Army.[73] The Western Squadron was thus in many ways an unusual operation, in that it involved the Navy in isolation. Thirdly, the nature of a ship on cruise, with its damp and crowded environment, and the lack of fresh provisions, was in itself the greatest challenge to the health of sailors during this period. Fourthly, there was no significant difference between the sick rates of military and naval troops. Whether on campaign for four months, or at sea for four months, both the Army and the Navy during the Seven Years War averaged morbidity rates of 20 per cent, and when campaigns or cruises continued for longer, rates dramatically

---

[71] SHB to Admiralty, enclosure in 4 January 1758, NMM, ADM F/17 (Sick and Hurt Board out-letters).
[72] Rodger, *Wooden World*, p. 346, chs 1, 6, and conclusion.
[73] Maxwell to Barrington, 16 March 1756, BL Add MS 73632 (Barrington Papers), ff. 1–2.

increased.[74] With archival material physically separated, historians of warfare tend to separate their studies of the Army and Navy, giving the illusion that during times of war, operations and conditions were also disparate.

Yet there were important differences between the Army and the Navy during this period. Most significantly, naval operations were clearly centralized around Admiralty offices, which is reflected in the structure of naval medical care. The establishment of permanent and large naval hospitals during the Seven Years War meant that almost all sick sailors were sent back to Britain for care, while sick soldiers were treated in field hospitals. As a result, the medical care for sailors and disabled sea veterans was more centralized and regulated than that of the Army; soldiers, in contrast, often settled in various colonial outposts upon the end of the war.[75] The structure of this medical care, and the power of the fiscal-military state that supported it, was also thus more clearly discernible, not least in the imposing naval hospital buildings.[76]

The British state is also made visible in the practice of these trials and experiments. As historians of science have pointed out, the development of experimental science depends not only on obtaining bodies on which to try methods, but also on the judgement and authority of the individual who conducts the experiment.[77] Douglas and other applicants whose trials were deemed failures by the Commissioners protested that this was because they had not been able to conduct the trial entirely as they had wished to. In this context, it was the British state that provided naval officers and ships' surgeons with the authority to oversee such trials, and this suggests the nascent development of later practices regarding state regulation and standardization, overseen by 'experts' acting as intermediaries between the state and theoretical knowledge.[78]

---

[74] E.M. Charters, 'Disease, War, and the Imperial State: The Health of the British Armed Forces during the Seven Years War, 1756–63' (Oxford University D.Phil. thesis, 2007), especially pp. 38–40, 88–94, 115–18, 131–2, 193, 197–8, 204–6.

[75] See S. Brumwell, *Redcoats: The British Soldier and War in the Americas, 1755–1763* (Cambridge, 2002), pp. 290–314; see also his 'Home from the Wars', *History Today*, 52:3 (2002), pp. 41–7. For India, see P.J. Marshall, *East India Fortunes: The British in Bengal in the Eighteenth Century* (Oxford, 1976), pp. 15–16; 'British Expansion in India in the Eighteenth Century: A Historical Revision', in his *Trade and Conquest: Studies on the Rise of British Dominance in India* (Aldershot, 1993), pp. 35–41.

[76] C. Stevenson, *Medicine and Magnificence: British Hospital and Asylum Architecture, 1660–1815* (London, 2000), chs 2–3.

[77] See, for example, Simon Schaffer, 'Self-Evidence', in J. Chandler et al. (eds), *Questions of Evidence: Proof, Practice, and Persuasion across the Disciplines* (Chicago, 1991), pp. 56–91; and notes 65–7 above.

[78] W.J. Ashworth, 'Quality and the Roots of Manufacturing "Expertise" in Eighteenth-Century Britain', forthcoming in *Osiris*; C. Rabier, 'Introduction: Expertise in Historical Perspective', in C. Rabier (ed.), *Fields of Expertise: A Comparative History of Expert Procedures in Paris and London, 1600 to Present* (Newcastle, 2007), pp. 1–34; E.H. Ash, *Power, Knowledge, and Expertise in Elizabethan England* (Baltimore, 2004). I am indebted to Dr William J. Ashworth on this point.

All this does not denigrate the importance of the Western Squadron and its achievements in 1759. As Lord Hardwicke recorded in his notes for the inquiry into Admiral John Byng's conduct during his unsuccessful mission to Minorca in 1757, when the Western Squadron was in place:

> The French Fleet was kept in, our coasts and colonies are unmolested, the French Trade, and the Succours intended for America have been in part intercepted, and our own Trade in the midst of War enjoyed all the Security of Peace.[79]

Yet Hardwicke also recognized the cost and dangers of the Squadron's implementation and maintenance. As he continued:

> These Benefits are not cheaply gained, a Fleet superior to what the Enemy can send out must be always employed … cruizers in all weather, and often with Tempestuous and contrary winds wears out the ships, the masts and rigging and it ruins the Health and costs the lives of the Seamen, it often disables a ship in a week which has been three months in preparing and it demands a great part of our naval Force.[80]

Hardwicke's notes were compiled to defend the decision not to send out a greater force with Byng, a decision which officials recognized had resulted in the loss of Minorca to the French.

Working with impressive, if still limited, resources, naval officials appreciated that keeping the Western Squadron constantly on cruise was of the utmost strategic significance in 1759. They accordingly directed resources into that which would ensure the Squadron's success, namely, the maintenance of sailors' health. Yet officials also recognized that such health provisions could only be supplied for short periods, that it was not a reliable or practical medium-term solution, and that it posed a great risk to Britain's naval capabilities in the long term, by undermining the availability of naval resources for years to come. Under these circumstances, the Sick and Hurt Board searched for a reliable and practical solution to ill health among seamen; in the process, it also developed a thoughtful and perceptive method of medical research.

79 BL, Add. MS 35895 (Hardwick Papers), f. 326.
80 BL, Add. MS 35895, f. 326.

2

Royal Navy Surgeons, 1793–1815: A Collective Biography

M. John Cardwell

Great Britain emerged from the great wars against Revolutionary and Napoleonic France between 1793 and 1815 as the world's foremost maritime and imperial power. Its ultimate victory in a struggle of unprecedented intensity owed much to significant advances in naval health.[1] Despite recognition of the seminal nature of this revolution, relatively little is known of the approximately two thousand surgeons who realised it through the daily care of the Navy's seamen and marines, often under the most adverse conditions.[2] Much of what has been written about the surgeons of the Georgian Royal Navy has been impressionistic in nature, given the limitations of source material. There are few surviving manuscript memoirs or collections of correspondence written by the surgeons themselves. Much contemporary printed commentary is often highly polemical in nature, and this has helped to create a negative image of their antecedents and ability, produced by reformers campaigning for improvements in Army and Navy surgeons' rank, pay, training and service conditions.[3] Popular fiction has also coloured perceptions, beginning with Tobias Smollett's caricature in *Roderick Random* (1748), while historical novelists such as C.S. Forester have at times portrayed the surgeon as a middle-aged sawbones, driven to the Navy by alcoholism or incompetence. At the other extreme, Patrick O'Brian's Stephen Maturin, skilled physician and world-renowned natural philosopher, embodies the highest attainments of a handful of elite practitioners, and is hardly more typical.

This essay presents a report of an ongoing research project, which seeks to provide a detailed and accurate collective biography of the naval surgeons of the

---

[1] Christopher Lloyd and Jack Coulter, *Medicine and the Navy 1200–1900. Vol. III. 1714–1815* (London, 1961), pp. 158–84; James Watt, 'Nelsonian Medicine in Context', *Journal of the Royal Naval Medical Service*, 86 (2000), pp. 64–71.

[2] Laurence Brockliss, M. John Cardwell and Michael Moss, *Nelson's Surgeon: William Beatty, Naval Medicine and the Battle of Trafalgar* (Oxford, 2005), pp. 1–34; J.C. Goddard, 'An Insight into the Life of Royal Navy Surgeons during the Napoleonic Wars', *Journal of the Royal Naval Medical Service*, 77–8 (1991–2), pp. 205–22, 27–36.

[3] J. Bell, *Memorial concerning the present state of military and naval surgery: Addressed several years ago to the Right Honourable Earl Spencer, First Lord of the Admiralty; and now submitted to the public* (London, 1800).

French Wars, and forms part of a wider study of the role played by the medical corps of the Army and Navy in promoting social opportunity, professionalisation and Britishness during the Industrial Revolution.[4] It is a work of social history, elucidating their origins, education, service careers, civilian practice, family, material welfare, intellectual interests, and wider contribution to contemporary British society. As it is impossible to treat all of these subjects here, attention will be concentrated upon the naval surgeons' background, medical training and professional expertise, as themes of most immediate interest to the naval historian. The project is made possible by the statistical analysis of a complex relational database of naval surgeons, supplemented by human insight gleaned from the testimony of the men themselves. Its foundation is a series of service registers, which were compiled from about 1825 for all medical officers who were warranted surgeon from the year 1774.[5] The registers were intended to assist in the settlement of questions involving seniority, and entitlement to half pay and retirement. With varying degrees of completeness, they record the medical officer's age, the date of his first warrant as surgeon, total years of service in that rank, declarations of physical fitness for duty, half pay addresses, and date of death. In the years following the rapid reduction of the Navy after the final defeat of Napoleon, the registers were also probably consulted to select the most capable officers for employment, since they summarize departmental correspondence denoting particular achievements, praise or censure.

Every second entry from the years 1793 to 1815 was entered into the database, giving an initial sample of 349 surgeons. For the purpose of comparison, the number was designed to be roughly equivalent to the sample of 454 surgeons which grounded the companion study of the British Army's medical corps. Therefore, eighty-one additional officers were added from the service register of naval assistant surgeons covering the period 1795 to 1815, making a representative sample of 430 navy medical officers.[6] A considerable number of other Admiralty archives were consulted to obtain the fullest possible picture of Navy surgeons' careers. These ranged from other service records, seniority lists, succession books, medical journals, and 'Black Books' listing appointments, the ships upon which they served, promotions and disciplinary breaches, to those dealing with full pay, half pay, other financial perquisites, prize money, superannuation, pensions for wounds or widows, compassionate allowances and probate.[7] This official data provides only the barest of skeletons from which to flesh out a vivid collective portrait of the contemporary naval surgeon. In order to investigate other vital aspects of his

---

4 See Marcus Ackroyd, Laurence Brockliss, Michael Moss, Kate Retford and John Stevenson, *Advancing with the Army: Medicine, the Professions, and Social Mobility in the British Isles, 1790–1850* (Oxford, 2006). I would like to thank my partners in this project, Laurence Brockliss and Michael Moss, for reading drafts of this paper.

5 TNA, ADM 104/12–15.

6 TNA, ADM 104/20.

7 See N.A.M. Rodger, *Naval Records for Genealogists* (Kew, 1998); Bruno Pappalardo, *Tracing your Naval Ancestors* (Kew, 2002).

experience, including his social origins, medical training, and family connections, it was necessary to mine an extensive variety of other archival sources in Great Britain, Ireland and abroad.

Origins

The most basic shortcoming of the Admiralty records is the lack of any source giving information about the surgeon's life before joining the Royal Navy, and in particular, his place of birth. Nonetheless, a reliable estimate of the national origins of naval surgeons can be obtained from the United Kingdom census records. The 1851 census was the first to record the country, parish and county of birth for those living in England, Scotland and Wales. The names of members of the cohort surviving to be counted in 1851, 1861 and 1871 were run through the census records, and one hundred were identified, nearly a quarter of the total.[8] The major weakness of the censuses lies in the absence of data from Ireland, where returns have not survived. This was compensated for by including the names of unidentified surgeons resident in Ireland, upon the likely surmise that the majority were Irish, in the same proportion of matches as found in the census records.

Table 2.1 Surgeons' country of origin

Country	No. of surgeons	Percentage of sample
Scotland	46	37.4
Ireland	41	33.3
England	31	25.2
Wales	4	3.3
Abroad	1	0.8 (Barbados)
Total	123	100

Source: The National Archives, HO/107, and RG9–10.

Although the Irish are probably now slightly over-represented, the results provide a sound estimate of the national make-up of the Navy medical service of the French Wars. According to the 1811 census, approximately 57 per cent of the population of the British Isles lived in England and Wales, 33 per cent in Ireland, and 10 per cent in Scotland. When these figures are compared to the nationality of Navy medical officers, the most striking features are the disproportionate number of Scots, who are over-represented by nearly four times, and the minority of English surgeons, who are under-represented by half. The small number of English naval surgeons is even more notable given that Englishmen formed the large majority of contem-

8   TNA, HO/107, and RG9–10.

porary British medical practitioners.[9] The number of Irish surgeons is roughly equivalent to their people's proportion of the entire population. The significant Scottish presence is emphasized by numbers of prominent officers, including the inspectors of hospitals and fleets, Sir James Clark (1788–1870) and Sir William Rae (1789–1873), and the long-serving Director-General of the Medical Department of the Navy, Sir William Burnett (1779–1861). Leading Irish figures included the inspector of hospitals, Sir George Magrath (1778?–1857), the assistant to the Director-General, Sir James Prior (1787?–1869), and the physician of Greenwich Hospital, Sir William Beatty (1773–1842).

It is possible to examine regional distributions where the census records the exact place of birth. The thirty-one English naval surgeons hailed from twenty different counties representing most of the country. The majority came from the south, where they were fairly evenly spread, with slight concentrations in Middlesex (4), and the maritime counties of Kent (4) and Hampshire (3). In Scotland, twenty-nine medical officers were drawn from a dozen counties, but nearly half hailed from two combined: Perth (8) and Aberdeen (5). There was a heavy concentration of Irish recruits in Ulster, which produced several senior officers, including Magrath, who was a native of Tyrone. A marked feature is the relatively small numbers who came from the three countries' capital cities. Only three of the thirty-one Englishmen were Londoners, only two of the twenty-nine Scots were natives of Edinburgh, and only two of the twelve Irishmen were born in Dublin. The number of surgeons who originated from London is slightly below the proportion of the national population who lived there (one in nine), while higher-than-average proportions were drawn from Edinburgh (which held one in twenty of the population) and Dublin (which held one in thirty).

Many of the English, Scottish and Welsh naval surgeons were born in ports, extending in size and significance from Bristol, Greenwich, Deptford, Scarborough, Aberdeen (the home of three) and Swansea, to smaller centres such as Wareham, Newhaven, Faversham, Kincardine and Cullen. Most others hailed from small market towns, villages, and rural parishes, some deep in the countryside. In England, examples included Northallerton in Yorkshire, Nantwich in Cheshire, Leigh-on-Mendip in Somerset, Radway in Warwickshire, and Wickham in Hampshire. Only one was born in a major county town, Hereford. The pattern is repeated in Scotland, particularly in the Perthshire cluster, which included the villages of Muthill, Abernethy, Callander and Methven. Notably, only two surgeons came from any of the industrializing areas of Britain: Stockport, near Manchester, and Hamilton in Lanarkshire.

Uncovering the social background of naval surgeons is perhaps the greatest challenge, given that official records offer few clues. There is one reliable source, however, which sheds light upon their fathers' occupations: the collection of wills deposited by servicemen in the Navy Office after 1786.[10] These are original wills

---

9   The accuracy of this data is confirmed by a close correlation with the geographic origins of Army surgeons; see Ackroyd *et al.*, *Advancing with the Army*, p. 61.
10   TNA, ADM 48.

listing the testator's name, rank, ship and disposable property. A search revealed the survival of nearly 190 wills, virtually all made by surgeon's mates or assistant surgeons. All were submitted between 1786 and 1807, except for one dated 1817. It is likely the wills were made by the surgeons immediately upon their first posting to active service. Many listed their parents as executors and beneficiaries, often providing their addresses, and in some cases including their fathers' occupations. Table 2.2 very broadly maps out the employment of all fathers recovered from ADM 48 (including those of surgeons not in the database) and all other sources.

Table 2.2 Occupations of naval surgeons' fathers

Occupation	No.
Agriculture	5
Professions	15
Administration	1
Architect/surveyor	2
Armed forces	1
Church	4
Medicine	7
Business/trade/service	19
Builders	1
Mariners	3
Manufacturers	3
Merchants	8
Labourers	1
Servants	1
Tradesmen	2
Independent gentlemen	1
Total	**40**

Source: The National Archives, ADM 48.

This sample gives a reliable general picture of the social background of the naval surgeons of the French Wars. Among members of the professional classes, medicine emerged as the largest occupation.[11] Significantly, all medical progenitors appear to have been simple surgeons or general practitioners. None was described as a physician – the position which occupied the height of medicine's professional and social hierarchy. Only one father, Thomas Billinghurst senior, an apothecary-surgeon, residing in Mayfair, London, seemed to have enjoyed an affluent practice or fashionable location. The fathers of two, Abraham Basson and Cuthbert Lee, worked as surgeons in the ports of Sheerness and North

[11] P.J. Corfield, *Power and the Professions in Britain, 1700–1850* (London, 2000), pp. 1–41.

Shields. Joseph Cornish's father was a country surgeon in Gloucestershire. Similarly, medical relatives, who may have influenced the cohort's choice of a career, rather than being well-connected members of the higher ranks of the calling, were also ordinary doctors employed in small towns or rural practices. These included Cuthbert Hillyars's uncle, who was a Portsea surgeon, and William Beatty's uncle, the naval surgeon George Smyth, who worked in the village of Buncrana near Londonderry. The overall impression is that these medical families lived in relatively modest circumstances, and that sons who wished to follow in the footsteps of their fathers or uncles had limited vocational prospects.

Other fathers who could claim the status of gentleman based upon their professional occupation included clergymen, but the identification of just four examples to date suggests that they were a very small minority. Of these, two belonged to the Church of Scotland, ministers of New Kilpatrick in Dunbartonshire and Liberton in Midlothian, while the third was a Church of Ireland cleric in Armagh. Other professionals included John Crofts's father, a surveyor of Margate, Kent, and Robert Dunlop's father, a builder and architect of Glaslough, Monaghan. Since Table 2.2 includes no lawyers, naval or military officers, university professors, or teachers, it is probable that they formed a very small fraction. Surgeon Forbes Chevers's father is listed under armed forces, but he was an army warrant officer, a master gunner stationed near Portsmouth. Government officials must also have formed but a minor proportion, since only one appears in ADM 48, the father and namesake of Charles Leith, who was an excise officer in Montrose.

The data collected so far suggest that the fathers of most naval surgeons were engaged in trade, business and manufacturing. The most successful of these was probably Sir John Richardson's father, Gabriel, a prosperous Dumfries brewer, who served as provost at one time and chief magistrate for many years.[12] The fathers of two other Scottish naval surgeons were also brewers. Assistant surgeon Neil Smith, who treated casualties on board HMS *Victory* at Trafalgar, was the son of an Aberdeen merchant. Fathers identified as merchants appear to have been small, local dealers. Two were based in Ireland, at Killybegs, Donegal, and Newcastle, county Limerick, and two more in Scotland, at Coupar Angus, Perthshire, and Bridgestown, Fifeshire. Tradesmen included Silas Wells's and Simon Brittons's fathers, linen drapers of Cheltenham and Bristol respectively. Several fathers were associated with maritime commerce. Sir Benjamin Fonseca Outram (1774–1856), a veteran of Sir James Saumarez's victory at Algeciras in 1801, and later inspector of hospitals and fleets, was born in Kilham, Yorkshire, the son of a merchant ship's captain.[13] John Booth described his father and namesake as an Aberdeen mariner.

Agriculture forms the final category of fathers' occupations. These men were most commonly minor landowners, estate managers and tenant farmers. They probably formed a larger percentage than reflected here, when one considers how

---

[12] J. McIlraith, *The Life of Sir John Richardson ... Inspector of Naval Hospitals and Fleets, &c.* (London, 1868), pp. 1–4.
[13] *Gentleman's Magazine*, 45 (1856), p. 429.

many naval surgeons were born in the countryside. The Australian pioneer Peter Cunningham's father, John, was a land steward and farmer of Dalswinton, and his mother, Elizabeth Harley, was the daughter of a merchant of nearby Dumfries.[14] The Irish surgeon John Gray, whose frigate *Majestic* captured the French frigate *Terpsichore* in 1815, was born into a farming family deep in rural Londonderry.[15] Some families earned their bread from associated activities, such as that of James Greig, whose father was a miller of Havant, Hampshire.

Few newly recruited medical officers apparently possessed any significant real or moveable property of their own, or had expectations of any from their family, according to the assistant surgeons' wills in ADM 48. This is not surprising, considering their relatively modest origins. Their prospects were probably further restricted by their place in the family hierarchy. Although the project has yet to examine naval surgeons' siblings in detail, what is known from English, Scottish and Irish probate records suggests that many were younger sons.[16] These included Magrath who was a third son, and Cunningham who was the fifth and youngest son. Naval surgeons' junior position is confirmed by comparison with their counterparts in the Army, who shared the same social make-up, less than a third of whom were the first born.[17] Inevitably, this must have influenced the cohort's prospects, both in families that were already members of the professional classes, and in the large group aspiring for their sons to join them.

Only one surgeon's father was described by that amorphous term 'gentleman', suggesting that he possessed an independent income: William Fuller senior of London. That some naval surgeons' origins were very humble indeed is suggested by Daniel McKechnie, born in Glasgow to Duncan, who is described as a 'labourer' and 'workman' on his marriage certificate and child's birth certificate.[18] The bulk of these families were materially well off, the most fortunate perhaps earning annual incomes of between £200 and £300, but they were by no means wealthy.[19] Preceding generations of small businessmen and tenant farmers would have had little formal schooling. Only a small minority, such as clergymen or doctors, would have enjoyed a liberal education or attended a university. In launching a son into the gentlemanly profession of medicine, many of these families were entering into uncharted waters.

---

[14] *Gentleman's Magazine*, 16 (1864), p. 799.

[15] I am grateful to Gray's descendant, Alistair Bodkin, for sharing his research with the project.

[16] Wills made by members of the cohort were consulted at the National Archives of England and Scotland, First Avenue House, London, a number of English local record offices, the National Archives of Ireland, and the Public Record Office of Northern Ireland.

[17] Ackroyd et al., *Advancing with the Army*, pp. 79–89.

[18] TNA, ADM 45/2/410.

[19] L. Davidoff and C. Hall, *Family Fortunes: Men and Women of the English Middle Classes, 1780–1850* (London, 1987), pp. 193–316.

Education

Paucity of source material has prevented the identification of the schools attended by most of the Navy sample. It can be assumed that the majority were educated locally, such as Sir James Clark, a native of Banffshire who attended the kirk session school at Cullen and later transferred to Fordyce parish school.[20] Among those to receive the best tuition were the students of grammar schools, such as John Richardson.[21] A few received private tuition, such as Archibald Robertson (1789–1864), the Northampton physician, who studied with a Mr Strachan in Berwickshire after leaving the Duns School.[22] Most students would have received a grounding in the classics, which was considered an important preparation for the study of medicine. Latin in particular was essential for those who wished to progress to the top of the profession. The University of Edinburgh required candidates for medical degrees to pass written and oral examinations in Latin, and to compose and publicly defend a thesis in the language as well. When the young Peter Cullen, another grammar school boy, consulted his relative, the eminent Dr William Cullen, professor of medicine at the University of Edinburgh, about his career preparation, the great man examined his Latin proficiency, and advised, 'it would be of great advantage ... to read chiefly Latin medical authors'.[23]

Latin was also the language of international scientific discourse. The Italian Augustus Bozzi Granville (1783–1872) joined the Royal Navy at Lisbon in 1807, as acting assistant surgeon of the sloop *Raven*. He wrote that the surgeon 'Francis Johnstone, a Scotchman, spoke Latin with a certain facility and a pronunciation analogous to that of the Italians. Indeed, our own official intercourse on board had been carried on in that language.' Because of his limited English, Granville's examination in physic at Haslar Hospital, required to confirm his appointment, was conducted largely in Latin as well.[24] In later writings, numbers of literary or scientific naval surgeons displayed the depth of their knowledge of classical languages and culture. Edward Harwood (d. 1814) became a noted collector of Greek and Roman coins, praised in an obituary for having 'the taste of a deep, elegant scholar'.[25]

Not all recruits reflected the same high standards of education, particularly during the early years of the wars. Surgeon Alexander Whyte of the *Atlas* complained in 1800 that his third mate knew no Latin and could barely spell in

---

[20] A. Cormack, *Two Royal Physicians: Sir James Clark, Bart., 1788–1870, Sir John Forbes, 1787–1861* (Banff, 1967).

[21] McIlraith, *Life of Sir John Richardson*, p. 4.

[22] *British Medical Journal* (January 1865), p. 16.

[23] H.G. Thursfield (ed.), 'Memoirs of Peter Cullen', in *Five Naval Journals, 1789–1817* (London, 1951), p. 46.

[24] Augustus B. Granville, *Autobiography of A.B. Granville: Being Eighty-eight Years of the Life of a Physician who Practised his Profession in Italy, Greece, Turkey, Spain, Portugal, the West Indies, Russia, Germany, France, and England* (London, 1874), I, p. 260.

[25] *Gentleman's Magazine*, 84 (1814), p. 200.

English.[26] Nevertheless, expectations of a solid early education were clear, and those possessing it were best equipped to prosper in their medical careers.

Apprenticeship to an apothecary-surgeon was the next step for those preparing for the medical profession.[27] Unfortunately, the naval surgeons' service records do not document any details, but sufficient individual testimony survives to set out their experience. Normally apprenticeship began between the ages of 14 and 16, although John Richardson was slightly younger, beginning his at 13.[28] Most contracts ranged from three to seven years. Many were indentured locally, such as Thomas Robertson, the son of an East Lothian farmer, who was apprenticed for three years to a surgeon named Cunningham in the small town of Tranent.[29] Apprenticeship to a relative was also common, which could reduce its cost. In November 1801, Richardson began his three-year training in Dumfries with his uncle James Mundell, a surgeon, before transferring after his death to another surgeon in the town, Samuel Shortridge. The value of apprenticeships varied considerably depending upon the expertise and commitment of the master. Relatives and family friends probably took greater pains than those with no connection to their charges. The early years of training usually consisted of mundane work, such as keeping the shop clean, running errands and compounding medicines; but if the master took his responsibility seriously, the apprentice would receive progressively more advanced instruction in the care of patients and routine surgical procedures. At the end of his indenture in 1788, Cullen was considered competent enough to be entrusted with the practice for three months during his master's absence.[30]

A medical apprenticeship represented a significant financial commitment for the families of future naval surgeons, considering that most were members of the middling orders. The great majority of future Army surgeons had paid between £50 and £100, indicating that they were indentured to reputable masters. Given that the apprenticeships of most naval surgeons appear to have been with modest, small-town practitioners, their expenses would have been similar.[31]

During the late eighteenth and early nineteenth centuries, an increasing number of prospective medical practitioners profited from the growing opportunities for formal medical instruction offered by the British Isles' universities, new teaching hospitals, and medical colleges. In addition, many physicians and surgeons, especially those associated with the leading London hospitals, organised private lectures. Independent lecture theatres also flourished during the period,

[26] TNA, ADM 101/88/4.
[27] Joan Lane, 'The Role of Apprenticeship in Eighteenth-Century Medical Education', in W.F. Bynum and Roy Porter (eds), *William Hunter and the Eighteenth-Century Medical World* (Cambridge 1985), pp. 57–104.
[28] McIlraith, *Life of Sir John Richardson*, pp. 4–6.
[29] William Watson, 'Thomas Robertson, Naval Surgeon, 1793–1828', *Bulletin of the History of Medicine*, 46 (1972), p. 131.
[30] Thursfield, 'Memoirs of Peter Cullen', p. 46.
[31] Ackroyd et al., *Advancing with the Army*, p. 113.

inspired by the example of William Hunter (1718–83), the prominent anatomist and man-midwife.[32]

Regrettably, there is no equivalent to the Army surgeons' questionnaires recording the details of the Navy cohort's educational *cursus*. It has been possible, however, to recover a good deal of information through careful research among surviving pupils' registers and class lists from some of the institutions they would have attended: the medical faculties of the University of Edinburgh and Trinity College Dublin, a number of the leading London teaching hospitals, and the Royal College of Surgeons in Ireland. Even these archives are incomplete for many of the relevant years and medical subjects, however, and they frequently fail to provide sufficient information to unmistakably recognize individuals. Naval surgeons with peculiar forenames or surnames such as Thraseclyces Clarke and Abraham Illingworth stand out among their fellows. Attempting to distinguish between the many common names such as William Bell and John Smith is at times difficult, even when the period of attendance is likely. The records do at times provide some helpful keys for recognition, indicating place of birth or whether a pupil is already a naval surgeon.

Before discussing the navy sample's medical courses, lectures and qualifications, it is important to emphasise that caution has been observed in compiling the database, and especially in determining the extent of the surgeons' medical training; hence the results reflect a reliable minimum rather than a hypothetical maximum. This work, too, is very much a fluid process, with data being added or amended in the light of ongoing research. Despite these caveats, sufficient source material survives to reconstruct an accurate general profile of the navy sample's institutionalized medical education.

Edinburgh University, with its flourishing and much-respected medical school, attracted large numbers of students. Searches to date have identified 101 members of the cohort who studied there. It is probable that approximately 102 more also attended, and the total figure rises to 232, or slightly more than half of the sample, if we include all potential matches from the surviving class lists and matriculation registers. The courses taken by the ninety-eight best documented students are listed in Table 2.3. The statistics illustrate how anatomy, surgery and clinical medicine formed the bedrock of contemporary medical education. Anatomy and surgery, taught during this period by the Professors of Medicine Alexander Monro *secundus* and *tertius*, was an essential prerequisite for the treatment of disease as it outlined the healthy state of the human body and demonstrated major surgical operations. 'Practice of medicine' concentrated upon pathology, discussing the causes, symptoms and cures of various diseases.

James Gregory, Professor of the Practice of Medicine from 1790, was heard by 85 per cent of students, emphasizing his status as one of the most influential medical educators of his generation. The popularity of chemistry owed much to

---

[32] Lisa Rosner, *Medical Education in the Age of Improvement: Edinburgh Students and Apprentices 1760–1828* (Edinburgh, 1991); Susan Lawrence, *Charitable Knowledge: Hospital Pupils and Practitioners in Eighteenth-Century London* (Cambridge, 1996).

Table 2.3 Edinburgh lectures 1789–1820

Course	No. of surgeons attending
Practice of medicine	83
Chemistry	66
Anatomy and surgery	65
Midwifery	51
Materia medica	42
Theory of medicine	30
Clinical lectures	29
Military surgery	19 (first established 1806)
Botany	14
Clinical surgery	12

Source: University of Edinburgh Library, Special Collections: Matriculation Records and Course Lists.

the charismatic teaching and impressive demonstrations of Thomas Hope, as well as indicating its importance in the field of pharmacy and for those contemplating scientific research. Most future naval surgeons seem to have spent between one and three years at Edinburgh. Most – like the majority of medical students – came to prepare for practice by consolidating their knowledge of the core elements of the medical curriculum, but with no intention of pursuing a medical degree.[33] There was considerable variation in the number of courses they took, ranging from as few as two or three, to as many as fourteen. Typical examples included John Gray, who studied anatomy and surgery, materia medica, the practice of medicine and midwifery during 1797–8, or Garden Milne, who attended military surgery, the practice of medicine, clinical lectures and chemistry during 1806–8. While in Edinburgh, members of the cohort also took advantage of tuition offered by private teachers outside the university. Thomas Downey, for example, under-took his training in the extramural classes offered by the Fellows of the Royal College of Surgeons.[34]

Walking the wards of Britain's great teaching hospitals and observing physicians and surgeons engaged in the daily care of patients provided excellent firsthand tuition for medical students. Statistics from the Army sample identify the large number of hospitals in London, Edinburgh, Dublin, Glasgow and other centres which offered instruction.[35] Although it is impossible to investigate the Navy cohort's participation on a similar scale, due to lack of sources, surviving pupil lists of four of London's leading institutions reveal that their experience

[33] Rosner, *Medical Education in the Age of Improvement*, pp. 104–18.
[34] William Watson, 'Two British Naval Surgeons of the French Wars', *Medical History*, 13 (1969), p. 220.
[35] Ackroyd *et al.*, *Advancing with the Army*, pp. 128–32.

was similar.[36] Approximately seventy-three naval surgeons attended classes at these hospitals, although the total number could be as high as 110 if all potential matches are included.

Table 2.4 Surgeons enrolled at London teaching hospitals

Hospital	No. of surgeons enrolled
St Thomas's and Guy's	22
London	29
St George's	25

Source: King's College London Archives: Student Records of St Thomas's Hospital Medical School, 1723–1986; Student Records of Guy's Hospital Medical School, 1725–1992; Royal London Hospital: Student Records of the London Hospital Medical College, 1740–1995; Library of St George's, University of London: Medical School Student Records.

Although Guy's was probably the most popular hospital for ward walking at this time, the naval surgeons' preference for the London Hospital clearly reflected their professional interests. The majority of those who patronized the London Hospital attended Sir William Blizard (1743–1835), one of its most eminent surgeons, who had co-founded its medical school in 1785. Blizard had military experience as a member of the Honourable Artillery Company and had been involved in the suppression of the Gordon Riots. He also had maritime connections. Blizard's expertise in military surgery was demonstrated in an influential treatise, *A Brief Explanation of the Nature of Wounds, more Particularly those Received from Firearms* (1798).[37] He also examined military and naval candidates for the Royal College of Surgeons, and those who anticipated facing him may have sought an edge by taking his classes.[38]

When treating casualties in 1797, George Magrath underscored the invaluable practical experience he had acquired by watching skilled hospital practitioners at work. Rather than amputate an arm as convention dictated, Magrath sutured the damaged artery and saved the man's limb:

> having had an opportunity of seeing a case nearly similar (during my attendance in the London Hospital as a pupil of Mr B[lizard] ...) attended with success it was a strong stimulus for me to attempt a trial in this case.[39]

There is evidence that surgeons also patronized London's popular private lecturers. One of the most successful was the army medical officer Joseph Carpue, who founded his own school of anatomy and surgery in Dean Street. While training

---

[36] See 'Source' for Table 2.4 above.
[37] William Cooke, *A Brief Memoir of Sir William Blizard* (London, 1835).
[38] 'Diary of Guy Alexander Acheson, 1799–1842', Royal Naval Museum, Portsmouth.
[39] Quoted in Goddard, 'An Insight into the Life of Royal Navy Surgeons', p. 30.

in London, the assistant naval surgeon Guy Acheson bought tickets for Carpue's classes as well as for admission to St George's.[40]

Naval surgeons attended other hospitals outside London as well. Edinburgh's Royal Infirmary was another major site of medical learning, and it would have been especially appealing to those with an interest in naval medicine, since the Commissioners for Sick and Hurt Seamen maintained two wards there as part of the contract system. These wards were used for teaching by the university, allowing students immediate observation of the treatment of the most common diseases and injuries plaguing naval seamen.[41] Many attending classes at the university also walked the wards of the infirmary, such as Thomas Robertson, who did both during 1789–93. As a promising senior student, he earned a coveted post as a dresser, assisting a staff member in the wards and the operating theatre, applying dressings, and carrying out minor surgery under his direction or at the request of other practitioners.[42] Other exemplary students gained similar experience, such as John Richardson, who worked as house surgeon of the Dumfries and Galloway Infirmary from 1804, also while studying at Edinburgh University.[43]

Dublin was the third major centre of medical education, and many of the cohort enrolled in the lectures on anatomy and surgery offered by its Royal College of Surgeons. Class registers before 1800 have been lost, but during that year and after, approximately thirty-one members of the sample attended its courses, although the figure could quite possibly be forty-five.[44]

Determining the precise number of naval surgeons who obtained university medical degrees or qualifications from the medical corporations is hindered by the same problems of matching names in graduates and members lists. Searches to date indicate that approximately sixty-five of the cohort (around 15 per cent) held an MD, while at least twenty-six more were also likely to have gained a degree. About two-thirds of the sixty-five earned their doctorates at Edinburgh, which had strenuous requirements, including three years' study at a medical faculty, written and oral examinations, and the submission and oral defence of a thesis.[45] Six acquired their degrees from Glasgow, which after 1802 had introduced stricter regulations similar to Edinburgh's (dissertation excepted).[46] Only a few gained MDs from Trinity College, Dublin, which insisted that students first must complete a BA there.[47] Most of the remaining degrees were granted by King's and

---

[40] 'Diary of Guy Alexander Acheson', 17 September 1810.

[41] Guenter Risse, 'Britannia Rules the Seas: The Health of Seamen, Edinburgh, 1791–1800', *Journal of the History of Medicine and Allied Sciences*, 43 (1988), pp. 426–46.

[42] Watson, 'Robertson', p. 132.

[43] McIlraith, *Life of Sir John Richardson*, pp. 4–6.

[44] 'An Account of the Class … under Mr Halahan and Dr Dease' and 'An Account of the Class under Dr Dease and Mr Colles', Royal College of Surgeons in Ireland.

[45] 'Edinburgh Graduates in Medicine', Wellcome Library, London.

[46] W.I. Anderson (ed.), *A Roll of the Graduates of the University of Glasgow* (Glasgow, 1898).

[47] 'Index of Matriculations in the School of Physic or Medicine, 1786–1838', Trinity College Dublin.

Marischal Colleges in Aberdeen, or St Andrews.[48] They were relatively easy to obtain upon the submission of recommendations from two respected physicians, and the payment of a fee, but hence carried less professional weight.

The naval surgeons' medical expertise is also reflected in the significant numbers who attained qualifications from the corporate medical bodies. A handful became Fellows of one or both of the London and Edinburgh Royal Colleges of Physicians and Surgeons. These were élite medical officers such as Sir William Rae, surgeon of the Plymouth and Chatham Hospitals, and Henry Parkin (1779?–1849), surgeon of the Woolwich Hospital, or high-flying figures in civilian medicine, such as Augustus Granville, who became a leading London physician, and the prominent Bolton and Manchester physician James Black (1788/9–1867). Many more of the sample achieved membership of the London and Edinburgh Royal Colleges of Surgery, which conferred considerable professional prestige. To date approximately a third have been identified.[49] The qualifying examination at the London college was more arduous than that required for a Navy or Army diploma, while in Edinburgh candidates had to prove that they had formally studied anatomy and surgery at university, or with a Fellow of one of the medical corporations or faculties.

Despite the limitations of the sources, which prevent the recovery of the sample's complete professional background, enough survives to demonstrate that the naval surgeon of the French Wars received considerable education and training, comparable to that of their fellows who went into civilian practice. In terms of its timing, it is important to stress that the bulk of this tuition was undertaken before entry into the Royal Navy's medical service. Accounts of examinations by the corporate surgical bodies, which approved candidates for admission as naval surgeons during the later eighteenth century, illustrate that they expected candidates to have undertaken study at the universities, corporate medical bodies and teaching hospitals.[50] That such study had become an almost universal prerequisite during the later stages of the French Wars is suggested by correspondence between the Royal Colleges of Surgeons in Ireland and England, and the Transport Board, in November and December 1810. When seeking clarification about assistant surgeons' previous training, the Irish corporation declared that it 'did not approve of examining any Candidate who has not attended Lectures and dissections for Two Seasons, and a Hospital for three months'. Although the English corporation did not specify its requirements, it implied that it insisted upon a minimum of six months of ward walking for officers seeking promotion to full surgeon, that period being 'the shortest for which pupils are entered at the hospitals in London'.[51]

---

[48] P.J. Anderson (ed.), *Fasti Academiae Mariscallanae Aberdonensis* (Aberdeen, 1898), R. Smart (ed.), *Biographical Register of the University of St Andrews* (St Andrews, 2004).

[49] 'Examination books', Royal College of Surgeons of England; 'Licentiates, 1815–1873' and 'Diplomates, 1770–1815', Royal College of Surgeons of Scotland.

[50] Watson, 'Two Naval Surgeons', pp. 213–14, Thursfield, 'Memoirs of Peter Cullen', p. 49.

[51] 'Resolutions of Examiners, 1763–1824, Vol. I', Royal College of Surgeons of England.

Many surgeons hungry to improve their professional knowledge took advantage of interruptions in their active service for additional tuition. John Gray's period of study at Edinburgh followed his first warrant as surgeon's mate, probably with a view to promotion as surgeon, which he achieved in 1801. After being invalided home from the Egyptian expedition, James Johnson (1777–1845), future medical writer and physician-extraordinary to King William IV, spent the winter of 1800–1 studying anatomy at the Great Windmill Street theatre in London, before returning to duty in June.[52] Richardson too invested in his continuing medical education when convalescing in London in the summer of 1812:

> I have laid out 20l. in taking perpetual tickets for surgical and anatomical lectures, so that, in the event of my being in London for a week or two at any future period, I can attend them free of expense.[53]

Only a few recruits, such as Sir William Rae, possessed medical degrees before entering the Navy, which was not surprising given that only a minority of contemporary civilian practitioners ever obtained them. A number of others gained their doctorates at Edinburgh during the war years, such as the deputy inspector of hospitals, James Veitch (1773–1856), who held appointments at the Norman Cross prisoner-of-war camp and the naval lunatic asylum at Hoxton. After 1815, however, when most surgeons were placed on half pay, there was a flurry of activity by those seeking to strengthen their professional hand for the transition into civilian medicine or to secure peacetime employment with the Navy. Between 1815 and 1820 a large cluster of naval officers received their MDs from Edinburgh, including Richardson, Clark, Robertson, Milne and Gray, many of whom were returning for a second period of study. Midwifery, meanwhile, was often taken by those contemplating family practice. A few, such as James Black, earned their MDs at Glasgow. In contrast, surgeons were more likely to have invested in a diploma from one of the surgical colleges before commencing their service career – Clark and Black were two notable examples. Membership of one of these colleges offered the option to join the Navy, the Army or the East India Company without a qualifying examination in surgery; and a diploma from the London college also conferred exemption from a further test for promotion to surgeon.

The cost of tuition, room and board, books and other expenses required for study in Edinburgh, London or Dublin would have placed a severe strain upon the finances of naval surgeons' families, especially given their limited means. The charge for a lecture course at Edinburgh during the early nineteenth century was three guineas, and admission to the Royal Infirmary was two guineas. When lodging and food were added to the costs of a respectable programme of courses, a minimum of £50 could easily be spent in one academic year. The annual expenses for attendance at a London teaching hospital have been estimated at £100. Many of the cohort would have spent more than one year taking courses in Edinburgh or

---

52 'James Johnson', ODNB.
53 McIlraith, *Life of Sir John Richardson*, pp. 41–2.

Dublin, or walking London hospital wards, and some did both. The full financial burden shouldered by their families to support their medical training, perhaps as much as £250, becomes clear when the cost of an earlier apprenticeship is added to the equation.[54] Conscious of their parents' saving and sacrifice, and that they had to rely primarily upon their own exertions to make their fortune, many students put their noses to the grindstone. John Richardson studied with his brother Peter at Edinburgh, and described their diligence: 'We have neither of us occasion to be out after four o'clock, and spend the evenings writing and reading on what we have heard through the day.'[55]

In many cases, given the need to share slender family resources with siblings, aid must have come from relatives who were more affluent, or who had no children of their own to provide for – hence the large number of hopeful practitioners apprenticed to their uncles. Acknowledgement of help from extended family is often recorded in Edinburgh thesis dedications. Outram thanked his uncle, Captain Sir Thomas Outram, who eventually left him a small estate in Kilham, Yorkshire.[56] Others must have relied upon the assistance of family friends or other benefactors. James Hall, the son of a struggling Quaker weaver in Spitalfields, attracted the notice of a local physician, Sir Daniel Williams, who paid for his medical education. When Williams died in 1831, a grateful Hall noted in his diary, 'My entrance into life began under his auspices when in my eleventh year of age.' He continued in Latin, 'In memory of this man I give thanks to God, and I know that I will never forget him as long as I live.'[57]

Naval Careers

It is impossible to quantify the combination of individual circumstances and motives which inspired the 430 members of the sample to join the Navy medical service at the outset of their medical career during the great wars against Revolutionary and Napoleonic France. Undoubtedly patriotism stirred many, who considered the Royal Navy to be 'the main bulwark of defence in the hour of emergency.'[58] Many young men who grew up in ports, or in mercantile families with connections to international trade, must have been fired by curiosity to sail the seas and explore a wider world they had only heard or read about. One naval surgeon described the fascination of travel,

> to view the manners and customs of strange nations, which flit before his eyes, and succeed each other, like the changing figures of the magic lantern … there

---

[54] Ackroyd et al., Advancing with the Army, pp. 146–7.

[55] McIlraith, Life of Sir John Richardson, p. 7.

[56] Benjamin Outram, Dissertatio medica inauguralis, de febre continua (Edinburgh, 1809).

[57] L. King-Hall (ed.), Sea Saga: Being the Naval Diaries of Four Generations of the King-Hall Family (London, 1935), p. 13.

[58] 'Extracts from the Diary of a Naval Surgeon', Colburn's United Service Journal, 3 (1843), p. 505.

is a certain indescribable charm in this changing life, which keeps its followers spellbound.[59]

For many, the decision to join the armed forces must have been a more pragmatic one, however, related to their distinctive geographic and social origins. When contemplating their future, these aspiring practitioners must have soberly weighed their chances of eking out an adequate livelihood in the small towns and villages where they were born. Prospects must have seemed particularly bleak for the vast majority who hailed from Ireland and Scotland, where affluent patients were few and far between, and already monopolised by existing practitioners. Furthermore, successfully establishing themselves in the national capitals and major provincial centres was extremely difficult for outsiders who lacked the backing of influential family, friends and patrons. This would have appeared more intimidating to the sons of modest merchants, tradesmen and farmers. Competition in the London, Edinburgh and Dublin medical marketplaces was severe, and Edinburgh and Dublin were to a large extent closed to those not already connected to their entrenched medical establishments. It was probably these unpropitious circumstances which inspired many to volunteer for the Navy, despite the hardships, hazards, and relatively poor pay – with some such as Beatty encouraged by relatives who were naval surgeons themselves.

Undoubtedly, the basic pay offered to naval surgeons was meagre during the early 1790s, made worse by the necessity of purchasing surgical instruments and many drugs out of their own pockets. Net pay was not so bad as it first appeared, due to a number of supplements – though half pay (a retainer for the unemployed) was restricted to senior surgeons. Furthermore, educated professional men considered their rank as warrant officers beneath them. Some of these problems were partially addressed in 1796, and in January 1805, an Order in Council significantly improved naval surgeons' pay, bringing it into line with that of their army colleagues, extended half pay to all who had served a minimum of two years, and provided medicines free of charge. To enhance prestige and *esprit de corps*, from 1805 surgeons were permitted to wear a distinctive uniform. In 1808, their status as officers and gentlemen was recognised when they became 'warrant officers of wardroom rank', or the practical equal of commissioned officers.[60] After 1805, as service conditions improved, and no end to the war seemed in sight, the pendulum swung in the opposite direction. The Navy became an increasingly appealing career opportunity rather than the refuge of the relatively disadvantaged, with the security of half pay and the prospect of a comfortable pension upon retirement. In 1813, John Richardson's old master Samuel Shortridge retired and invited his former pupil to return home and succeed him. Although Richardson was beginning to tire of the rigours of duty afloat, the advantages of naval service, including his right to six shillings per diem half pay, were superior to what he could expect as a small-town apothecary-surgeon: 'I think that too much to

[59] Ibid., p. 505.
[60] For a full discussion of service conditions, see Brockliss et al., *Nelson's Surgeon*, pp. 15–18.

throw away without better prospects than even full practice at Dumfries holds forth.' His entitlement to half pay, increased by further employment, 'will be no contemptible addition to my income, should I begin to practice on shore.'[61]

Prize money was always one major incentive which the Navy alone held out to the impecunious young practitioner.[62] The power of its allure is suggested by the wills of many newly recruited assistant surgeons bequeathing their hopes to beneficiaries. While few could expect the phenomenal gains of fortune's favourites such as William Beatty, who made £2,468 from the capture of Spanish bullion ships, fresh hope rose with every dawn.[63] Newly warranted surgeons usually spent the first few years of their career serving upon small cruisers, which snapped up the lion's share of prizes. Contemporary diaries and correspondence emphasize how many surgeons' incomes were steadily augmented by the capture of prizes, yielding money which could be spent upon further professional education, or invested and later used to purchase a civilian practice. Between 1805 and 1808, while serving as surgeon of the frigate *Sirius* in the Mediterranean and the North Atlantic, Thomas Robertson recorded the capture of at least seventeen prizes. An excellent example of what could be earned from just a single coup is illustrated by the auction of a Greek merchantman and her cargo in 1807. The ship sold for £2,000, and the sugar, hides, cocoa, coffee and tobacco she carried went for another £7,825. Robertson received £98 from the sale of the vessel, and although he does not state what he gained for her cargo, a share in the same proportion would have brought in another £384. All together this one windfall added up to a bonus of nearly two years' pay.[64]

The data collected from the naval surgeons' service records provide the basis for a detailed analysis of the structure of careers during the period. The first warrants issued to surgeon's mates/assistant surgeons confirm that the vast majority were young men in their late teens and early twenties, who had recently completed their formal medical training. Hands-on experience under a veteran medical officer formed a vital second apprenticeship, in that they encountered diseases infrequently met with in civilian training, such as typhus, typhoid, dysentery and yellow fever, and acquired experience of combat surgery. Joseph Emerson emphasised this crucial process of in-service instruction when joining Horatio Nelson's *Agamemnon* as second mate to her surgeon J. Roxburgh in 1793: 'He is very communicative & has much professional merit. I am happy, that I can learn something from him.'[65]

The amount of time surgeons served as mate/assistant was influenced by a host of factors, including wartime developments and levels of recruitment. Promotion to surgeon for the talented, diligent and ambitious usually occurred within three years, especially during the early stages of the war, when the Royal Navy expanded

[61] McIlraith, *Life of Sir John Richardson*, pp. 48–9.
[62] J.R. Hill, *The Prizes of War: The Naval Prize System in the Napoleonic Wars* (Stroud, 1998).
[63] Brockliss et al., *Nelson's Surgeon*, p. 75.
[64] Watson, 'Robertson', p. 143.
[65] Joy Lody, 'Treasure in a Parish Chest', *Nelson Dispatch*, 6 (1999), p. 435.

rapidly and prolonged campaigning in the West Indies caused heavy losses from disease. During the later years of the conflict, the period was often longer. A sample of those warranted surgeon reveals that most achieved the rank in their twenties (Table 2.5). Early appointments were usually to the navy's smaller vessels, and progression to ships of the line occurred as surgeons gained experience and proved their merit.

Table 2.5 Age beginning active service as a surgeon, 1793–1815

Age	No.	Percentage of sample
17–19	12	4.9
20–24	131	53.0
25–29	81	32.7
30+	23	9.3
Total	247	100

Source: Research Project Database on Navy Surgeons, Oxford University.

One is struck by the sheer amount of active service many of these surgeons completed. Nearly half served a minimum of ten years, and a quarter more than fifteen. This is an even more remarkable achievement of physical and mental endurance when it is remembered that this was mostly time afloat, much of it during wartime. Moreover, most of the minority who eventually achieved coveted posts ashore as hospital surgeons or physicians were veteran officers, who had demonstrated their worth by prolonged sea service.

Table 2.6 Surgeons' years of service

Years	No. of surgeons	Percentage of sample
5 or more	319	91.4
10 or more	151	43.3
15 or more	84	24.1
20 or more	51	14.6
30 or more	13	3.7
40 or more	5	1.4

Note: These figures are likely to underestimate total time served as they only include up to three years' tenure as surgeon's mate/assistant surgeon.

Source: National Archives, ADM 104/12–15.

The number of appointments some veteran surgeons accumulated was truly remarkable. During a twenty-seven-year career covering 1793–1833, Forbes Chevers, a veteran of the Glorious First of June and Trafalgar, was warranted to no less than twenty-four vessels, including several ships more than once.[66] The global nature of some surgeons' service and the sheer number of sea miles they clocked

---

[66] TNA, ADM104/12, sub Forbes Chevers.

up were also extraordinary. During the first seventeen years of his career, Thomas Robertson served in the West Indies between 1793 and 1796, in the Channel and off the coast of West Africa during 1796–8, in Chinese and Indian waters and the Red Sea between 1798 and 1803, and in the Mediterranean from 1803 to 1810.[67]

After 1815, when opportunities for naval appointments were drastically reduced, many officers were employed as surgeons-superintendent of vessels transporting convicts to the Australian penal colonies. The replacement of poorly qualified private contractors' surgeons with experienced Navy medical officers resulted in significant improvements to the health of passengers.[68] Approximately forty members of the cohort had completed a combined total of about 120 voyages by the mid 1840s. Several served for many years, including Alick Osborne, who made the arduous journey ten times.[69] Many were noted for their humane treatment of their charges, including John Rodmell, who ran a successful school for boys on the *Medina*.[70]

Several surgeons also took medical charge of emigrant ships. During 1836–8, Osborne, a native of Tyrone, organised the re-settlement of an Irish party in New South Wales on behalf of the Colonial Office.[71] James Rutherford became an advocate of pauper emigration to New South Wales, and helped to sponsor an initiative after consultation with the colonial secretary, Earl Grey, in 1848.[72] Public inquiries investigating the transportation of emigrants also praised the conscientious care provided by naval surgeons.[73] At times they often provided medical aid in civilian maritime emergencies, as in the case of John Stirling, who travelled to Orkney in 1837 to treat the crews of whaling ships buffeted by severe storms.[74]

In 1831 Sir William Burnett, Director-General of the Medical Department of the Navy, stated that surgeons suffered the highest mortality rates in the service, and this is probably correct given their intimate exposure to a range of potentially lethal diseases.[75] The members of the cohort were survivors of the French Wars, of course, and there is no easy way to estimate how many of their brother officers perished during the conflict. One survey records the death of eighty-five surgeons between 1799 and 1815 from accident, illness and unspecified causes, but there is no straightforward way of judging its completeness.[76] The service registers, however, are important sources for a study of the health of the medical men themselves, and emphasize the grave physical and psychological impact of so many years of dangerous and demanding active service in varied climates and disease environments. Even during peace, death or invaliding from accident and

---

[67] Watson, 'Robertson', p. 132.

[68] C. Bateson, *The Convict Ships, 1787–1868* (Glasgow, 1985), p. 276.

[69] TNA, ADM 104/14, sub Alick Osborne.

[70] http://www.medicalpioneers.com/ sub John Rodmell.

[71] TNA, ADM 104/14, sub Alick Osborne.

[72] *The Times*, 18 August and 26 September 1848.

[73] *Freeman's Journal and Daily Commercial Advertiser* (Dublin), 6 March 1843.

[74] *Freeman's Journal and Daily Commercial Advertiser* (Dublin), 1 February 1837.

[75] Sir William Burnett, 'Report on Medical Officers of the Navy, 1831', NMM, ELL/245.

[76] TNA, ADM 104/60–77.

illness remained a constant threat. The registers record the deaths of twenty-four members of the sample after 1815, including three who drowned by shipwreck and foundering, two who died on convict ships, and one who was reportedly captured by pirates.[77] Over the course of their careers, many contracted serious diseases including typhus, tuberculosis, pneumonia, malaria, yellow fever, dysentery, cholera, hepatitis, opthalmia and paralysis. Some were stricken by more than one serious illness, such as Granville, who contracted malaria in 1809 and yellow fever in 1810.[78] Surgeons of the Navy's 'coffin squadron', which fought a sustained campaign to suppress the trans-Atlantic slave trade off the pestilential coasts of western Africa after 1807, were especially vulnerable. Fatalities included Duncan McNicoll, who died of fever in Sierra Leone in 1828.[79] Ten surgeons were struck off the list for refusing appointments, many to avoid service in unhealthy stations, such as the West Indies, where four died during the 1820s and 1830s. Several surgeons, including Magrath, claimed pensions for wartime wounds, the loss of limbs, or the effects of imprisonment. Routine injuries included hernias, and fractured ankles, thighs, arms and ribs. Damaged eyesight and crippling rheumatism were other common occupational hazards. Henry Plowman complained of mercury poisoning.[80] Finally, the question as to why the Navy apparently suffered from such high rates of mental illness deserves further investigation, emphasized by the total of twenty-six naval surgeons who suffered some form of instability during one time in their life. Even this brief overview of surgeons' medical histories makes it clear that an iron constitution was required to bear lengthy service within the 'wooden world'.

A naval surgeon, emphasizing the high professionalism of the medical service, declared that there was no civilian equivalent to the strict supervision of surgeons which fostered that professionalism: 'from the moment of his entering the service to the date of his leaving it, he is required to submit a daily journal of his practice, giving a minute description of the disorders of the sick, and detailing every variation of symptom and treatment to the superior medical officers …'.[81] Until 1806, surgeons were required to keep two journals, a surgical one which they submitted to the Surgeons' Company/College, and a medical one, deposited with the Sick and Hurt Board or the Physician of Greenwich Hospital. After that date, only one had to be delivered to whichever administrative body was then overseeing the service. In 1810, Richardson wrote that part of each morning was spent writing a 'daily report of each case for the Transport Board'.[82] During the French Wars, Physicians of the Fleet were also responsible for monitoring the performance of surgeons under their eyes. Surgeons' service registers suggest how closely medical journals were scrutinized during the later period they cover. From

[77] The following discussion is derived from ADM 104/12–15, 20–21.
[78] Granville, *Autobiography of A.B. Granville*, I, pp. 279–81
[79] TNA, ADM 104/20, sub Duncan McNicoll.
[80] TNA, ADM 104/12, sub Henry Plowman.
[81] *The Times*, 8 June 1833.
[82] McIlraith, *Life of Sir John Richardson*, p. 32.

1832 this became one of the duties of Burnett as head of the medical department. Functioning something like a personnel file, the registers preserve examples of professional shortcomings or personal misconduct. In 1837, Burnett reacted with 'great surprise and displeasure' to the incompleteness of John Armstrong's journal for the *Thalia*, and when he received an unsatisfactory explanation, warned that it 'would operate to his disadvantage'.[83] In 1838, Francis Logan was censured for failing to issue sufficient lemon juice during an outbreak of scurvy aboard the convict ship *Mangles*, and for keeping his journal in an 'unscientific manner'.[84]

Alcohol abuse among medical officers appears to have been exceptional. Four members of the cohort were dismissed from their ships for drunkenness, and the intoxication of two others prompted complaints from commanding officers. In 1825, Robert Marshall, a hospital mate at Haslar, was nearly expelled from the service for 'introducing a woman of ill fame into the hospital' and being absent without leave.[85] The registers also reveal occasional irregularities in accounting. Edward Bromley, who was a foundation shareholder in the Bank of Van Diemen's Land while enjoying a civilian appointment, perpetrated a notorious embezzlement of public funds, which was exposed in 1824.[86] The impression left by comments upon the surgeons' practice is that professional failings were rare, and that exemplary standards of moral rectitude were expected of officers and gentlemen.

The registers also contain considerable praise of surgeons' clinical excellence and devotion to duty from Burnett and many of their commanding officers. The role of patronage in advancing a Navy surgeon's career is a factor which resists quantification, but its importance is emphasized by numerous examples where employment, favourable postings and the opportunity for promotion depended upon the intervention of a powerful benefactor. John Richardson, for example, was fortunate to enjoy the backing of an influential naval officer – Sir William Hope, one of the Lords of the Admiralty (1807–9) and MP for the county of Dumfries (1804–30) – early in his career, probably as a result of his father's political support. Richardson was dismayed by the cavalier treatment he received from the Secretary of Transport when he called to request his first warrant in the spring of 1807. He visited Hope, who sent him back armed with a letter requesting appointment to a frigate, and Richardson was immediately assigned to *La Nymphe*. Hope later recommended him for transfer to the flagship of a squadron blockading the mouth of the Tagus in 1808, which soon led to a promotion as acting surgeon.[87]

In Corfu in 1803, before joining the Royal Navy, Augustus Granville had met William R. Hamilton, private secretary to Lord Elgin. They renewed their friendship in 1812 after Hamilton returned to England, where he became an undersecretary of state at the Foreign Office. Hamilton acted as an energetic patron, and soon after, Granville was transferred from a small vessel to the *Maidstone* frigate,

[83] TNA, ADM104/15, sub John Armstrong.
[84] TNA, ADM104/13, sub Francis Logan.
[85] TNA, ADM104/20, sub Robert Marshall.
[86] TNA, ADM104/14, sub Edward Bromley.
[87] McIlraith, *Life of Sir John Richardson*, pp. 16–17.

a 'station which the personal influence of my friend … had procured for me, was one likely to yield what sailors look for in war – a good share of prize money'.[88] In 1813, 'Mecaenas' arranged for the surgeon to be placed on half pay, so that he could 'instruct his two eldest sons, William and Alexander in the Latin language, and to teach them to speak it fluently'.[89] In a final example, the last years of Thomas Robertson's career were made more comfortable by the interest of unidentified patrons, who facilitated his appointment as surgeon to the Commander-in-Chief of the Nore's flagship. This allowed him to live much of the time with his family on shore.[90]

The service registers contain many examples of officers requesting the appointment or re-appointment of skilled surgeons to their ships, since operational efficiency and fighting capacity depended so much upon a fit and healthy crew. It was also often by successfully treating ailing commanders, officers and their families that a surgeon gained lifelong friends and patrons, there being few stronger bonds of gratitude. Magrath earned Nelson's confidence by his conscientious personal care while surgeon of the *Victory*. Nelson praised him as 'by far the most able medical man I have ever seen', and promoted him to surgeon of the Gibraltar Hospital in 1804.[91]

These contacts also prepared surgeons for a successful post-service civilian career anchored by naval patients and their connections. In 1802, Peter Cullen's private practice at Sheerness included the port's admiral, commissioner, and many senior officers.[92] The Edinburgh thesis dedications suggest the identity of some of the cohort's patrons, or those they hoped to cultivate by demonstrating their commitment to the pursuit of professional knowledge. They included leading figures at the Admiralty such as the First Lord, Viscount Melville, Richardson's patron Hope, more than twenty admirals including Viscount Keith, Viscount Exmouth and Baron Gambier, and senior figures in the medical department, such as Burnett, and John Weir, a Commissioner of the Sick and Hurt Board. Those with an eye to their future outside the Navy dedicated their theses to leading figures in civilian medicine, including court physicians, and practitioners at major London and Edinburgh hospitals.

Conclusion

As many as three-quarters of naval surgeons warranted during the French Wars came from the Celtic fringe of Scotland, Ireland and Wales. They revealed a diverse range of middling backgrounds in commerce, the professions and agricul-

---

[88] Granville, *Autobiography of A.B. Granville*, I, p. 303.

[89] Ibid., I, p. 323.

[90] Watson, 'Robertson', p. 147.

[91] Nelson to Baird, 30 May 1805, in Nicholas Harris Nicholas (ed.), *The Dispatches and Letters of Lord Nelson* (London, 1845–6), vi, p. 41.

[92] Thursfield, 'Memoirs of Peter Cullen', p. 114.

ture, and many were younger sons. Their decision to begin their medical career by joining the Navy owed more to their relatively disadvantaged position than to any inferiority of intellect, education, or ambition when compared to the majority of their fellow practitioners, who probably had access to easier avenues into civilian medicine. Wartime service as a naval surgeon provided a window of opportunity for many sons of modest merchants, tradesmen and farmers to enter the medical profession, and to acquire the tastes and manners of an officer and gentleman by wide reading during hours of leisure, and by mixing with their social superiors in the wardroom and at the captain or admiral's table.

The social prestige of the Royal Navy rose considerably during the late eighteenth century, typified by King George III's decision to send his teenage son, the future William IV, to sea as a midshipman in 1779.[93] Augustus Granville suggested the potential for social mobility the service offered. A tireless networker, he emphasised the invaluable contacts surgeons could make among their fellow officers: 'persons of birth, education, and whose higher qualities were in course of further development, would probably form friendly relations with one another that might last through life'.[94]

After 1815, the considerable number of the cohort who successfully set up their plates throughout the United Kingdom as physicians and surgeons is a testimony to the quality of their initial education, often improved by subsequent study, the value of their naval service, which provided a clinical experience unparalleled in civilian practice, and their inherent determination and ability. Some medical practitioners whose careers began in the Navy reached the highest echelons of nineteenth-century British medicine and society. Sir James Clark, the son of the earl of Findlater's butler, tended the dying John Keats in Rome, became the trusted physician and confidant of Queen Victoria and Prince Albert, and was rewarded with a baronetcy.[95]

Clark is but one example of the most notable members of the cohort, many of whom were based in London and other large cities, but searches through medical and trade directories reveal the presence of large numbers of half-pay naval surgeons providing medical care in a host of smaller communities across the United Kingdom, some as factory, mine, prison or Poor Law medical officers. Not all thrived, and the struggles of the less fortunate are recorded in requests to the Navy for compassionate allowances from surgeons or their widows, and even imprisonment for debt. Probate valuations, however, which have been collected for nearly half of the sample, demonstrate that the majority lived comfortably, and that a quarter were truly affluent, enjoying the fruits of successful practice.[96] A small but significant number of surgeons, whose travels had suggested the pros-

---

93 N.A.M. Rodger, *Command of the Ocean: A Naval History of Britain, 1649–1815* (London, 2005), p. 388.
94 Granville, *Autobiography of A.B. Granville*, I, p. 308.
95 *The Lancet*, 9 July 1870, pp. 66–7.
96 Navy Surgeons Database: Wealth 1 Table.

pect of a better life in Australia, New Zealand, Canada or other colonies or coun-tries, emigrated and usually became pillars of their new home societies.

Naval surgeons made significant contributions to nineteenth-century science, particularly as naturalists, exemplified by John Richardson, who earned great fame as an explorer and pioneering naturalist of the Arctic.[97] Medical officers were active members of national and regional learned societies, including the Royal Society, where Granville was a moving spirit in the mid-century reform move-ment. Many were also involved in philanthropic and voluntary projects attempting to improve the quality of life for all and to broaden intellectual horizons, such as James Black, who was instrumental in the formation of a free library in Bolton in 1853.[98] Finally, a number of the sample were also avid authors, publishing on surgery, tropical disease, the impact of climate and topography, and a range of other medical and scientific subjects gleaned from their service experience. A few naval surgeons also made their mark as men of letters, including Sir James Prior, who published poetry, literary editions, and well-regarded biographies of Edmund Burke and Oliver Goldsmith.[99] By the mid nineteenth century, British naval surgeons had earned widespread public gratitude and respect, not only for their dedicated service in national defence, but for their wider achievements in medicine, science, philanthropy and the world of letters.

---

[97] Robert Johnson, *Sir John Richardson: Arctic Explorer, Natural Historian, Naval Surgeon* (London, 1976), pp. 101–7.
[98] James Black, *A Few Words in Aid of Literature and Science, on the Occasion of the Opening of the Public Library, Bolton* (Bolton, 1853).
[99] 'James Prior', ODNB.

3

Surgery in the Royal Navy during the Republican and Napoleonic Wars (1793–1815)

Michael Crumplin

> I say that where the learned physician is not to be had, be it either by sea or land, far or near, I will then use all honest and lawful means, both in physic and surgery, to the utmost of my knowledge and skill, before I will in any way permit and suffer my patient to perish for want of all help.
>
> William Clowes, *'A Right Fruteful and Approoved Treatise'* (1602)[1]

In 1540 Henry VIII granted a charter that joined the Surgeons' Guild and the Company of Barbers. William Clowes (1543/4–1604) – one of the most eminent, innovative and controversial members of this amalgamated Barber-Surgeons Company – served as a military and naval surgeon from 1563 to 1588, and he constantly strove to improve the low standards of surgical treatment that he observed in the services. But over two hundred years later, there still remained concerns over the standard of surgery in Britain's armed forces. Three months after the Battle of Camperdown in October 1797, John Bell, a master Edinburgh surgeon serving at the naval hospital at Yarmouth, composed a 'memorial' to the Right Honourable Earl Spencer, First Lord of the Admiralty, in which he expressed his concern at the low state of surgical practice and the poor training of many naval surgeons. A large part of the document was a plea for a military school of surgery; just as important, however, was a commentary on the plight of contemporary naval surgeons. 'To the life of a navy surgeon there are, God knows, no seductions', Bell wrote. 'Nor will men ever delight in a profession which is not made respectable, honourable, and useful.' Reflecting on the under-provision of surgeons, he continued:

> Perhaps in the whole fleet there are few Surgeons Mates, not one may be, who is able to perform the greater operations of surgery. It has happened, that, after the most earnest entreaties of the Officers, of the Surgeon, of everyone concerned, a ship of the line has gone into battle without one assistant on board; no, not

---

[1]   Quoted in J.J. Keevil, *Medicine and the Navy, 1200–1900. Vol. 1: 1200–1649* (Edinburgh and London, 1957) pp. 135–6.

one to screw a tourniquet, to tie an artery, to hold a shattered stump, to put a piece of lint to a bleeding wound![2]

The messages taken from this perceptive missive seem to have been that there were few opportunities for learning, advancement, further education and remuneration to recruit the better practitioner surgeon into the Royal Navy. In due course, some of these issues would be addressed, and the situation (and abilities) of surgeons were certainly improved by the end of the wars with France in 1815.

Nevertheless, and despite the lack of antisepsis and anaesthesia, competent Royal Navy surgeons in the early nineteenth century could perform a remarkable range of procedures to benefit their patients. Although the everyday shipboard clinician in the Georgian Navy was known as a surgeon (as were his assistants or mates), it is apparent that only a small part of his life was spent in exercising his operative skills. He acted not only as a surgeon, but also as physician, apothecary, confidant and health adviser to the ship's crew. While a ship in combat often called for sustained and frenetic medical activity that would often stretch a surgeon's ability to the limits, most of his time was taken up treating day-to-day diseases, contagion, climate-induced problems or 'civilian' types of trauma. Ship surgeons' log records bear witness to this. Of the total naval losses incurred in the war against France, figures gleaned from the researches of Professor M. Lewis (in 1960) and the statistician W.B. Hodge (in 1855 and 1856) vary slightly from 92,386 to 103,660 deaths. For the 144,558 seamen registered in 1801 (from a population of around nine million), by far the most frequent threats to life were the risks of disease, accident, foundering, fire and explosion. The proportion of deaths from battle strikes was low: merely 6,663 (7.2 per cent, according to Hodge) or 6,540 (6.3 per cent according Lewis).[3] This limited level of exposure to mass trauma offered only graduated opportunity to acquire medical or surgical skills in the cockpits of line of battle ships. This problem would be, to some extent, ameliorated by the constant demands on a ship's surgeon to practise his operative skills on seamen when on blockading, escort or patrol duties – accidents or injuries were relatively commonplace on board a crowded sailing vessel, and a surgeon might be called upon to set simple fractures and treat compound fractures, undertake occasional herniotomies (that is, the surgical treatment of a hernia), manage venereal disease, drain sepsis, and undertake the occasional amputation or (rarely) trephining of a head fracture.

A ship's surgeon's skills in the craft of surgery, the diagnosis of illness and the prescription of correct medicines varied widely. As John Cardwell observes in Chapter 2 in this book, they often 'received considerable education and training, comparable to that of their fellows who went into civilian practice,'[4] and many

[2] J. Bell, *Memoir on the Present State of Naval and Military Surgery addressed to The Right Honourable Earl Spenser, First Lord of the Admiralty* (Yarmouth, 20 January 1798), pp. 6–7.
[3] C. Lloyd and J.L.S. Coulter, *Medicine and the Navy, 1200–1900. Vol. 3: 1714–1815* (Edinburgh and London, 1961), p. 182.
[4] See Chapter 2, p. 51.

surgeons certainly had extensive exposure to maritime disease and trauma. The reasons for these somewhat uneven standards included the fact that surgery was a yet undeveloped science; that both the preservice training for and experience of surgery were haphazard and often unsuited to maritime practice; and that the relatively low pay and status of the naval surgeon (together with the hardships of a life at sea) did not always attract – especially during times of war, when the demand for surgeons was high – the highest-quality candidates. Furthermore, surgeons were (with apothecaries) considered merely craftsmen. However able a surgeon was, his status was considerably inferior to that of a physician. Physicians were considered gentlemen and, having attended university, were more learned; they often possessed a doctorate in medicine, and many were members or licentiates of the Royal College of Physicians. As one of the 'warrant officers of wardroom rank', the surgeon was, before the reforms of 1805, inferior in status to the master (though he was paid more), but (along with the chaplain) superior to the purser. Furthermore, before the reforms of 1805, he did not wear a uniform. As Chapter 2 in this volume reveals, a high proportion of ship's surgeons were (as in the British Army) the younger sons of farmers, ministers, merchants or other professional men, many of them emanating from Celtic backgrounds.[5]

Although often poor in means, many surgeons had a superior education compared to other service officers, and in understanding the nature of a naval surgeon's work, it is useful to explore their origins. Most surgeons' schooling would have been at a village, church, private or charitable institution, and usually ended at around 12 to 15 years old. The young man was then indentured to a physician, surgeon or even an apothecary in a town, city or hospital. There were clearly potential problems in such a practice: if the apprentice was attached to an apothecary, his surgical grounding might be deficient; likewise if the pupil was apprenticed to a surgeon, his diagnostic and therapeutic skills were limited.[6] Apprenticeship was an honourable agreement between master and pupil, whereby the apprentice would learn as much about surgery and physic as he could in a diligent, committed and sober manner. The master provided teaching and assistance, and offered his apprentice increasing responsibilities as appropriate. He often also supplied accommodation – though at a price. The costs of an indenture varied between £50 and £300, depending on the master and the location. Costs of individual instructive courses given by surgeons were high in London but less so in many Scottish universities, hospitals and schools, so encouraging a trail of students northwards over the border, where accommodation was cheaper and some university lectures were given gratis.[7]

5   Laurence Brockliss, M. John Cardwell and Michael Moss, *Nelson's Surgeon: William Beatty, Naval Medicine and the Battle of Trafalgar* (Oxford, 2005), pp. 19, 23; and ch. 2 in this volume.
6   See Charles Dunne, *The Chirurgical Candidate; Or Reflections on Education Indispensable to Complete Naval, Military and Other Surgeons* (London, 1808).
7   Matthew H. Kaufman, *The Regius Chair of Military Surgery in the University of Edinburgh, 1806–1855* (Amsterdam and New York, 2003), p. 59.

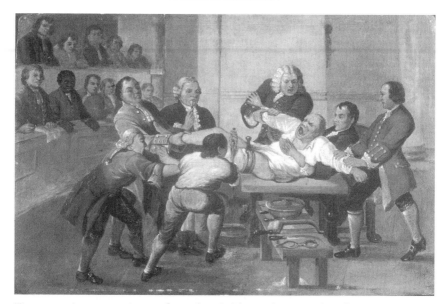

Figure 3.1 An amputation performed at St Thomas's Hospital in the mid eighteenth century. The Royal College of Surgeons of England.

Following three to five years of blinkered training with primarily one teacher, the freed apprentice would then walk the wards of a provincial or city hospital, as a ward walker, dresser, 'plaister-man' or house surgeon, for a year or two.[8] For the privilege of undertaking the bulk of the chores in the wards, dead room and operating room, he would pay around £20 to £30 per annum, but was granted certain allowances for essentials such as coal and candles. Concurrently with these hospital or infirmary duties, he would attend courses of lectures at extramural schools or in a hospital. Such courses were held in a range of subjects, including anatomy, surgery, midwifery, materia medica, etc. These would run in the winter and spring terms and the costs were generally between £2 and £5 for each course, with reductions for attendance at several sessions.

There would be ample chance in such civilian training to study infections, venereal diseases, complications of labour, fractures, contagion and a smattering of head injuries. However, what the aspiring naval surgeon was rarely exposed to were outbreaks of typhus, typhoid, dysentery and yellow fever – nor how to manage a deluge of casualties. Neither could he, at such a junior age, be a competent operative surgeon. Much could be learned, however, from books, anatomical preparations and attendance at dissections. From these sources he could certainly gain some confidence in surgical anatomy (for example, where to find major arteries, the action of muscles and the position of abdominal organs, etc.). There

[8] Michael Crumplin, *Men of Steel: Surgery in the Napoleonic Wars* (Shrewsbury, 2007), pp. 152–4.

remained mammoth challenges in acquiring in civilian practice skills that would be required for combat surgery. For instance, relatively few amputations would be performed each year by individual surgeons, and the view students had of their trainers undertaking operations on patients, usually with necessary haste, was frequently distant and obscure, as can be seen in Figure 3.1 which shows an amputation performed at London's St Thomas's Hospital in the mid eighteenth century. Finally, the supervision provided was often of patchy quality.

A young mate might, therefore, be able to prescribe and recognize some common ailments and bleed a patient, but would have little inkling of the techniques required for more advanced surgery at sea. How able a surgeon's mate would become depended on his commitment to learn, discuss, and attend all the useful sessions he might, and (most importantly) on further instruction from a competent surgeon, who could teach hands-on in the sick bay and cockpit. Lessons had to be learnt at every opportunity, because the best 'postgraduate school' was that of learning on service.

There are essential differences between military surgery and civilian practice, since management of war injuries was frequently delayed, and untreated wounds could be easily and quickly contaminated. A system of triage (sorting cases into order of importance) was required in combat, as well as successful control of haemorrhage and the proper timing of safe and simple procedures. Most importantly, the surgeon had to learn when to operate and when not to. Speedy surgery was essential as there was no anaesthesia, a need to limit haemorrhage and often a high caseload.

Books could provide some guidance, and popular contemporary surgical texts included John Ranby's *Treatise on Gunshot Wounds* (1744), William Northcote's *The Marine Practice of Physic and Surgery* (1770), Benjamin Bell's *System of Surgery* (1780), John Bell's *Discourses on the Nature and Cure of Wounds* (1793–5) and *The Principles of Surgery* (1801–6), William Turnbull's *The Naval Surgeon: Comprising the Entire Duties of Professional Men at Sea* (1806), and, towards the end of the war, Charles Bell's *A Dissertation on Gun-Shot Wounds* (1814). In due course, the experiences of army surgeons in the Napoleonic Wars would produce an important set of treatises for future use by naval practitioners, in particular John Hennen's *Observations on Some Important Points in the Practice of Military Surgery* (1818) and George James Guthrie's *Commentaries on the Surgery of the War in Portugal, Spain, France, and the Netherlands, 1808–1815* (1853).

Whilst medical men could graduate in London, Edinburgh, Glasgow, Aberdeen or Dublin, the right to examine candidates for the Royal Navy was initially restricted by long tradition to the Company of Surgeons of London (from 1800 the Royal College of Surgeons). The essential requisites to sit for the qualifying diploma (such as the membership of the Company or College of Surgeons) varied, according to the year and also according to the need for new recruits in the Royal Navy. Certificates of attendance at appropriate courses of lectures, attendances in hospital, the recommendation of Masters, and an appropriate age, were all demanded by the Company of Surgeons' Court of Examiners. The Company held on jealously to its monopoly on the examination of naval candidates, and

388. Q. What are the favourable symptoms that point out success from trepanning?

A. The favourable symptoms are, the patient becoming less stupid. his breathing less oppressed, and the pupils contracting upon exposure to strong light.

389. Q. If, after trepanning, a collection of fluid should be found between the dura and pia mater, how is it to be removed?

A. Under such circumstances, a small hole may be cautiously scratched on the dura mater, to evacuate it.

390. Q. When the parotid duct is wounded, what is the consequence?

A. The consequence of wounding the parotid duct is a fistulous opening which discharges saliva, particularly during meals.

391. Q. What is ecchymosis?

A. Ecchymosis is an extravasation of blood in the cellular membrane, occasioned by a rupture of the small vessels of the part.

392. Q. What is meant by exfoliation?

A. Exfoliation is a separation of a dead portion of bone from the living.

393. Q. What method is to be taken to prevent exfoliation that is likely to occur from a wound?

A. In attempting to prevent exfoliation that may take place from a wound, all that is to be done is to cover the exposed bone as soon as possible with the flesh that has been detached.

394. Q. Where is the fluid in hydrocele situated?

A. The fluid in hydrocele is situated between the tunica vaginalis and the tunica albuginea of the testicle.

395. Q. How are fistulæ in perinæo to be dressed after they have been laid open?

A. Fistulæ in perinæo, after being laid open, are to be dressed quite down to the end, to allow of granulations shooting up from the bottom before reunion of the parts takes place.

396. Q. What is meant by simple fracture?

A. By simple fracture is meant a breach of continuity of bone, without an external wound.

397. Q. What regimen do gun-shot wounds require?

A. Gun shot wounds generally require the antiphlogistic regimen.

398. Q. How is the operation for phymosis performed?

A. This operation is performed by introducing a directory under the prepuce, then passing a curved pointed bistoury, and slitting open the prepuce.

399. Q. Where do strictures most frequently take place in the urethra?

A. Strictures most commonly occur at the membranous part of the urethra; from its being more acted upon by the salts of the urine; the urine, after being expelled from the bladder, remains at this part of the urethra to be thrown out by the accelaratores urinæ.

400. Q. From whence does the discharge of gonorrhœa flow?

A. The discharge of gonorrhœa flows from the mucus lacunæ of the urethra.

EXAMINATIONS

IN

ANATOMY, PHYSIOLOGY,

PRACTICE OF

PHYSIC, SURGERY, MATERIA MEDICA,

CHEMISTRY, AND PHARMACY;

FOR THE USE OF

STUDENTS,

WHO ARE ABOUT TO PASS THE

COLLEGE OF SURGEONS, OR THE MEDICAL OR

TRANSPORT BOARD.

BY ROBERT HOOPER, M.D.

LECTURER ON MEDICINE, &c. IN LONDON.

NEW-YORK:

PRINTED FOR AND SOLD BY COLLINS AND CO.

NO. 189, PEARL-STREET.

1815.

Figure 3.2 Title and sample pages from Dr Hooper's revision handbook. Michael Crumplin

until 1797 thwarted efforts by the Edinburgh Royal College to share this privilege. Many Scottish practitioners, of course, including James Lind, Thomas Trotter, Robert Robertson, Andrew Baird and Tobias Smollett, had been taught and had qualified in their native land – at Edinburgh, Glasgow or Aberdeen – before travelling to London for examination and going on to serve in the Navy.[9] Indeed, by the period 1800 to 1850, over 95 per cent of British medical graduates had attended a university in Scotland.[10]

Having found no evidence of a strategy to lower the standard of examination, consequent on the demands of war, there may have been directives to admit more candidates. Examinations were held more frequently during the wars with France – twice a week instead of once. Interestingly, a revision handbook for the College of Surgeons examinations was published in 1815 (Figure 3.2); it was written by a most competent teacher, Dr Robert Hooper, who had started his career as apothecary to the Marylebone workhouse infirmary, before going on to study medicine at the University of Oxford. Hooper directed his handbook's model questions and answers not only to candidates for the armed services and East India Company, but also to those sitting the MRCS (Member of the Royal College of Surgeons) diploma. The handbook made no differentiation between the types of examination question, whether the qualifications were military or civilian.

The qualifying diploma for the Navy, Army, East India Company or civilian service was conducted by *viva voce* only, with each candidate standing in front of a panel of ten examiners, one of whom was a senior naval doctor (Figure 3.3). The President (or Master), two Wardens (or Governors) and seven members of the Court could ask questions of the candidate. Rather than rely on Tobias Smollett's well-known and derisory vignette of the examination presented in his novel *Roderick Random* (1748), it would be instructive to relate the account of Peter Cullen (a relation of Dr William Cullen of Edinburgh), who attended the London examination on 27 November 1789. As he reports, in the third person,

> The examiners were seated at a semi-circular table, where were two or more candidates standing before it, and answering such questions as were put to them. Mr Cullen having walked up to the table, and made his bow, was asked his name, from whence he came, and for what purpose he meant to be examined? On answering that it was for the Naval Service, one of the examiners arose, and taking Mr. Cullen to the side of the room, enquiring his age, his apprenticeship, studies and practice in his profession. [Sometimes, more than one candidate could thus be examined on a one-to-one basis.] To all these Mr. Cullen having returned a satisfactory reply, the examiner proceeded to question him on anatomy, physiology and surgery. Then stated some more of the important surgical cases or diseases, and how he would treat them. This gentleman was quite satisfied with Mr. Cullen's proficiency, and taking him to the centre of the table, where the President was sitting, said, 'I find this young gentleman fully

---

9   Crumplin, *Men of Steel*, p. 158.
10   Kaufman, *Regius Chair of Military Surgery*, p. 18.

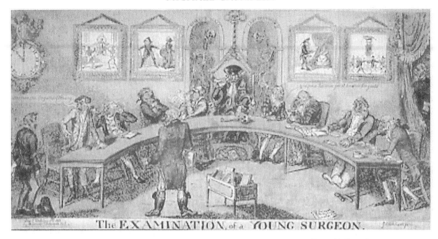

Figure 3.3 *The Examination of a Young Surgeon*, by George Cruickshank.
The Royal College of Surgeons of England.

Note: This is a cartoon of an examination in the College of Surgeons, London (1811).

qualified as an assistant surgeon for His Majesty's Navy'. The President bowed
to Mr. Cullen, and desired him to pay one guinea as a fee, and to call the next
day at the Navy Office, where he would find a certificate of his having passed.[11]

Having obtained a certificate, the successful candidate would proceed to obtain
a warrant from the Sick and Hurt Board, appointing him to serve as first, second,
third, fourth or fifth mate (later termed an assistant surgeon) on an appropriately
rated ship of war or at a shore hospital. For this appointment, the young surgeon
would be further assessed by the Board on his training, experience and abilities.

In 1808 Charles Dunne, a junior army surgeon, took a Smollett-like stand
against the inexperienced junior surgical appointments and laid the fault firmly at
the feet of the Royal College of Surgeons (of London). He railed,

> I cannot pass over in silence the absurdity of employing such a number of raw
> apothecaries' boys as hospital mates, or assistant surgeons, in His Majesty's
> army or navy, whose whole education has been acquired, in the course of a year
> or two, behind the counter of some obscure apothecary or barber-surgeon, nay,
> in the cockpit of a man of war, as loblolly boy.[12]

It is not easy to assess the veracity of such criticism. The juniors criticized by
Dunne might have been perfectly able, and would rarely have been given significant initial responsibility. Well-educated trainees were often hard to come by in a
volunteer service. Each year of the war, examiners in London alone (other colleges
in Edinburgh, Glasgow and Dublin examined fewer) passed between 250 and

11   Lloyd and Coulter, *Medicine and the Navy*, vol. 3, p. 14.
12   Dunne, *The Chirurgical Candidate*, p. 20.

350 candidates as suitable to receive a service diploma (to the Navy, Army or East India Company).[13] Edinburgh also issued diplomas, both from the university Faculty of Medicine and the Royal College of Surgeons of Edinburgh, but it was not until 1797 that the Sick and Hurt Board recognised the Edinburgh diploma – even later for the British Army.

Before considering the life of the ship's surgeon at sea (a few would serve on shore or on a fleet hospital ship as hospital mates), it is relevant to mention the other responsibilities of the licensing corporations, principally the London College of Surgeons. The Court of Examiners of the College was, by an edict of 1731, required to inspect the capital instruments (i.e. large sets) for the ship's surgeon (which he had to pay for himself) before they were sent on board. Another of the College's requirements (until 1816, when the practice ceased) was to examine naval officers for disability pensions – which were awarded on the basis of a wound equivalent to the loss of an eye or limb. Captain John Harvey's family, for example, was allowed £74 4s 6d for expenses after his death consequent to a wound received on the Glorious First of June 1794.[14] The final requisite of the Court of Examiners was, in conjunction with the Physician of the Navy Board, to occasionally peruse the ship's surgeons' journals and their accounts. These were submitted by the surgeon at the completion of a voyage, and could give considerable insight into quality of care, diagnostic, operative and therapeutic skills and also economy. The physician Sir Gilbert Blane would note in 1815 that he had perused 'several hundreds of surgeons' journals', using information contained in them to help compile his study, 'On the Comparative Health of the British Navy'.[15]

The number of surgeons on board a ship was based on the rating of the vessel, as Table 3.1 shows. There was rarely a full medical complement on board, however, since not infrequently surgeons or their assistants were indisposed, absent, or sometimes incompetent – or vacated positions had simply not been filled. As in the Army, it was the surgeon's mates that were often in short supply. There were 1,250 surgeons in a British Army around 300,000 strong by the end of the French Wars. In the Royal Navy, there were between 1,400 and 1,450 doctors for about 130,000 sailors, which was an approximate allocation of one surgeon for every hundred men: over twice the proportional provision for the Army.

As we have noted, over the course of the twenty-three years of the Revolutionary and Napoleonic Wars with France, the situation of the surgeons on warships was to improve. Dr Thomas Trotter's *Review of the Medical Department in the British Navy, with a Method of Reform proposed* (1790) suggested some sensible changes, bringing more control over medical practice within the powers of

[13] S.C. Lawrence, *Charitable Knowledge: Hospital Pupils and Practitioners in Eighteenth-Century London* (Cambridge, 1996), p. 93

[14] Lloyd and Coulter, *Medicine and the Navy*, vol. 3, p. 18.

[15] Gilbert Blane, 'On the Comparative Health of the British Navy, from the Year 1779 to the Year 1814, with Proposals for its Further Improvement', in Christopher Lloyd (ed.), *The Health of Seamen: Selections from the Works of Dr James Lind, Sir Gilbert Blane and Dr Thomas Trotter* (London, 1965), p. 179.

Table 3.1 Allocation of naval surgeons by rate of ship

Rate	Guns	Men	Surgeon	Surgeon's assistants (mates)
1	100	880	1	5
2	84	750	1	4
3	74	600–700	1	3
4	60	400–435	1	2
5	36	240	1	2
6	28	200	1	1
Sloop	12	80–110	1	1
Bomb ketch	8	60	1	0
Fireship	8	45	1	0
Yacht	8	40	1	0

Note: The allocation of surgeons was in ideal peacetime circumstances, also assuming that there were sufficient fit surgeons available.

Source: Michael Crumplin, *Men of Steel: Surgery in the Napoleonic Wars* (Shrewsbury, 2007), p. 146.

the Navy. Sir Gilbert Blane, in the 1799 edition of his *Observation on the Diseases of Seamen*, called for a change in attitude in the service, towards doctors, as well as for improved pay, as only then could the Navy attract men of the right calibre. A significant shortage of naval surgeons, consequent on losses (principally to disease) in the West Indian campaigns of 1793–8, caused surgeons in the year of the naval mutinies (1797) to petition the Admiralty to give them parity with the Army. This followed a Royal Warrant of 1796, which had given improved pay and allowances to Army doctors. A further such Warrant was issued in 1804 to attract surgeons into the Army. Trotter's 'memorial' of 1801, concerning naval salaries, the iniquity of fining seamen for suffering venereal complaints, the free provision of drugs and instruments, and eligibility for half pay, coupled with a lack of pay increases for chaplains and doctors in 1802, led to an Order in Council of the Sick and Hurt Board dated 23 January 1805. This encompassed some long-overdue reforms. The Order's introductory paragraphs emphasised the needs:

> Your Majesty's Naval Service having suffered materially in the present war from want of surgeons and surgeons' mates, and the Commissioners for Sick and Wounded Seamen having represented to us that the difficulty of procuring qualified persons being in great measure attributed to the more liberal provision made for the same description of officers in Your Majesty's land forces, we directed the said Commissioners to propose to us a plan for the better encouragement of Surgeons and Surgeons' Mates of Your Majesty's Navy …
>
> And the Commissioners having further submitted to us the propriety of allowing Medical Officers to wear a distinguishing uniform during the time of their actually being employed, and giving them a comparative rank in the service suitable to their situation, to which consideration it is believed they attach much importance, especially as regimental Surgeons are allowed to rank with Captains,

and their Assistant with subaltern officers, having taken the plan into consideration, we are of the opinion that the adoption of the proposal contained therein will be of great advantage to Your Majesty's Naval Service …[16]

The surgeon was, however, to be subordinate to lieutenants in His Majesty's ships. The cost to Britain of these proposals was – for drugs supplied gratis, uniforms and increased pay – £41,726 9s 2d (around £2.6 million in today's money).

A summary of these long-overdue reforms consisted of the following important details for surgeons:

1. All surgeons to be eligible for half pay (after thirty years' service).
2. Hospital Surgeons to be paid fifteen shillings a day.
3. Any practitioner appointed to serve as Physician of the Fleet or in a shore hospital must have served five years as a surgeon; emoluments to be one guinea *per diem* rising to one and one half at three years and two guineas at ten years (plus residence gratis).
4. A pay increase to eleven shillings a day for surgeons on active service – eighteen shillings after twenty years service (fifteen shillings for serving on a hospital ship).
5. Surgeon's Mates to be renamed Assistant Surgeons and paid eight shillings and sixpence a day. All to be fully qualified (i.e. properly examined after suitable training).
6. Drugs to be provided by the service, but surgical instruments to be purchased (i.e. by the surgeon himself – a capital set might cost fifteen to twenty guineas; a pocket set five to ten pounds).
7. Various types of assistants in hospital, including surgeons, to be called Hospital Mates; these to be paid six shillings and sixpence a day if 'unqualified' (i.e. not yet examined by a licensing body) and if warranted, four shillings per day.
8. Every surgeon to wear a 'distinguishing' uniform. This would be a Captain's undress uniform with a stand-up collar. Physicians to wear gold lace on their sleeves.[17]

The aforementioned memorial sent by John Bell to the Admiralty in 1800 commented on the lack of a school of military medicine – something never established in England, though found elsewhere in Europe – and also on the lowly status and pay of naval surgeons. In 1806, however, the University of Edinburgh established a Regius Chair of Military Surgery – the only such appointment in Britain at that time – and appointed, after some competition, John Thomson. For those entering the Navy, Army or the East India Company the Edinburgh lectures were given gratis. This prestigious Chair was abolished in 1855.[18]

As well as the naval surgeon's surgical duties (which we will examine in detail), there were certain other general health responsibilities which he shared with the captain and other senior crew-members. Issues of diet, water supply,

[16] Sick and Hurt Board (preliminary paragraphs), NMM, 8 December 1804, F/36.
[17] Lloyd and Coulter, *Medicine and the Navy*, vol. 3, pp. 33–4.
[18] The Chair was latterly held by George Ballingall. See Kaufman, *Regius Chair of Military Surgery*.

Figure 3.4 Daily sick rates, new cases and deaths on board the American frigate *New York* – outward bound from Virginia to the Mediterranean, 2 September to 10 December 1802

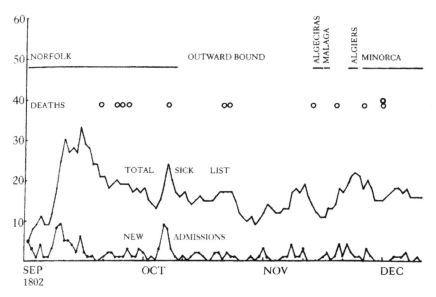

Source: J. Worth Estes, *Naval Surgeon. Life and Death at Sea in the Age of Sail* (Massachusetts, 1998) p. 93.

clothing, ventilation and fumigation, and the dispatch by 'smart ticket' of seriously ill patients ashore, would frequently involve the surgeon. He would hope to have the sympathetic ear of a good commander, to whom such matters could be addressed. The surgeon was required to visit his patients twice daily, and to provide a daily sick list to his captain. He kept a day book of all sick therapies and operations; each of these was to be entered in two separate journals: the journal of his 'Physical Practice in Disease' was to be shown to the Commission of Sick and Wounded or the Physician of Greenwich Hospital, and the journal of his 'Chirurgical Operations' was to be perused by the Governor of the Surgeon's Company.[19] The records of a large American frigate, *New York* (38 guns, crew complement 346), patrolling the Mediterranean in 1802–3, provide an informative example of sick rates at sea (see Figures 3.4 and 3.5). Before sailing from Norfolk, Virginia, there was an outbreak of dysentery and fever (possibly malaria and hepatitis). As can be seen from Figures 3.4 and 3.5, the number of men sick on a daily basis fluctuated between ten and thirty, with up to ten new patients presenting per diem.[20]

---

[19] Lloyd and Coulter, *Medicine and the Navy*, vol. 3, pp. 22–3.
[20] J. Worth Estes, *Naval Surgeon: Life and Death at Sea in the Age of Sail* (Massachusetts, 1998), pp. 93, 123.

Figure 3.5 Daily sick rates, new cases, deaths and injuries in the frigate *New York* cruising the Mediterranean, 20 March to 30 June 1803

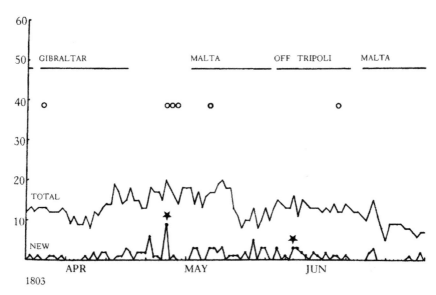

Note: The circles denote fatalities and the two stars, powder explosions.

Source: J. Worth Estes, *Naval Surgeon. Life and Death at Sea in the Age of Sail* (Massachusetts, 1998), p. 123.

Although the Royal College of Physicians of London had some influence on the choice of medications for the Royal Navy, it was the Society of Apothecaries who, since 1703, held sole rights of supply.[21] According to William Turnbull's *Naval Surgeon* (1806), there were around sixty-five medications, which had been recommended by Blane and were provided by the Society of Apothecaries. These included cordials, emetics, cathartics, stimulants (e.g. hartshorn and camphor) and sedatives (tincture of opium and laudanum). There were drugs for use in the anti-phlogistic regimen (to combat sepsis, contagion and febrile illnesses), blistering agents for counter irritation and mercurial preparations for gonorrhoea and syphilis.[22]

A frequent scheme of therapy (the anti-phlogistic regimen) to combat infections such as pneumonia, wound sepsis, typhus, cystitis, etc., was to bleed the patient with a thumb lancet, extracting twenty to thirty fluid ounces (600–900 ml) of blood each session, and then to administer a purgative (or cathartic) medicine

---

[21] J.J. Keevil, *Medicine in the Navy, 1200–1900. Vol. 2: 1649–1714* (Edinburgh and London, 1958), p. 272.
[22] William B. Turnbull, *The Naval Surgeon: Comprising the Entire Duties of Professional Men at Sea. To which are Subjoined, a System of Naval Surgery, and a Compendious Pharmacopoeia* (London, 1806).

Minutes of the Court of Examiners of the Royal College of Surgeons of England referring to the matter of approval of surgical instruments supplied to HM ships of the line - 1813.

1813

January 15th. Resolved that the master and Govenors be desired to communicate to the Hon'ble the transport Board the Sentiments of this Court relating to the Instruments of Naval Surgeons as expressed in the following Minute.

Mr Evans, of the Old Change, Chirurchigal Instrument Maker, having delivered at the College for examination, agreeably to the request of the Court, Specimens of Instruments, according to the Copy of a List, by the Director of the Hon'ble the Commissioners for Transports, etc. Viz;

Three Amputating Knives.
One Do. Saw, with spare Blades.
One Metacarpel (sic) Do. with Do.
Two Catlins.
Pair of Artery forceps.
Two Dozen curved Needles.
Two Tenaculums.
Two Pettit's (sic) screw Tourniquets.
Pair of Bone Nippers è Turnscrew.
Three Trephines.
Saw for the Head.
Rugine.
Pair of Forceps.
Elevator.
Brush.
Two Trocars.
Two Silver catheters.
Two Gum Elastic Do.
Six Scalpels.
Small Razor.
Key-tooth Instrument.
Gum Lancet.
Two Pairs of Tooth Forceps.
Punch.
Two Seton Needles.

Pair of Strong Probe Scissors.
Curved Bistory (sic) with a Button.
Long Probe.
Pair of Bullet Forceps.
Scoop for extracting Balls.
Two Probangs.
Half a pound of ligature thread.
One Paper of Needles.
Case with Lift out.
Apparatus for restoring suspended anima – do.
Set of Pocket Instruments.
Two Lancets in a Case.
Two Dozen Bougies, in a Case.
Two Pint Pewter Clyster Syringes.
Two Sets or Bundles of common Splints.
Set of Jappaned Iron Do. For legs.
Twelve Flannel or Linen Rollers.
Two Eighteen-Tailed Bandages.
Twenty yards of Keb for Tourniquets
Sixty yards of tape, different Breadths.
A Cupping Apparatus, consisting of One Scarificator and Six glasses --

Figure 3.6 Transcription of a list of instruments prescribed for the Royal Navy in 1813 by the Royal College of Surgeons of England

Source: Minutes of the Court of Examiners, Royal College of Surgeons of England.

(such as a mercurial agent), an emetic (e.g. tartar or ipecacuanha), or perhaps an antimonial solution. Fumigating agents, soap, wormwood and no doubt many an idiosyncratic choice of medicament were provided or purchased by the surgeon. Adequate knowledge of the properties and mixtures of medications was essential, as pastes, ointments, cordials and tinctures often had to be freshly prepared. Questions from a revision book for the London College membership examination underline the significant quantity of chemistry that was required for the prescription and dispensing of contemporary remedies. These included, 'What is meant by deliquescence?' 'What combinations does sulphur form with oxygen?' 'What does an acid consist of?' 'How is benzoic acid made?'[23] Of particular importance were two drugs, Peruvian bark (cinchona) and varying preparations of opium. The former was employed to combat many febrile illnesses, often with an unpredictable outcome, but it was clearly of importance in the management of malaria, since the bark contained quinine. Opiates were essential for analgesia, but were also sometimes used in efforts to prevent dysentery and diarrhoea, since they had a constipating effect.

Although surgical instruments had to be purchased by the surgeon, there may well have been a prescribed set of instruments for each warship. The chosen instruments were selected at the College of Surgeons of London by a triumvirate of surgeons appointed annually from the Court of Examiners – usually the Master and two Wardens. An appropriate manufacturer was also selected by the Court to supply them. Any useful, ineffectual or obsolete instruments were recommended or expunged respectively.[24] The list for 1813 is shown in Figure 3.6; the manufacturer was John Evans and Co. of 10, Old Change, London. After approval, the metal-bound mahogany (or oak) felt-lined boxes were sent directly onto His Majesty's vessels, sealed in canvas bags to avoid tampering.

Most of the duties of a ship's surgeon were the day-to-day drudge of treating sailors' injuries, ailments and other concerns. Bowel complaints, catarrhal illnesses, rheumatism, soft tissue and bony injuries and venereal diseases all took up much time. Venereal diseases were frequent, accounting for around 60 to 70 per cent of problems affecting the urinary tract, and were considered shameful.[25] Until 1795, the sailor could be fined fifteen shillings, paid to the surgeon, if they presented with a venereal infection.[26] This, inevitably, discouraged crew from consultation.

The surgeon's quarters and his small dispensary were situated near the sick berth or often the cockpit on the orlop deck. Although in the eighteenth century the sick berth might be placed anywhere – at the whim of the captain – it was, between 1790 and 1800, commonly sited under the forecastle, placed amid two

---

[23] R. Hooper, *Examinations in Anatomy, Physiology, Practice of Physic, Surgery, Materia Medica, Chemistry, and Pharmacy, for the use of Students, who are about to Pass the College of Surgeons, or the Medical or Transport Board* (New York, 1815), pp. 103, 108, 109.

[24] Minutes of the Court of Examiners, Royal College of Surgeons of England, 15 January 1813.

[25] J.C. Goddard, 'An Insight into the Life of Royal Naval Surgeons during the Napoleonic War, Part 1', *Journal of the Royal Naval Medical Service*, 77 (1991), pp. 205–22, p. 218.

[26] Lloyd and Coulter, *Medicine and the Navy*, vol. 3, pp. 357–8.

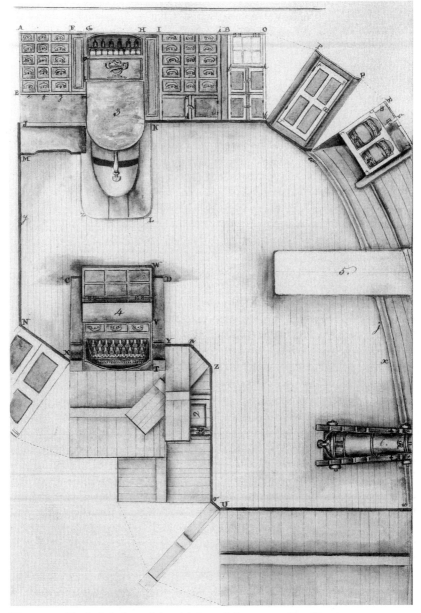

Figure 3.7 Exploded plan of the sick bay of the 74-gun *San Domingo*.
National Maritime Museum

Note: Commencing at the bow of the ship (top of picture), notice the apothecaries' drawers, containing medications, and a cupboard straddling the bowsprit, on which rests a table for making up prescriptions, resting instruments, etc. The door leads to the sick bay roundhouse (toilet or head). Between the door to the heads and the cannon were situated two large containers, one for water the other for vinegar. A board has been laid over a starboard gun, for dressings and surgery. Board screens, which were dismantled in action, are shown laid flat for descriptive purposes. In the centre is the apothecary's chest and drug store.

or three of the starboard ordnance, with reasonable ventilation and access to a roundhouse. Lord St Vincent mandated this arrangement in the Mediterranean fleet in 1798 and later in the Channel fleet.

The bay contained a small dispensary, from which the loblolly boys doled out medication morning and evening, announced by the beating of pestle on mortar. Here there was also storage space for splints, razors, wash-bowls, rollers and instruments; there were washing facilities and sometimes a small stove. The sick berth could be partitioned off from the rest of the deck by temporary wooden or canvas screens. A hinged board lowered over a cannon served as an operating platform, and square-ended frame cots were suspended from the deck beams. The sick berth facility could be expanded along the deck in the event of an epidemic, or for convalescent battle casualties who could not be evacuated to a shore hospital. A rare surviving deck-plan of the sick berth on board HMS *San Domingo* (74 guns) gives some idea of the typical layout (see Figure 3.7). The exploded sketch is taken from a watch bill of the ship, under command of Captain J.B. Pechell in 1814.

In combat, the sick berth would have been exposed and vulnerable. Thus it was cleared for action and a temporary space was provided for the surgeon, his assistants and the wounded in the cockpit on the orlop deck. This was below the waterline (unlike on some French line of battle ships), and was a safer location for battle surgery. The price for such relative security was a lack of ventilation, space, light and headroom. The last of these problems made the ergonomics of surgery particularly uncomfortable. In addition to the pandemonium of the cockpit and the supplications of the wounded, the noise and reverberation of the largest ordnance overhead must have imposed severe restriction and discomfort. One challenge for the naval surgeon was that most of the casualties were, in contrast to the Army, very near to hand. Thus, many hopeless cases were delivered to the surgeon speedily and would, despite small chance of success, take up time, whilst patients with greater chance of survival waited. Sorting casualties into order of importance (the concept now known as triage) was not formally taught, but one mid-seventeenth-century naval surgeon based at Plymouth, James Yonge, strongly believed in methodical working and hygiene, and is on record as carrying out this important practice.[27] Another naval surgeon, Edward Ives, followed an alternative and innovative course of action. Finding the orlop cockpit cramped and noisy, he moved his operation area into the hold and merely used the cockpit for casualty accumulation.[28]

A striking vignette of work on the orlop is well described in a report written by the surgeon on board HMS *Ardent*, Robert Young, working alone during the Battle of Camperdown in 1797. His poignant account highlights pragmatic issues for the surgeon:

---

[27] John Atkins, *The Navy Surgeon; or, Practical System of Surgery* (London, 1742), pp. 147–9.
[28] Edward Ives, *A Voyage from England to India: In the year MDCCLIV: And an Historical Narrative of the Operations of the Squadron and Army in India* (London, 1773), p. 453.

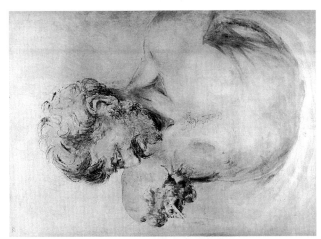
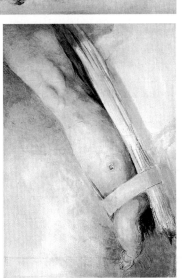
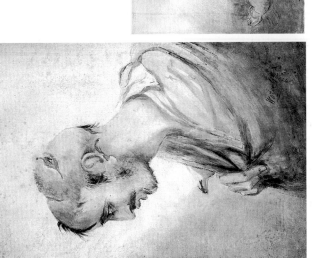

Figure 3.8 *Wounded after Waterloo*, by Sir Charles Bell. Army Medical Services Museum

Note: Notice the slicing wounds to the head (left); musket ball injury of a leg; and avulsion of an arm by round shot.

All of these were wounded in the action of October 11, in which I had no mate (many were driven out of the service by the mutinies), having been without one for three months before. I was employed in operating and dressing till near 4.0 in the morning, the action beginning about 1.0 in the afternoon. So great was my fatigue that I began several amputations under a dread of sinking before I could secure the blood vessels.

Ninety wounded were brought down during the action. The whole cockpit deck, cabins, wing berths and part of the cable tier, together with my platform and my preparations for dressing were covered with them. So that for a time they were laid on each other at the foot of the ladder where they were brought down, and I was obliged to go on deck to the Commanding Officer to state the situation and apply for men to go down the main hatchway and move the foremost of the wounded further forward into the tiers and wings, and thus make room in the cockpit. Numbers, about sixteen, mortally wounded, died after they were brought down, amongst whom was the brave and worthy Captain Burgess, whose corpse could with difficulty be conveyed to the starboard wing berth. Joseph Bonheur had his right thigh taken off by a cannon shot close to the pelvis, so that it was impossible to apply a tourniquet: his right arm was also shot to pieces. The stump of the thigh, which was very fleshy, presented a dreadful and large surface of mangled flesh. In this state he lived nearly two hours, perfectly sensible and incessantly calling out in a strong voice to me to assist him. The bleeding from the femoral artery, although so high up, must have been very inconsiderable, and I observed it did not bleed as he lay. All the service I could render this unfortunate man was to put dressings over the part and give him a drink. … Melancholy cries for assistance were addressed to me from every side by wounded and dying, and piteous moans and bewailing from pain and despair. In the midst of these agonising scenes, I was able to preserve myself firm and collected, and embracing in my mind the whole of the situation, to direct my attention to where the greatest and most essential services could be performed.[29]

Such arduous service could take its toll. Robert Young was soon invalided out of the service, having contracted typhus and developed a hernia.

Civilian and inexperienced witnesses to hasty battle surgery could, not unexpectedly, often be disturbed by what they saw. A poignant and vivid example of this is found in an account by Samuel Leech, a boy sailor on board HMS *Macedonian*, which was forced to surrender by the US frigate, *United States*, in October 1812 following a fierce action. Leech observed: 'Such scenes of suffering I saw in that wardroom I hope never to witness again.' Assisting in a below-the-knee amputation of one of his mess mates, Leech wrote: 'The task was most painful to behold, the surgeon using his knife and saw on human flesh and bones as freely as the butcher at the shambles.'[30] Leech's observations, however, must not detract from recognising the necessity of inflicting intense suffering on those whose lives might only be saved by this controlled mutilation. Such sights often seemed to upset servicemen more than the destructive injuries of combat. Despite significant

[29] Surgeons' journals, National Archives, ADM 101/58.
[30] Lloyd and Coulter, *Medicine and the Navy*, vol. 3, p. 61.

Table 3.2 Causation of army combat injuries compared with those suffered by naval personnel

Type of injury	Land forces (%)	2 French ships at Trafalgar (%)	HMS *Shannon* 1813 (%)
Musket/carbine/pistol	449 (61.7)	14 (13.5)	19 (31.6)
Sword/sabre	98 (13.5)	–	2 (3.3)
Round shot/canister/common shell/spherical case (Army)	126 (17.3)	–	–
Round shot/grapeshot/splinter (Navy)	–	69 (66.4)	37 (61.7)
Lance/pike/spontoon	28 (3.9)	–	–
Bayonet	9 (1.2)	12 (11.4)	1 (1.7)
Blunt injury/burns	8 (1.1)	9 (8.7)	1 (1.7)
Ramrod	5 (0.7)	–	–
Knife	4 (0.5)	–	–
Musket feather spring	1 (0.1)	–	–
Total	728	104	60

Sources: Army casualties: Crumplin, *Men of Steel*, p. 41. Naval casualties: Sir James Watt, personal communication (Trafalgar data); and H.F. Pullen, *The Shannon and the Chesapeake* (Toronto/Montreal 1970), appendices A, D and E.

danger of death from shock or infection, men often survived the amputation of one or more limbs: as early as 1676, Samuel Pepys calculated that there were up to forty 'double-maimed' men (that is, missing two limbs) eligible to claim naval pensions.[31]

Combat wounds on board ship were of several common types. On board the two French ships of the line *L'Algeçiras* and *L'Argonaute*, at Trafalgar, around 69 out of 104 wounds (66 per cent) were caused by ship's ordnance (round shot, grapeshot and splinters). As a rule, only those hit on the limbs by round shot would survive. A common sequela of round shot strike on a ship's hull was the detachment of wooden debris. These jagged splinters, potentially impregnated with salt water, bacteria, excrement, vomit and dirt, led to inevitable sepsis, and mortality from such injury was consequently high. The kinetic energy of round shot was greater close to than when fired from some distance and thus resulted in less splintering at close quarters. During the engagement on 1 June 1813 between HMS *Shannon* and the United States frigate *Chesapeake*, grapeshot injury was most frequent; this reflected the attempts of American gunners to clear the exposed enemy deck prior to boarding. Thus, although mainly anti-personnel ordnance was used here, injuries from ship's guns and the consequent splinters still accounted for 62 per cent of inflicted wounds.[32] Other potential types of wounding in naval actions included

[31] Keevil, *Medicine and the Navy*, vol. 1, p. 138.
[32] H.F. Pullen, *The Shannon and the Chesapeake* (Toronto, 1970), appendices A, D and E.

penetration of the body by musket balls, pikes, tomahawks, cutlasses and dirks. Chopping wounds were generally inflicted on the upper part of the body – the head, neck, shoulders and arms (see Figure 3.8). Stabbing wounds often fell about the neck and torso. Then there were also the 'civilian' types of trauma with which a new surgeon might be more familiar – fractures, burns, rope burns, drowning, blunt head wounds and sprains.

Injuries sustained during actions at sea can be informatively contrasted with the wounds received by land forces. Table 3.2 compares the causation of 728 wounds received by soldiers, presenting alive to surgeons of the Army Medical Department between 1808 and 1814; 104 French naval injuries on board *L'Algeçiras* and *L'Argonaute* (both ships with naval and infantry complements of 755) at Trafalgar; and 60 wounds inflicted during the above-mentioned engagement between the *Shannon* (complement 330) and the *Chesapeake*. These data show that injuries suffered by land forces were proportionally different – two-thirds were caused by small arms fire, rather than by ordnance (17 per cent).

Surgical treatment consisted of first aid and definitive treatment. As noted, because of the proximity of their casualties, naval surgeons were rapidly deluged, resulting in some patients bleeding to death whilst awaiting treatment. There was general approval for the procurement and provision of tourniquets, since around 10 per cent of the ship's company were required to be proficient in first aid.[33] Initially, all surgeons could do was to staunch bleeding, bandage wounds, splint fractures, administer water (wounded men have an intense thirst), reassure, and also assess those who had no chance of survival. Pain relief was not generous, neither before nor after surgery.

When the casualty had been manhandled down to the orlop deck, definitive surgical decisions and therapy could be meted out (see Figure 3.9). Operations were capital (major) or minor procedures. Essential definitive surgery in the Navy consisted of partial or complete limb ablation (that is, amputation); retrieval of foreign debris from the body; the management of thoracic and abdominal wounds; draining purulent material (pus) after sepsis had set in; tissue repair and the treatment of fractures; and finally, occasional trephining of the skull to relieve pressure or stem bleeding. There was no anaesthesia. Laudanum and opium were prescribed sparingly after surgery (not before), or for those in severe discomfort. Alcohol was likewise not used during operations, since it is a sedative and anxiolytic (i.e. anti-anxiety) drug, and not an analgesic. Also, it could make patients more uncooperative, and it increased their tendency to bleed. Doses of laudanum or tincture of opium large enough to remove the pain of surgery would prove dangerous to the patient, inducing respiratory depression and vomiting, with the serious risk of inhalation.

Many operations, aside from some cranial, abdominal and thoracic procedures, were carried out in an upright position, both for access and speed (see Figure 3.10). This gave the surgeon the best access for a swift operation. For upper limb

---

[33] Lloyd and Coulter, *Medicine and the Navy*, vol. 3, p. 63.

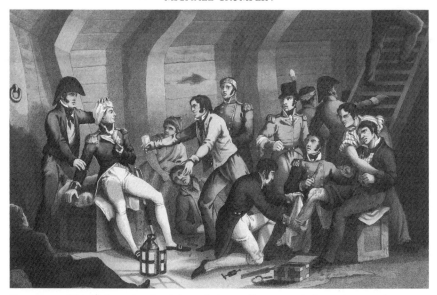

Figure 3.9 *The Cockpit, Battle of the Nile*, by William Heath [artist], M Dubourg [engraver], 4 June 1817. National Maritime Museum

Note: Nelson's head wound is being dressed during the Battle of the Nile in the cockpit of HMS *Vanguard*. Notice the drink being handed to the patient, and the surgical operation about to be performed on the sailor on the right.

surgery and ablation, the patient would be seated on a chair, and for lower limb procedures, a chair or the sailcloth-covered end of a platform, sea chest or table was employed. Assistants, usually loblolly boys or lightly wounded or convalescent sailors, restrained the patient, and a mate would steady the limb on which surgery was to be performed.

The most capital of operations, and one with many technical controversies, was amputation. This was performed in cases of mutilation, where there was severe muscle and bone damage, continued bleeding or open major joint injury. Primary amputation refers to surgery carried out soon after wounding, and secondary amputation was a delayed procedure, usually performed in cases of infection in an injured limb. Secondary amputation doubled the mortality of surgery. The success of amputation was dependent on many factors, including general fitness of the patient, delay, sepsis, quantity of blood loss, site of injury and (not least) the experience and skill of the surgeon. (The latter certainly varied, but John Ring's 1798 claim that it was 'a notorious truth, that at sea they amputate like the barbarians of Abyssinia; only with this difference, they use a knife instead of a hatchet'[34] was only occasionally correct.)

[34] John Ring, *Reflections on the Surgeon's Bill* (London, 1798), p. 36, quoted in Margarette Lincoln, 'The Medical Profession and Representation of the Navy, 1750–1815', in Geoffrey L. Hudson (ed.), *British Military and Naval Medicine, 1600–1830* (Amsterdam and New York, 2007), pp. 201–26, p. 202.

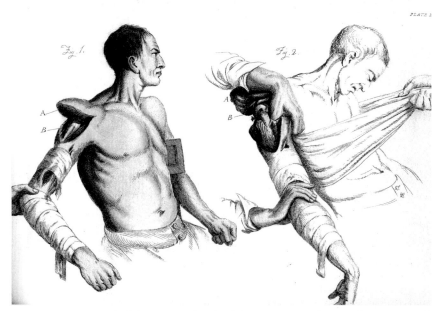

Figure 3.10 Removal of the arm at the shoulder-joint. Note the upright position of the patient and almost inevitable syncope (fainting). Michael Crumplin

Given a fit enough patient, and a reasonable surgeon, mortality after a mid-thigh amputation was about 40 to 50 per cent, after a below-knee amputation 25 to 30 per cent, and after a foot amputation 15 per cent, and so on.[35] There was less risk incurred in the amputation of an arm when compared with a lower limb. A thigh amputation would last about fifteen to twenty minutes, since surgery did not just entail removal of the limb (which could be accomplished in a few minutes) but also ligating the blood vessels, trimming the tissues, and then closing and bandaging the wound. Either a screw tourniquet was applied above the site of amputation or firm digital pressure could be applied over the main artery. The patient was firmly held and supported. After separation of the soft tissues with a sweep of a large curved blade, the bone was divided with a tenon or bow saw, the soft tissues being retracted out of the way of the saw teeth. The wound was then closed with adhesive tapes or sutures, after securing the blood vessels with linen or silk ligatures (see Figure 3.11). Less severe battle wounds were trimmed, closed and dressed, and any haemorrhage was controlled by ligatures or linen bandages. Stitching was again carried out with linen or silk sutures, using a semi-curved hand-held needle, or alternatively, a wound might be closed with adhesive tapes, freshly prepared before the action. Splinters or bone fragments were removed with fingers or forceps.

35 Crumplin, *Men of Steel*, p. 301.

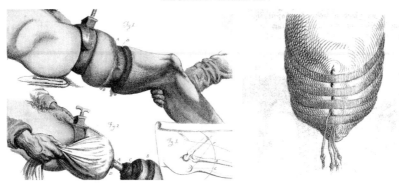

Figure 3.11 Above knee amputation (left); closure of stump after surgery (right): note the ligatures left long, for later removal. Michael Crumplin

Searching wounds for in-driven debris was a common procedure. There was less concern at leaving a lump of inert metal buried in the patient's body than there was with the fact that often fragments of wood, cloth or other debris were driven deep in the tissues, and being impregnated with bacteria would cause infection. First the surgeon would ascertain whether or not the missile or splinter had exited the body part. If not, then some attempt at retrieval was necessary, and the surgeon's finger would be introduced. Thus, in a body cavity or a limb, the presence and position of the missile could be determined and the extent of bony and soft tissue damage revealed. If the missile was not detected by a finger, it was unlikely that it could be retrieved using (bullet) forceps. Digital exploration in the abdomen or chest gave the surgeon clues as to the extent of visceral damage. The problems with deep wound exploration were that access and illumination were limited, and soft debris was difficult to retrieve. Damage to nerves or blood vessels was easily inflicted by exploring instruments.

Bleeding and infection were the most frequent complications of wounds and surgery. Another adverse outcome of amputation was impaired healing, resulting in bone protrusion and possible further uncomfortable surgery. Bleeding was of great concern to surgeons and was categorized in three particular ways. Primary haemorrhage was simply uncontrolled continued bleeding. If accessible, this was controlled with pressure from hand, tourniquet, bandages or ligature. If the source of bleeding was inaccessible, such as in the cranial cavity or abdomen or chest, it became impossible to deal with. Sometimes in a shocked patient, the bleeding would slow or stop by dint of low blood pressure and vasoconstriction (narrowing of the bore) of the arteries. Reactionary haemorrhage occurred when, initially, there appeared to be a cessation of blood loss, but as the patient's blood pressure rose, bleeding recommenced. Finally, secondary haemorrhage occurred when infection eroded and 'digested' the healing blood vessels, whose integrity was destroyed, thus causing haemorrhage, which was difficult to control by ligature.

Early nineteenth-century surgeons had no concept of bacteriology, but there had to be some way of managing an infected patient. The Galenic theory of imbalanced humours was then considered, but the management of sepsis required some vigorous antidote to the 'heightened response' of inflammation. The septic patient was observed to be feverish, sweating, ill, delirious, and to have a rapid pulse rate. The body part affected might be red and swollen. This necessitated some reduction in these observed responses, and the anti-phlogistic (anti-inflammatory) regimen was called into play. This consisted of bed rest; a low (that is, simple) diet; the letting of blood (venesection) three or four times a week; emesis (vomiting) induced with a medicine such as tartar, ipecacuanha or salt water; and purgation of the bowels with a drug such as calomel or jalap. This regimen usually made the patient weak and faint, and inevitably diverted his attention from irritating symptoms. Venesection was liberally prescribed in the armed services, most especially for cranial and thoracic wounds.

Infection was manifest frequently and the event was so common as to produce the term 'laudable pus'. This inferred that if the patient survived long enough to form a purulent discharge or a 'collection' (i.e. an abscess), he might well survive. Aside from tetanus (a relatively rare problem), infection with intestinal bacteria, streptococcus or staphylococcus, or a mixture of many organisms, was often present to challenge the patient's immune response. This itself was frequently depressed by the effects of malnutrition, scurvy, anaemia or intercurrent infection, such as diarrhoeal illnesses, tuberculosis or venereal disease.

In the Navy there was the occasional case of tetanus (also known as lockjaw), which occurred most commonly with wounds of the lower limb. This was as a result of wooden decks and footwear being heavily (microscopically) contaminated with horse or other animal manure. The causative bacterium, *Clostridium tetani*, secretes a neurotoxin which produces intense bodily muscular spasms. This can even impede the ability to eat, as a result of the clenched jaw. The outcome at this time was usually fatal. In one series of nineteen amputations in a hospital in Bermuda in 1780, nine cases succumbed to tetanus.[36] Since even proffered food or water excited intense muscular spasms (opisthotonus or emprosthotonus), occasionally the heavily sedated patient might have some front teeth extracted in order to be fed with a gum-elastic catheter passed into the stomach.

Burns were also frequent on board warships, often as a result of loose powder and blow-back of hot dry wadding. Men were often told to remove loose clothing to prevent it catching alight. Treatment was with cold dressings, linseed oil, vinegar and analgesics. Severe pain, sepsis and fluid loss were the immediate problems, with disfiguring scars being the end result. Impaired wound healing was a frequent occurrence and was usually a consequence of infection, poor blood supply to the affected body part, general debility, malnutrition, retention of foreign material and lack of essential nutrients. (The scourge of scurvy in the Royal Navy barely requires relating. Wounds that had previously healed soundly often broke down in the presence of what is now known to have been vitamin C deficiency.)

---

[36] Lloyd and Coulter, *Medicine and the Navy*, vol. 3, p. 361.

One of the hardest issues to research is the general standard of surgical ability. Whilst a ship's surgical log would record outcomes for a surgeon and his assistants (mates), there is insufficient detail to pronounce on an audit consensus on a mass of surgical cases. However, one large survey of surgeons in the British Army after the Battle of Toulouse at the end of the Peninsular War (1814) provides some helpful statistics. Of 1,242 badly wounded men admitted to one general hospital in Toulouse, 88 per cent walked out to convalesce or rejoin their units.[37] Such good surgical results could not have been obtained at the commencement of the war in 1793. It is arguable that surgical skills in the Royal Navy would likewise have improved over the twenty-three-year period of the war. Less able surgeons could be weeded out if they failed to cope with injury and contagion, and the sick berth and cockpit provided the best and most relevant classroom.

The first rate, HMS *Victory*, was certainly in the forefront of combat on 21 October 1805. At Trafalgar the ship's company suffered 132 casualties from a muster of 822 – a rate of 16 per cent; total Royal Navy casualties during the battle were 9.5 per cent.[38] This is comparable with land force casualty rates in action, which were around 10 to 25 per cent. Notably, of eight amputations performed on board *Victory* and afterwards, at Gibraltar, only one patient died; this was a mortality rate of 13 per cent, and compares favourably with larger series in the land forces of around 20 per cent overall. Also, of those retrieved from combat alive but hurt, on HMS *Victory* only four out of twenty-three dangerously ill servicemen died (17 per cent) – a remarkable achievement for the ship's surgeon, William Beatty, and his two assistants.

We should, however, recall the occasional advantage sailors had of being a good deal closer to surgical assistance, as compared to those injured on the battlefield. Excluding the casualties from HMS *Prince* (for which casualty rates are not available), 439 Royal Navy men were killed at Trafalgar and 1,213 wounded, around a 3:1 wound-to-kill ratio (though on board the *Victory*, which was closely engaged in the battle, this ratio was closer to 2:1). By contrast, the combined French and Spanish fleet sustained very approximately 3,600 killed and 3,400 wounded, almost a 1:1 wound-to-kill ratio. This high death rate incurred reflects high-quality British ship handling, superior gunnery at close range, and a large number of enemy men dying from burns or drowning.[39]

The extent to which these figures were influenced by the skills of Royal Navy surgeons cannot be accurately assessed, but it is worth addressing some of the innovations brought in by serving naval surgeons, which contributed significantly to the craft. These included cutting short ligatures for placing around blood vessels

[37] George James Guthrie, *Commentaries on the Surgery of the War in Portugal, Spain, France, and the Netherlands, 1808–1815. Sixth edition, with additions relating to the Crimea* (London, 1855), p. 154.
[38] James Watt, 'Surgery at Trafalgar', *The Mariner's Mirror*, 91 (2005), pp. 266–83, p. 272.
[39] John D. Clarke, *The Men of HMS Victory at Trafalgar* (Darlington, 1999), pp. 75–6: Watt, however, suggests that the number of French and Spanish sailors wounded must be an underestimate: Watt, 'Surgery at Trafalgar', p. 271.

(Surgeon Lancelot Haire, 1786); the first successful ligation of the common carotid artery (following a suicide attempt, Surgeon David Fleming, 1803); primary repair of the trachea (windpipe) after another suicide attempt (Surgeon Nathaniel Bedford, 1783); some attempt at triage, (see above); and finally, possibly the first surviving naval service forequarter amputation performed in Antigua, following a round shot strike (Surgeon Ralph Cuming, 1808). A tribute to these increasingly able surgeons and naval medical care is recognised by the fact that in 1782, hospital admissions were 1 in 3.2 and deaths 1 in 45, whereas in 1813, near the conclusion of the French Wars, comparable figures were 1 in 10 and 1 in 143 respectively.[40] Looking at improvements in sanitation, victualling and general medical provision in the period between 1779 and 1814, Gilbert Blane conjectured that 6,674 lives had been saved in 1813, compared with mortality in the Royal Navy in 1779.[41] Undoubtedly the improvements in health of the Navy were better controlled than in the mobile land forces, but the surgical skills acquired and improved upon could progress little further until the advent of antisepsis (in 1865) and anaesthesia (in 1846).

Despite the progress made by His Majesty's service surgeons, many of the fundamentally important tenets of surgery, so hard learnt in these wars, such as the management of contaminated wounds, the sea transport of battle casualties, and the timing and indications for surgery, were to be forgotten during the Crimean campaigns, forty years on. Unfortunately, there were many lessons that would have to be re-learnt.

---

[40] James Watt, 'Health in the Royal Navy During the Age of Nelson: Nelsonian Medicine in Context', *Journal of the Royal Naval Medical Service*, 86 (2000), pp. 64–71, pp. 70, 71.
[41] Blane, 'Comparative Health of the British Navy', p. 176.

4

The Sick and Hurt Board: Fit for Purpose?[1]

Pat Crimmin

The Sick and Hurt Board (formally titled the Commissioners for taking Care of Sick and Wounded Seamen and for the Care and Treatment of Prisoners of War) had first been created during the Dutch Wars of the mid seventeenth century. Fresh commissions were formed at the beginning of the succeeding wars, and dissolved at the peace. From 1715 the commissioners (there were only two) were members of the Navy Board, who were assigned these additional duties, though there was little work for them to do in these years of peace. It was not until 1740 that a new commission was established to deal with the increasing business created by the war with Spain. Henceforth the Board, though reduced in peacetime, remained a permanent department of the Royal Navy – though this permanence seems rather to have been the result of regular eighteenth-century wars than any deliberate decision by the government. But as the French Wars of the late eighteenth century progressed, and the size of the Royal Navy increased, it came under increasing strain and gathering scrutiny and criticism from the Admiralty and the government, with accusations that it was 'unfit for purpose'. In 1806 it was abolished. This chapter re-examines the history of the Sick and Hurt Board and the role it played in maritime health, and suggests that the perceived failings of the Board had, in fact, much to do with departmental policies and practices in the Royal Navy, and their political considerations, than with a lack of vision on the part of its commissioners.

In the early years of permanence the commissioners were bureaucrats whose earlier careers were formed within naval administration, and they had no medical qualifications. The Board was responsible for the care of sick and wounded seamen ashore, making regular returns of the numbers of such men to the Navy Board (which was responsible for administrative matters, such as the dockyards, pay and victualling) and the Board of Admiralty (which was responsible for appointments and opera-

---

[1]   This chapter is based on the series of original letters at the National Maritime Museum, Greenwich (hereafter NMM), between the Sick and Hurt Board (hereafter SHB) and the Admiralty Board, and material from The National Archive (hereafter TNA): NMM ADM/F/3–37, 1742–1806, SHB to Admiralty; ADM/FP/1–49, 1756–1806, SHB to Admiralty; ADM/E/5–52, 1715–1806, Admiralty to SHB; TNA ADM 1/3528–29, 1727–1742, SHB to Admiralty.

tional matters). The Sick and Hurt Board was responsible for overall supervision of the contracts made for sick quarters ashore, negotiated locally through their agent, or abroad by the senior sea officer; it was also responsible for the furnishing and equipping of contract hospitals and hospital ships, and later, when the Navy started building its own hospitals from the 1740s, for their supervision. The commissioners carried out visitations and inspections of such quarters and hospitals – either themselves, or through their agents or the local commander-in-chief who was instructed to visit as often (and unexpectedly) as possible. The office also examined and cleared the accounts of surgeons and those who had made contracts or engaged quarters for sick seamen.

Only when a surgeon received his warrant and was appointed, by the Admiralty, to a ship, did he come under the supervision of the Sick and Hurt commissioners, having to deliver to them at the end of his voyage his accounts, vouchers and receipts, without which he could not receive his pay. Only in 1796 did the granting of warrants to surgeons and their mates pass from the Navy Board to the Sick and Hurt commissioners, together with the care of sick seamen afloat and the superintendence of medicines and necessary extra items of diet and care for sick seamen, afloat and ashore.[2] The Board also supervised the salaries of its officials in London and at the outports, and its own office expenses.

Prior to 1796, the Board had little to do with the actual care of sick seamen afloat; communication with ships, squadrons and fleets was by letter and infrequent. Nor did it have much more than a token supervision of foreign-based hospitals or quarters; indeed the further away from London, the less supervision it could exert. This could cause difficulties in Britain; it was a major problem abroad. The Board could not control or dictate treatment, apart from issuing general instructions. These formed part of the General Printed Naval Instructions issued to sea officers by the Admiralty, and were revised fairly regularly, as a result of wartime experiences. When a revision was contemplated the Admiralty wrote to the Sick and Hurt Board asking if they had any changes they wished to make or articles they wished to add, but at first these were infrequent. In July 1748 the commissioners wished to amend instructions about sending sick seamen ashore, but the details they inserted were not medical but financial, concerning how captains were to provide for such men at the rate of 12d per man per day, and how they were to draw on the commissioners for money and keep proper accounts and receipts.[3]

From 1702 the Board was also responsible for the care and treatment of prisoners of war and their exchange. For non-commissioned men, prison depots were established at specially built prisons, at Plymouth and Portsmouth, or in hired buildings with some aspect of security, such as Portchester castle or Edinburgh castle. Officers were parolled and sent to nominated parole towns where they lived subject to certain restrictions. A Board agent, often a local surgeon, superintended both prisons and prisoners on parole. For most of the eighteenth century, prisoners were exchanged

---

[2]   Admiralty to SHB, 29 July 1796, ADM/E/45.
[3]   SHB to Admiralty, 1 July 1748, ADM/F/11.

fairly quickly according to mutually recognised rules of exchange. Numbers increased dramatically from the outbreak of war with France in 1793, however, and the breakdown of regular exchanges resulted in administrative problems. In 1796 the care of healthy prisoners was transferred to the Transport Board. The Sick and Hurt Board clerks dealing with prisoners were also transferred to the Transport Board, and were not replaced at the Sick and Hurt Office, though that Board still retained supervision of sick prisoners.

Office Record Keeping

One of the accusations levelled against the Sick and Hurt commissioners when the Board's abolition started to be discussed early in the nineteenth century was that absenteeism and office business were left in the hands of clerks. There is little evidence for this, though the office was organized in a particular way. There were 'Board days', when the available commissioners attended to sign letters and deal with current business. In peacetime this was infrequent, perhaps once or twice a week. In wartime, attendance was much more frequent and at very busy times it was daily. Commissioners were indeed absent, but on visits to hired sick quarters and hospitals. Those at Deptford and Woolwich, within easy reach of London, involved a day's visit. Visits to those further afield in Kent – the Medway towns, Deal or Dover – usually took two to three days, while visits to Portsmouth and Plymouth on the south coast, or to Great Yarmouth on the east, often took a week or more. The first commissioner and chairman of the Board usually stayed in London to deal with immediate Board business, whilst other commissioners took it in turn to visit. In 1742, out of 142 Board days, William Bell, first commissioner, attended all of them, Robert Allix attended 103, and Nathaniel Hills 91. In a typical war month, November 1745, out of twenty-one working days Bell again attended all, Allix attended twelve (but he was absent on visits to Gosport and Great Yarmouth), and Hills attended two days (but he too was absent at Deal, and at Dover investigating sick prisoners held at the castle).[4] This pattern was broadly repeated through the century.

The commissioners were also summoned to the Admiralty for discussions on important matters. On 14 April 1755 they were asked to attend 'tomorrow at 12.0 noon to discuss the subject of Haslar hospital', a discussion which took three days, and must have concerned the preparation of the partially completed hospital for the admission of sick seamen in the imminent war.[5] There were similar requests to attend the Navy Board, and though, in the earlier years of the century, this meant a brief walk to the Navy Office in Crutched Friars, a visit to the Admiralty involved a coach – or more probably a boat – to Westminster. The great move of the naval offices, from Tower Hill to the remodelled Somerset House in the Strand, in the late 1780s,

---

4   1741–2, ADM 1/3529; November 1745, ADM/F/7.
5   Admiralty to SHB, 14 April 1755, no. 71, ADM/E/13.

certainly shortened such journeys. Established on Tower Hill from 1714, the Board had overflowed into another house there in the 1740s. By 1770 the commissioners were complaining that their offices were too cramped, but it was not until March 1775 that the Admiralty began to consider moving the Navy, Navy Pay and Victualling offices from Tower Hill and Broad Street 'to a situation nearer the Admiralty'. On hearing this, the Sick and Hurt commissioners were anxious to be included, arguing, rightly, that the constant connections of their business with other naval departments necessitated their proximity.[6] The establishment did not move until May 1787, into modest offices, tucked between the more splendid suites of the Navy and Victualling Boards.[7]

The Work of Clerks

In common with most naval offices, though unlike all government offices, the Sick and Hurt clerks attended the office daily. The chief work of the majority was copying. Careful record keeping was a feature of the office, and this involved the handwritten duplication of every letter, order, form, instruction, warrant and contract, sometimes several copies, sent to all other naval offices and to the Surgeons' Company, the Society of Apothecaries, the Board's own agents, contractors and hospitals, and in wartime the Army departments. Reference was frequently made to past records when quoting precedents. In July 1744, for example, the Board's officials at Plymouth (the surgeon, physician, dispenser and their assistants) were being threatened by the Treasury with distraint on their goods for non-payment of the Land Tax. The commissioners appealed to the Admiralty, since they had no authority to deal directly with the tax officials, and referred their Lordships to records of 1703 (a war year), when these salaries had been exempted from tax. Armed with this argument the Admiralty was able to gain a rebate for these officers, though not until 1746.[8]

Letters received into the office were numbered and indexed, at least in peacetime, though indexing sometimes broke down in wartime because of pressure of work. But each letter usually had the Board's minuted decision, dated and written on the turned-over corner of the original letter. These minutes are the Board's immediate response, in abbreviated form, before it was translated into the formal reply. Clerks also recorded, in red ink, the date the letter was received, usually the same day or within two days at most. The Admiralty's request of 1755, to discuss Haslar Hospital, was received at 11.30 p.m., some clerks still being on duty until the business of the day was completed. The time of receipt was always recorded if it was after normal working hours, and other letters, received in wartime, are often marked 'past midnight' or 'received at 1.0. in the morning'.

---

6 SHB to Admiralty, 9 and 16 March 1775, ADM/FP/18.
7 SHB to Admiralty, 29 May 1787, ADM/FP/30.
8 SHB to Admiralty, 9, 11 July 1744, ADM/F/4; Admiralty to SHB, 21 January 1746, no. 7, ADM/E/12.

The number of letters sent and received depended on whether it was war or peacetime. In 1751, a peace year, there were only nine letters sent to the Admiralty, and seven received from their Lordships. The commissioners had been reduced to two at that time, and there was no secretary and only three clerks – a skeleton staff. But in 1755, when hostilities with France had already begun, there were 131 letters from the Sick and Hurt Board to the Admiralty, and 132 letters in reverse. There are twenty-four volumes of letters between the two boards during the period of the Seven Years War. In 1795, another war year, there were 334 letters sent from the Board, and just over 300 received from the Admiralty.

Commissioners and Clerks

Though in peacetime the number of commissioners was reduced to two, in war years it varied between three and five. Most were long-serving. Lewis Guiguer, appointed in 1756, served until his death in 1771; Robert Lulman from 1780 to 1795 after 'nearly thirty six years in various naval departments'; William Gibbons from 1789 to 1806.[9] Over the years the professional composition of the Board changed. In the 1740s and 1750s the commissioners were men trained in other naval departments without medical qualifications. When they needed medical advice they consulted the Physician of Greenwich Hospital, or leading experts of the day. In 1744, when the Board asked for an extra commissioner to deal with increasing business, they required not a doctor but someone who could help with the growing number of visits to the ports, and the man appointed was a sea officer, Captain Cayley.[10] But by the 1790s the professional balance had tipped in favour of a majority of doctors as commissioners. Between 1740 and 1799 the annual salary of the first commissioner and chairman of the Board was £465, and the other commissioners had a salary of £300 each. By 1800 these salaries had increased: the first commissioner now earned £565 annually, the other commissioners £500, and this rate remained fixed until the Board's abolition.

The Sick and Hurt Board's clerical establishment was small compared with those of the Navy and Victualling Boards. There was no permanent secretary until 1755, peacetime duties being performed by one of the senior clerks, and the secretary's annual salary remained at £200 between 1755 and 1800, when it increased to £500. Until the 1770s there were only three established (that is, permanent) clerks, with annual salaries ranging from £40 to £100 according to seniority, as well as a number of extra, non-established clerks, paid at a daily rate of 2s 6d and employed as needed. Their numbers varied according to peace or war: three in peacetime, rising to ten or more during the war years of the 1760s. After 1763 the annual salaries of all the established clerks were increased to £100, while those of extra clerks were established at an annual rate of £50. Clerical numbers rose to sixteen during the American war,

9 Lulman to Nepean, 6 April 1795, ADM/F/25.
10 SHB to Admiralty, 6 April 1744, ADM/F/3.

but fell back to thirteen during peace, only to rise to twenty from 1794 – an indication of the growing business at the Board.

In 1795 ten clerks were removed when the sub-department responsible for the care and exchange of healthy prisoners of war was transferred to the Transport Board.[11] Sick prisoners remained the responsibility of the Sick and Hurt office and the clerical gap was filled by between two and three new junior clerks. When the Board was abolished in 1806 there were three commissioners and twenty-three clerks. Four of them were chief or senior clerks whose annual salaries now ranged from £300 to £400. The annual salaries of the clerks and extra clerks ranged from £80 to £150 according to their seniority.

Compared with similar increases in staff numbers and salaries in the Navy Office, this was not a large establishment. Throughout these years the number of clerks was proving insufficient to cope with the labour of bringing old accounts up to date and liquidating them. In 1796, in reply to an Admiralty query about the number of clerks needed to solve this problem, the commissioners considered the answer lay not merely in appointing more extra clerks, but in appointing an accountant, 'holding rank next to the Secretary', with the sole duty of dealing with the overdue accounts and preventing further accumulations. He would report regularly to the Board and would have a small staff of six clerks, which would be reduced as the accounts were settled. The commissioners also recommended the whole system of accounting should be changed to simplify and shorten the process, which required vouchers and receipts, since

> the present minutely circumstantial mode of investigation tho' extremely well calculated to prevent the smallest abuse or fraud at a time when the service was on a less extensive scale than at present and the methods of eluding the detection of frauds less known and practiced, puts it in the power of persons so inclined to protract almost infinitely the period of the final settlement of their accounts.[12]

Such suggestions hardly support the contemporary view – later adopted by historians – of a board of doctors unable or unwilling to confront accounting problems.

The government of the period was more occupied with war and a grave financial crisis than with the appointment of an accountant's department for the Sick and Hurt Board. Yet the problems the Board tried to address did not go away. In 1799 the commissioners again expressed their serious concern over the number and size of unsettled accounts in the office. They did not blame their clerks, who were dealing with current business and trying to prevent the accumulation of fresh debts, but they blamed too small a clerical establishment and salaries which were too low to encourage both recruitment and promotion. Once again they drew attention to

[11] SHB to Admiralty, 5 October 1795, ADM/F/26, acknowledging the Admiralty order to transfer of 1 October. At the Transport Board's request the handover was postponed to January 1796.
[12] SHB to Admiralty, 4 July 1796, ADM/F/27.

the dismissal of staff in peacetime when the office was 'capable of little more ... than carrying on the current business of the peace'.[13]

The situation was made worse in 1796 by the transfer of the ten clerks employed in dealing with healthy prisoners to the Transport Board, but leaving the whole of those unsettled accounts with the Sick and Hurt Office, something contemporary critics did not mention and later historians have also ignored. This had left one chief clerk and three assistants to deal with sick prisoners and cope with accumulated debts of over one million pounds. But the government did not respond to these pleas. Peace again intervened in 1801; and the problem was shelved and left to the investigating commissions and their recommendations.

Finance and Naval Credit

Since another of the criticisms levelled against the Sick and Hurt Board was the number of large debts the department had accumulated through the century and seemed unable to liquidate, the system of naval credit must be briefly described.[14] Every year the Navy Board, under Admiralty direction, prepared estimates of the money needed for the service during the coming year. To do so it wrote to all naval offices, asking for their estimates. Once the Navy Board had received these, it drew up the general naval estimates, and sent them to the Admiralty, who accepted them and laid them before the Crown, for formal royal approval. Copies were then sent to the Treasury for information, and the estimates were presented to Parliament, by the First Lord of the Admiralty, all as a matter of regular office and parliamentary business. The estimates were open to inspection by MPs, but few bothered to look at them and fewer still could understand what the items referred to.

The Admiralty always took care to keep the quoted figures unalarmingly low, and the estimates were presented in general, traditional terms. They were divided into three: Ordinary estimates, dealing with fixed costs, mothballed ships, salaries, pensions and half pay (after 1745 Haslar and other naval hospitals also came under this heading); Extraordinary repairs; and Sea Service estimates. The Sea Service estimates took most of the money, and were reckoned in terms of the number of seamen employed and their wages. There was no debate on these estimates, nothing was itemized and so nothing could be investigated. The only figure which changed annually was that of the number of seamen required.

The Sea Service estimates were significant since they contained the money for paying bills, amongst them those of the Victualling Board and the Sick and Hurt Board. Naval bills were the largest part of the naval debt and were paid using money

---

[13] SHB to Admiralty, undated letter, probably 1799, ADM/FP/42.

[14] This section owes everything to Daniel A. Baugh, *British Naval Administration in the Age of Walpole* (Princeton, 1965), pp. 452–93; N.A.M. Rodger, *The Command of the Ocean: A Naval History of Britain, 1649–1815* (London, 2004), pp. 291–3, appendix VII, pp. 640–6, appendix IV, pp. 618–28.

voted by Parliament, held by the Treasurer of the Navy and passed, via the Navy Pay Office, to departments as they requested it. Bills were payable 'in course' (that is, in chronological order), according to their date of registry in the bill book of every naval office. The larger the debt, the longer the course or waiting time for maturity; and the longer the course, the higher the discount a holder of a bill had to accept if he wished to sell his bill, before maturity, for immediate cash. There was a regular market in such discounted bills since many holders often needed to do this. Most Navy bills yielded 4 per cent interest six months after registry. Victualling Board bills apparently did not. I do not yet know whether Sick and Hurt bills did.

Regular payment of bills 'on the course' was essential to maintain naval credit, since interruptions in regular payment led to cash shortages and damaged confidence. So when, in 1760, the Sick and Hurt Board complained there was no money at the Navy Pay Office for their bills and that their credit was in danger, this was a serious issue not only for the Board but also for the government.[15] Any failure to continue regular payments saw discount rates increase and contractors raise their prices to offset the higher discount. In July 1745, for example, Alexander Campbell in Jamaica had contracted to victual sick seamen for a fixed sum. It was always difficult for West Indian islands to feed themselves, and in wartime it sometimes became impossible also to feed the large numbers of soldiers and sailors sent there. The price of provisions, already quite high during the war with Spain from 1739, rose more steeply from 1744 when France entered as Spain's ally. Campbell soon complained that he could not fulfil his contract: butter and cheese had risen from 1s 3d a pound to 5s, beef and mutton from 5d to 1s 3d a pound. He therefore asked permission to dissolve the contract, and for some compensation for the losses he had suffered. The contract had been for three years, with a proviso that either party might withdraw at the end of the first year, giving sufficient notice. When this dispute came before the Admiralty, the Sick and Hurt Board argued that Campbell had broken this proviso, and that the contract could not be voided. But their subsequent argument is interesting for the light it sheds on the power of contractors and the Board's dilemma. It declared that on consideration, and being convinced that the public rather than Campbell should bear the increased costs, Campbell should be repaid the money he had spent since August 1745, when prices rose. The commissioners recommended that the contract be cancelled and no new one drawn up, and that Campbell should continue to supply provisions in an *ad hoc* manner, being paid the real cost if he could support his claims with sworn affidavits, receipts and proper accounts. The Admiralty agreed with this proposal.[16]

The advantage here was wholly with Campbell. Contractors abroad were not numerous. It was rare for government departments to have a choice – particularly in the West Indies. To whom could the Board turn, quickly, if Campbell had refused? It was clearly necessary to make accommodations with contractors, and to attempt to control them through insisting on affidavits and receipts, though this was a slow,

---

[15] SHB to Admiralty, 18 November 1760, ADM/F/21. There was a similar complaint sent 22 April 1796, SHB to Admiralty, ADM/F/27.
[16] SHB to Admiralty, 1 October 1746, ADM/F/8.

cumbersome business. Moreover, there were political pressures. The contractor and business interest in Parliament was strong and well organised. Between 1715 and 1754, 198 MPs were business men, many of them holding government contracts.[17] Domestic politics too played their part. In October 1754 the corporation of Plymouth appealed to Lord Anson, First Lord of the Admiralty, that one of their aldermen might be recommended to the Sick and Hurt Board as a contractor for victualling sick seamen at the port. Plymouth was a naval town returning two MPs who were government supporters, and Lord Anson, in his letter to the Board, wished the corporation to be answered 'by this night's post'. The Board's minutes record this speed. Anson's letter was received on the evening of 31 October, an answer was written and sent within the hour and the following day the necessary contracts were made out in favour of the alderman.[18]

Foreign contracts also involved rates of exchange, another stumbling block in the rapid settlement of accounts and payment of bills. In West Indian accounts it is plain that some sums quoted are in sterling ('English money') and others in Jamaican pounds. Throughout the Caribbean and Mediterranean pieces of eight and the Spanish silver dollar, an international currency, were in general use, while the East India Company used both sterling and Indian currencies. In 1746 Commodore Curtis Barnett agreed a price for the care of his sick seamen at the East India Company's Fort St David on the Coromandel coast, putting them under the care of the Company surgeon there at a cost of 18d per man per day. He sent home properly attested accounts for a total of just over £648. But the Sick and Hurt Board refused to accept and pay them because the Company had later insisted on a rate of payment of eight *fanams* per day, which equalled 2s per man per day, the price the Company paid for the cure of its own men. After some argument the Board was compelled to pay this, though it regarded the rate as too high.[19] But the Admiralty overruled them; the Company was too powerful to offend, commercially and politically. Such sums were not very large, but they were outside the amounts the Board had established and on which it had based its estimates, and such sums could amount to formidable totals.

Because of the insistence on proper accounting with receipts and vouchers duly attested, and because of inadequate numbers of clerical staff to deal with backlogs, the settlement of accounts was very slow. Sometimes sheer accident made it impossible for claimants to provide proper vouchers and receipts. One surgeon, at Newfoundland, lost all his possessions, including his vouchers, in a warehouse fire in 1773. Dr White at Boston in 1776 and Dr Polhill at Leghorn in 1796 were caught up in the hasty evacuation of their hospitals in wartime and were unable to produce receipts.[20]

---

[17] Romney Sedgwick (ed.), *The History of Parliament: The House of Commons, 1715–54* (2 vols, London, 1970), I, p. 148.
[18] SHB to Admiralty, 31 October 1754, no. 53, ADM/E/13.
[19] Admiralty to SHB, 14 and 25 April 1749, nos. 2, 3, ADM/E/12; SHB to Admiralty, 17 April 1749 and 24 July 1751, ADM/F/11.
[20] Admiralty to SHB, 23 February 1773, ADM/E/41; White to SHB, 19 March 1776, ADM/FP/19; Polhill to SHB, 17 October 1796, enclosed in SHB to Admiralty, 21 October, ADM/F/27.

In such cases the Board could be humane, especially if the sums were small, and paid the bills on the supporting evidence of the captain or commanding officers of the station. Yet the debts owed to the Board in 1795 totalled £1,240,000. The major part of this sum, over £700,000, consisted of debts concerned with prisoners of war and those owed by foreign governments. Accounts of over £500,000 concerned sick seamen – over £400,000 for men treated abroad, chiefly in the East and West Indies. Only £62,500 was for sick seamen in home service. But these are staggering sums, and make the Board's pleas for an accounting department to clear them understandable.[21]

Sick Quarters, Hospitals and Hospital Ships

At the beginning of the century sick seamen ashore were cared for in sick quarters or contract hospitals, run by individuals who contracted with the Board to supply buildings, food, clothing, bedding and nurses at a fixed price. Sick quarters were established in most ports and were usually local inns or ale houses where seamen were inevitably tempted (and even encouraged) to drink and delay their recovery; desertion was also a common problem. There are endless complaints, which were passed from the Board to the Admiralty, from sea officers about the ill-treatment and neglect of their men in such places, and of desertions from them. One of the chief problems for the Board and its local agents was the lack of ready cash to pay quarters regularly. In 1740 those who offered quarters at Gosport had only been paid to the end of 1738.[22] Under such circumstances, quarters of any sort were difficult to hire.

The contract system threw the trouble and expense of caring for sick and hurt seamen onto private individuals, and it saved the government the permanent expense of building and maintaining hospitals and their establishments in peace as well as war. It worked, after a fashion, in peace, but the eighteenth-century wars revealed the system's faults. The serious typhus epidemic in the winter of 1740–1, which caused numerous deaths, completely overwhelmed the contract hospitals. The naval authorities thus began to consider other, permanent methods of caring for sick seamen and curbing desertion.

Sir James Barclay, physician at Gosport contract hospital, dismissed for negligence in 1741, declared that a black picture was painted of contract hospitals because 'the whole bent of the dockyard commissioner and the captains' who inspected the Gosport hospital was for building a royal hospital, that is a hospital built using public money for and run by the Navy.[23] As a result of these numerous complaints from senior sea officers, supported by the Board, in the spring of 1741 the Admiralty asked the commissioners whether the present system should continue or whether

---

[21] SHB to Admiralty, 4 July 1796, ADM/F/27.
[22] SHB to Admiralty, 2 May 1740, ADM 1/3528.
[23] Barclay to SHB, 1 May 1740, enclosed in SHB to Admiralty, 2 May 1740, ADM 1/3528; Admiralty to SHB, 5 May 1741, no. 33, ADM/E/8b.

hospitals should be built at public expense to care for sick seamen.[24] Discussions produced a scheme to build three such hospitals, at Portsmouth for 1,500 men, and at Plymouth and Queenborough (on the Medway) for 750 men each. Though a memorial was presented by the Admiralty to the Crown in October of that year nothing was achieved until 1744, when the Earl of Sandwich, First Lord of the Admiralty, presented a similar memorial for the building of three hospitals to preserve sick seamen from 'death and destruction' as a matter of urgency. An Order in Council directing them to be built was issued shortly after.[25] The Board was asked to consider plans, costs and necessary staff numbers, and from this developed the building of Haslar Hospital. By 1753 part of it was ready to admit 100 men, still managed on the contract system, but by 1755, as admissions increased, the Board proposed that the management be taken into the hands of the Crown, and the Admiralty agreed. When completed in 1758, Haslar was the largest contemporary brick building in Europe. The final cost of £100,000 was a sign of the Navy's commitment to seamen's health.

In the same decade a naval hospital was built at Stonehouse, near Plymouth. Similar complaints of neglect, confusion and desertions familiar from Portsmouth had been made against the contract arrangements there. In 1755 the mayor and corporation of Plymouth, afraid of disease and disorder, wrote to the Admiralty about the dangers threatening the town from the great number of sick seamen, and asking that a royal hospital be built, offering to give all the assistance in their power.[26] A hospital was begun the following year and was fully opened in 1762. Haslar Hospital was then running at an annual cost of £13,500, so the responsibilities, work and costs of the Sick and Hurt Board were greatly extended by these new establishments. The medical staff – physicians, surgeons, dispensers, nurses and assistants – were appointed by the Admiralty on the Board's recommendation, though the Admiralty sometimes decided on particular men to fill these posts. James Lind was appointed surgeon at Haslar Hospital through Lord Anson's intervention.

The expense was justified since the new hospitals were successful in reducing deaths from disease, promoting cures and reducing desertion. Future commissioners wished to extend that success by building more of them. The proposed hospital at Queenborough lapsed because of costs. The idea was revived in the 1760s, but protracted and unsuccessful negotiations over leases and costs meant no hospital was built in the Chatham area until the 1820s. The Board had supported the scheme throughout, despite the Admiralty's suggestion of hospital ships as a cheaper alternative. Plans to build a Medway-sited hospital may have been deferred by the Admiralty's decision to buy the existing contract hospital and adjoining land at Deal to expand it and run it as a naval hospital.[27] The commissioners also suggested a purpose-built naval hospital at Falmouth in 1795 when that port was a centre for sick seamen and returning sick British prisoners of war. But the Admiralty rejected

---

[24] Admiralty to SHB, 21 March 1741, no. 15; Admiralty to SHB, 4 April 1741, no. 21, ADM/E/8b.
[25] C.C. Lloyd and J.L.S. Coulter, *Medicine and the Navy, 1200–1900. Vol. III, 1714–1815* (Edinburgh, 1961), pp. 194–5.
[26] Admiralty to SHB, 31 December 1755, no. 120, ADM/E/14.
[27] SHB to Admiralty, 21 October, 18 November 1795, 27 February 1796, ADM/F/26.

the idea on the grounds of cost, and thought a hospital ship adequate and cheaper. The commissioners disagreed in both cases and in much firmer terms than previous commissioners had used. The medical majority at the Board supported their professional case with statistical evidence of sick numbers, and with costings. They proved hospital ships were more expensive to run than hospitals over the long term, and they thought the lowness of the decks made it difficult to maintain the purity of air essential to health. They declared that, 'if their Lordships stick to their determination not to establish a hospital at Falmouth', they would recommend using two-deck ships, rather than the less healthy single-deck frigates normally used. The Admiralty agreed over ship size but government finances did not allow the building of more hospitals at that time.[28]

Though the Navy did build hospitals abroad, as at New Greenwich, Jamaica, in the 1740s, they were run by contract. The New Greenwich hospital was doomed from the beginning, being built near a marsh. Malarial attacks regularly killed staff and patients and the hospital had to be moved back to Port Royal.[29] In 1761 the Board proposed building a hospital in Antigua, base for the Leeward islands, to answer the continual complaints of sea officers about the existing inadequate buildings used for their sick seamen. But the Admiralty was unwilling to spend the estimated £13,000 that building a hospital would cost in the middle of a war, and nothing was done. In the early 1770s a hurricane destroyed the wooden buildings of the contract hospital and the Board again proposed a stone-built naval hospital. But it was now peacetime; the immediate need for a hospital was no longer evident, and once more nothing was done.[30]

Naval hospitals in the Mediterranean – at Minorca and Gibraltar, the chief naval bases, and later at Malta – were contract hospitals, as were the temporary hospitals at Baia in 1718, and Leghorn or Ajaccio in the 1790s. Minorca's hospital, rebuilt in the mid 1720s to hold 2,000 men, and Gibraltar's, rebuilt in the mid 1740s for 1,000, were paid for by government but continued to be run by contract, despite complaints, for most of the period.

The position of hospital ships was anomalous. In war they formed part of fleets and squadrons; in peace they were established at ports to hold sick seamen, often as a cheaper alternative to established hospitals there. The Navy Board was responsible for assigning ships to act as hospital ships, and for fitting them out, while the Sick and Hurt Board supplied their medicines and necessaries and the appointed surgeon. Yet sick seamen sent to such ships had never been under the direction of the Board; rather, they were the responsibility of the commander-in-chief of the port where the ships were moored. Here was another example of divided authority and responsibilities which limited efficiency and certainly weakened the Board's authority

[28] Admiralty to SHB, 27 July 1796, ADM/E/45; SHB to Admiralty, 16 September 1796, ADM/F/27.
[29] Lloyd and Coulter, *Medicine and the Navy*, vol. 3, pp. 101–3.
[30] Admiralty to SHB, 6 July 1748, ADM/E/12; SHB to Admiralty, 7 July 1748, ADM/F/7; SHB to Admiralty, 7 March 1761, ADM/F/21; SHB to Admiralty, 4 December 1772, ADM/FP/15; SHB to Admiralty, 11, 21 April 1786, ADM/FP/29.

over medical care. The Admiralty was ignorant of this division of authority when, in 1748, it ordered the Sick and Hurt Board to take charge of patients and medicines aboard hospital ships then being paid off at the peace. In this case the Board had to ask for special Admiralty orders to move the sick into quarters ashore, where they would become the Board's responsibility. But nothing seems to have been done to resolve this anomaly.[31]

Hospitals and hospital ships were, in general, as well run as the Sick and Hurt Board could achieve, but its authority was never absolute. The naval hospitals of Haslar and Stonehouse were run by a council of the medical staff and the Board's appointed agent, but the Board had insufficient immediate control and the situation attracted mounting complaints of maladministration, neglect and poor discipline from sea officers during the 1770s. Admiral Barrington had investigated defects at Haslar in 1780, recommending the appointment of a resident Governor, and though the commissioners did not agree to this they did appoint a resident Commissioner in 1781. Even so, complaints continued, and they culminated in a board of inquiry in 1794, established by Admiral Lord Howe, commander-in-chief at Portsmouth. As a result, from 1795 Haslar and Stonehouse were put under the command of a resident Governor of the hospital, who was to be a sea officer appointed by the Admiralty. All non-medical decisions were now transferred to him and the Board was ordered to correspond only with him on non-medical affairs concerning the hospital.[32]

Surgeons

Until 1796 it was the Navy Board, and not the Sick and Hurt commissioners, who granted warrants to surgeons and their mates entitling them to practise in the Royal Navy. Aspiring surgeons and mates had to apply to the Navy Board for a letter to Surgeons' Hall, requesting an examination.[33] Here they were examined on their competence in surgery, and, if successful, given a certificate. They underwent a similar examination of their medical competence by the Physician of Greenwich Hospital, and received a similar certificate. Thus provided, they returned to the Navy Board to be granted a warrant, and to seek a vacancy on board a ship. This choice was made at the Navy Board, and was based on where there were vacancies, where there was the greatest need, and (as discussed in Chapter 2) sometimes patronage. Only when they had received a warrant did surgeons and mates come under the supervision of the Sick and Hurt Board.

[31] SHB to Admiralty, 13 May 1748, ADM/F/10.
[32] Admiralty to SHB, 22 July 1796, ADM/E/45.
[33] Though the name of the examining body changed over the years, there was a degree of continuity: between 1540 and 1745 it was the Barber-Surgeons' Company; in 1745 they were once more split in two, with the new Company of Surgeons taking responsibility for the examinations. The Company in turn became in 1800 the Royal College of Surgeons of London, and in 1843 the Royal College of Surgeons of England.

By 1795, three of the four Sick and Hurt commissioners were professionally qualified doctors: surgeons James Johnston and Robert Blair, and Gilbert Blane, a distinguished physician who had joined the Board that year at the suggestion of Earl Spencer, First Lord of the Admiralty (1794–1801). This was a board able to judge medical qualifications far better than medically ignorant Navy Board clerks. Thus in October 1795 the Admiralty ordered the granting of surgeons' warrants, the care of sick seamen on commissioned ships, and the superintendence of medicines and necessary extras to be transferred from the Navy Board to the Sick and Hurt Board. Bureaucratic delays meant the actual transfer was not made until August 1796, after an Order in Council of 29 July authorised the Board to make appointments henceforth, as the commissioners 'from their education and habits are likely to be better acquainted with the characters and qualifications of men of that profession than any other public board …'.[34] This was a public recognition of professional competence, and it strengthened the Board's authority.

The shortage of surgeons – and, even more, of surgeons' mates – was particularly felt in wartime, and had long been complained of. The principal reasons were poor pay and prospects and the lack of status (particularly compared with the Army). Surgeons serving on ships received £5 a month, 2d a head for every crew member, £5 a year for every 100 men treated for venereal disease, and (in wartime) Queen Anne's Free Gift. This ranged from £16 to £62 a year, according to the size of the ship, and was provided to help supply medicines for their chests. They were required, however, to provide their own instruments. In earlier periods of peace, shore-based surgeons, in contract hospitals and quarters, had earned 6s 8d per man, per cure. During war, at the Board's suggestion, they were paid a fixed annual salary.[35] Only when the contract hospitals at Haslar and Stonehouse became entirely naval hospitals were permanent salaries paid to their surgeons in war and peace.

Surgeons' mates were divided into classes; first mates, with the most experience, earned £2 10s a month, second mates £2, third mates and below £1 10s. At times of necessity mates could be appointed by the captain from the ship's crew, and they did not necessarily require any formal training. They received no other allowances. Before 1805 only 200 senior surgeons received half pay when unemployed, so at the end of a war most surgeons and mates lost their livelihood and returned to civilian life. Though they might rejoin at the beginning of a new war, many were permanently lost to the Navy.

Low wages did not encourage men to become surgeons' mates; nor did low status. Their early association with barbers was unhelpful to surgeons' efforts to establish themselves as professionals and gentlemen. The job itself was regarded as manual, dirty and socially low. Unlike sea officers, before 1805 surgeons had no distinguishing uniform. They were appointed by warrant, like the practical officers of a ship, and though classed with the master, purser and chaplain, they were not commissioned

---

[34] SHB to Admiralty, 4 January 1796, ADM/F/26; Admiralty to SHB, 17 August 1796, ADM/E/45, enclosing the Order in Council, 29 July 1796.
[35] Admiralty to SHB, 16 July 1740, no. 66, ADM/E/8a; SHB to Admiralty, 14 May 1755, no. 77, ADM/F/12.

officers enjoying the status and privileges of gentlemen, as sea officers were. Yet the Sick and Hurt commissioners of the 1790s made successful efforts in improving the conditions of surgeons and mates, arguing for their enhanced professional status. In November 1796 they persuaded the Admiralty to agree to supplying some of the most expensive and useful medicines free to surgeons. Later that month the Admiralty agreed to pay the travelling expenses of candidates successful in their examination at Surgeons' Hall, and in 1797 permitted candidates who feared to incur travelling expenses to London if they failed the examinations, to take them at the Surgeons' Companies of Dublin and Edinburgh.[36]

While the Navy Board was engaged in the transfer of their traditional medical duties to the Sick and Hurt Board, the commissioners were beginning a similar transfer of responsibilities for healthy prisoners of war to the Transport Board, together with the existing clerks.[37] These upheavals resulted not only in the commissioners drafting new instructions for their office duties but, more significantly, in August 1796, receiving an urgent Admiralty directive proposing further regulations governing the conduct and duties of surgeons at sea. These were aimed at establishing 'a regular system ... in that very important department'. An argument between Blair and Blane over details disrupted the Board's work on this code of practice, but discussions with the Admiralty, more particularly between Blane and their Lordships, led to a draft of these instructions being approved by the Admiralty on 25 November 1796.[38] Though modifications delayed their issue to surgeons until March 1797,[39] the instructions mark an advance in the increasing professionalism of naval surgeons.

The response to the fleet mutinies of 1797 brought pay increases to seamen and a flat rate increase to surgeons' mates of 5s 6d a month. There was no increase for surgeons, however. When other warrant officers received an increase in 1802 surgeons again did not benefit, nor was anything done to improve half pay or pension provision. Thus, on the renewal of war, in May 1803, few surgeons or mates rejoined the service. Their petitions for the correction of these inequalities, protests at their unequal treatment compared with Army surgeons, and pleas for recognition of lengthy professional training, eventually brought change. In January 1805 an Order in Council produced many of the long-desired improvements. Surgeons were now to be 'warrant officers of wardroom rank', equal to lieutenants though ranked behind them, and to have a distinguishing uniform. Their pay, now assessed according to their seniority and not according to the rate of the ship, was to range from a monthly £25 4s to £15 8s. Surgeons' mates, renamed assistant surgeons, had their pay increased

---

[36] SHB to Admiralty, 2 November 1796, ADM/F/27; Admiralty to SHB, 4 November 1796, ADM/E/45; SHB to Admiralty, 17 November 1796, ADM/F/27; Admiralty to SHB, 19 November 1796, ADM/E/45; SHB to Admiralty, 7 March 1797, Admiralty minute 8 March 1797, ADM/F/27.

[37] SHB to Admiralty, 5 October 1795, ADM/F/26; SHB to Admiralty, 15 December 1795, 20 July 1796, ADM/F/27.

[38] Admiralty to SHB, 17 August and 25 November 1796, ADM/E/45.

[39] SHB to Admiralty, 1 February 1797 and 13 March 1797, Admiralty minute 14 March, ADM/F/27.

to £11 18s a month in all ships. All medicines and drugs for surgeons' use were to be issued free, though they still had to provide their own instruments.[40]

Closure of the Sick and Hurt Board

In the last decade of its existence the Board was willing to express opinions on medical matters and naval health in more forthright terms. It was vigorous and active in proposing improvements in medical care, in suggestions for controlling costs, in improving the professional standing of surgeons, and trying, with some success, to achieve a better medical service at sea. All this was not enough, however, to save it from abolition. In 1801 the Prime Minister, William Pitt, resigned and his place was taken by Henry Addington. Lord Spencer was succeeded as First Lord by Admiral Earl St Vincent. He headed a vengefully reforming Admiralty that was determined, through a newly established Parliamentary Commission of Naval Enquiry, to find and root out abuses in the civil departments of the Royal Navy. That these abuses had been committed by and under the regime of political opponents made their extirpation all the more urgent and satisfactory.

St Vincent's Admiralty and Addington's administration fell from power in May 1804, to be succeeded once more by William Pitt as Prime Minister and Lord Melville, formerly Henry Dundas, as First Lord of the Admiralty. His naval adviser was Sir Charles Middleton, formerly Comptroller of the Navy Board and a great reforming administrator in his own right. Pitt and Melville established a Royal Commission for Revising and Digesting the Civil Affairs of the Navy, with Middleton as its chairman. This, they hoped, would neutralize St Vincent's reforms and propose alternative restructuring.

Meanwhile, the Parliamentary Commission of Naval Enquiry continued to bring out its reports on various naval departments. The tenth report, in 1805, on the Treasurership of the Navy, produced evidence of a former Paymaster of the Navy speculating with public money, apparently with the connivance of the then Treasurer, Henry Dundas, now Lord Melville. Calls for Melville's resignation and a House of Commons vote of censure on his conduct led to his resignation on 10 April 1805. On 29 April Pitt announced Middleton as Melville's successor at the Admiralty, and in May Middleton (now ennobled as Lord Barham) entered office. The summer session was spent in pursuit of Melville, who was threatened with criminal prosecution by the Opposition. The government was seriously weakened by resignations in the new session, and Pitt's death in January 1806 led to its immediate resignation. A new government, labouring under the nickname of 'All the Talents', took office on 1 February. Lord Barham, who had resigned the Admiralty to the Honourable Charles Grey, remained head of the Board of Naval Revision, but his influence was reduced.

---

[40] Lloyd and Coulter, *Medicine and the Navy*, vol. 3, pp. 32–4. For a fuller account of surgeons and the Sick and Hurt Board see P.K. Crimmin, 'The Shortage of Surgeons and Surgeons' Mates, c.1740–1806: An Evil of a Serious Nature to the Service', *Transactions of the Naval Dockyards Society*, forthcoming.

The Sick and Hurt Board's future was thus examined in an atmosphere of intense reforming zeal and political partisanship, with two investigating commissions being used as weapons by opposing political groups in Parliament. In such political battles the Board needed weighty friends. It had none. The commissioners, now Dr John Harness, Dr John Weir and Sir William Gibbons, lacked the political and even the social weight to mount a convincing rebuttal of the charges against the Board. In November 1805 Barham proposed its abolition on the grounds that its deplorable state of business had long been known and needed to be put under the management of a Board 'accustomed to the investigation of accounts.' This was the Transport Board, Barham's own creation of 1794. Evidence was drawn from the two commissions already described. Irregularities and abuses in the Board's medical duties were not produced. The accusations were that medical men, by their training, could not be expected to transact the business of accounts, and on 6 January 1806 an Admiralty order to transfer the office books, papers and instructions to the Transport Board finalised the Sick and Hurt Board's abolition.[41] The expanded Transport Board now consisted of seven commissioners, only one of whom, Dr Harness, was medically qualified, and whose duty would be to control the entry of surgeons into the Navy and examine their journals.

Conclusion

No one has examined the Sick and Hurt Board since *Medicine and the Navy, 1200–1900* was published in the late 1950s. The authors of volume 3, C.C. Lloyd and J.L.S. Coulter, subordinated eighteenth-century administration to the important advances in medicine and improvements in health. They correctly labelled the eighteenth-century commissioners as generally undistinguished. Yet the commissioners of other naval administrative offices were not always men of distinction. They quoted Dr Robertson, physician at Greenwich Hospital, later senior physician in the Navy, who in 1781 referred to 'the indigent and penurious establishment of the medical department of the Navy', as evidence of the Board's inefficiency. But Robertson was here criticizing the under-staffing of the office and its inadequate financial establishment, rather than the Board's inefficient handling of business. These were the Board's own arguments which it advanced, unsuccessfully, to the Admiralty from the 1790s. Absenteeism, inattention to duty and financial slackness were other criticisms voiced by contemporary critics in 1804 and repeated by Lloyd and Coulter. 'The immense accumulation of arrears' in the Board's accounts was criticized in terms which implied it was administratively unique in this regard,[42] but such allegations, coupled with those of inefficiency and corruption, were frequently levelled at other areas of naval administration.

Healthcare, the improvement of health and its supervision is not, perhaps, a subject readily responsive to bureaucracy. This was especially true in the eighteenth

---

[41] Lloyd and Coulter, *Medicine and the Navy*, 3, pp. 3–7.
[42] Ibid., pp. 3–9.

century when causes and cures for disease were unknown, often unknowable, or clinically undefined, and when a small bureaucracy still conformed to the checks and balances of seventeenth-century practice in many areas, particularly finance.[43] Though non-interventionist government was an eighteenth-century ideal, antipathy to government interference clashed with the need to reduce costs and tackle the Royal Navy's manning problems, which grew more acute each year. One solution was to try to keep men healthy. This meant investigations into the efficiency of medical practice and of the department tasked with the responsibility for these things. It meant investigations into costs.

The Sick and Hurt Board had been required to do more throughout the century, and it responded well. In 1700 there were around 7,000 naval seamen; by 1796 there were around 114,365; by 1812, a peak year, there were around 145,000. Yet the Board's clerical staff and number of commissioners had not increased in proportion. With its abolition in 1806 only one medically qualified commissioner sat on the Transport Board, which was now responsible for the former Sick and Hurt Board's duties. It is questionable whether this new configuration was a recipe for either greater medical efficiency or improved accounting. Contemporary criticisms of the Sick and Hurt Board appear – as far as my reading of the evidence is concerned – to have been partial. The commissioners, though not well known to historians, were not absentees. The department was hardworking; its staff – particularly with peacetime cuts – was insufficient to deal with the backlog of accounts. Other boards faced similar problems and criticisms, but none was totally abolished in wartime.[44] Furthermore, Sir James Watt has argued that the Sick and Hurt Board served the interests of Royal Navy surgeons (and thus the men under their care) better than the comparable system in the French Navy.[45]

But as a lesser branch of naval administration the Board was unable to inaugurate reforms independently; every decision had to be referred to the Admiralty for approval and the Board's areas of responsibility often overlapped with more senior, powerful naval departments. Though improvements in naval health were largely due to preventive medicine, the Board's part in these improvements has still to be fully explored. It does not deserve the censure it has, until now, earned for supposed inattention and inefficiency. A re-assessment of its historical role is overdue.

[43] Roger Morriss explores this point in illuminating detail in *Naval Power and British Culture, 1760–1850: Public Trust and Government Ideology* (Aldershot, 2004).
[44] R.J.B. Knight, 'Politics and Trust in Victualling the Navy, 1793–1815', *The Mariner's Mirror*, 94 (2008), pp. 133–49.
[45] James Watt, 'Surgery at Trafalgar', *The Mariner's Mirror*, 91 (2005), pp. 266–83, p. 270.

5

An 'Important and Truly National Subject': The West Africa Service and the Health of the Royal Navy in the Mid Nineteenth Century

Mark Harrison

At the end of the Napoleonic Wars the health of the Royal Navy was a matter for celebration. Two decades of reform in hygiene and victualling had conferred great advantages on the British during the recent wars with France.[1] As head of the Naval Medical Board, the physician Gilbert Blane presided over most of these initiatives.[2] Yet, in his view, there remained much to be done: a sentiment echoed by the vast majority of naval surgeons. At the conclusion of the wars, the most pressing issue in the medical realm was the health of impressed men. Some former naval officers saw the system of impressment as an evil on a par with slavery, and they drew attention to the poor health and morale of sailors who had been forcibly recruited.[3] But the broader issue of naval health attracted little interest until the 1830s and 1840s, when it began to be highlighted by naval medical officers and their supporters in the medical press. Backed by the crusading editor of *The Lancet*, Thomas Wakley, naval surgeons began to demand better pay and conditions while demonstrating their role in maintaining the health and efficiency of their service. Although their claims were disputed and even bitterly opposed by conservative interests within the Navy and the royal colleges, they were ultimately successful, and their efforts contributed materially to improvements in health from the 1850s.

---

[1]   Gilbert Blane, 'On the Comparative Health of the Royal Navy, from the Year 1779 to the Year 1814, with Proposals for its farther Improvement', in Gilbert Blane, *Select Dissertations on Several Subjects of Medical Science* (London, 1822), pp. 1–64.

[2]   Christopher Lawrence, 'Disciplining Diseases: Scurvy, the Navy and Imperial Expansion, 1750–1825', in D. Miller and P. Reill (eds), *Visions of Empire* (Cambridge, 1996), pp. 80–106.

[3]   See for example Thomas Urquhart, *Substance of a Letter to Lord Viscount Melville, written in May 1815, with the Outlines of a Plan to Raise British Seamen, and to form their Minds to Volunteer the Naval Service when required; to do away with the Evils of Impressment, and Man our Ships effectually with Mercantile Seamen* (London, 1815); Thomas Trotter, *A Practicable Plan for Manning the Royal Navy, and Preserving our Maritime Ascendency, without Impressment: Addressed to Admiral Lord Viscount Exmouth, K.G.B.* (Newcastle, 1819).

This chapter examines this campaign for professional and hygienic reform in the light of mounting concern over the health of sailors in the Navy's West Africa Squadron. During the 1840s several well-publicised incidents drew attention to the appalling mortality of crews involved in anti-slavery operations along the West African coast. The first of these was the ill-fated Niger Expedition of 1841–2; the second involved the steam-sloop, the *Éclair*, which returned to Britain from West Africa in 1845 via the Cape Verde Islands, apparently infecting one of them with yellow fever. The heavy mortality suffered during the Niger Expedition and the plight of the *Éclair* and the Cape Verde islanders focused public attention on the health of the Navy and, in particular, the conditions endured by seamen in the hot and ill-ventilated conditions of steam vessels. The issue of naval health benefited from the increased publicity given to naval anti-slavery operations and led to demands that government pay as much attention to the welfare of sailors as it apparently did to the slaves they were sent to liberate. Comparisons also began to be drawn between the sufferings of sailors in steam vessels – which were often unbearably hot – and those of workers in steam-powered mills and factories at home. While the working conditions of sailors had received little attention, those of factory hands had been improving for some time, partly as a result of the Factory Acts passed in 1833, 1844 and 1847. If the welfare of workers and slaves was worthy of attention, then why not the health of those upon whom the nation depended for its security?

A Neglected Service

The more assertive attitude of naval surgeons during the 1830s and 1840s was largely due to the backing they received from professional organs such as *The Lancet*. Under its founding editor, Thomas Wakley (1795–1862), this weekly journal acquired a reputation as the mouthpiece of a new breed of surgeon-apothecaries (prototype general practitioners) who were challenging the monopoly of power formerly held by the royal colleges of physicians and surgeons.[4] Although it did not endorse all the demands made by naval medical officers, *The Lancet* laid their grievances before the profession at large, giving them a mouthpiece outside service journals such as the *Naval and Military Gazette*. By giving publicity and, generally, support to naval surgeons in their battles with the Admiralty and the royal colleges, *The Lancet* simultaneously raised the profile of the naval medical service and of naval health and medical care.

Of the many grievances felt by naval surgeons, the one which gave rise to most complaints in the late 1830s was their unfavourable position in relation to surgeons in the Army. It was argued that Army surgeons were paid more, were promoted

---

[4] See Irvine Loudon, *Medical Care and the General Practitioner 1750–1850* (Oxford, 1986); Christopher Lawrence, *Medicine in the Making of Modern Britain 1700–1920* (London, 1994), ch. 2.

faster, and enjoyed more and better privileges than their naval counterparts.[5] There appears to have been some basis for these complaints, as rates of pay were somewhat lower in the Navy. A surgeon in the Army with less than ten years' service received a daily pay of thirteen shillings, whereas his naval equivalent received only ten or eleven.[6] Some surgeons also contended that the supply of medicines and equipment to naval surgeons was deficient by comparison with that given to surgeons in the Army,[7] but others thought these criticisms exaggerated.[8] The Lancet refused to support the more outlandish claims made by naval surgeons but it strongly backed their campaign for improvements in pay and for an end to the anomaly whereby naval surgeons were listed among non-commissioned officers, despite being given the rank of commander. Indeed, it was The Lancet which had first raised the matter with the English Royal College of Surgeons in 1831, only to see it buried for another seven years, apparently because of the obstructive attitude of some senior figures on the college's council.[9] The issue was also raised in the House of Commons by Sir Edward Codrington (1770–1851), a former naval officer and long-time friend of the naval surgeon.[10]

In early 1838 the pressure stoked up by Codrington and The Lancet culminated in the appointment of a parliamentary commission of inquiry which examined the complaints of naval surgeons. One of its members was Wakley, who had been elected to Parliament as an independent MP for Finsbury in 1835. As a parliamentarian, Wakley was inevitably preoccupied with medical matters, but his reformist politics were also evident in his support for the Tolpuddle Martyrs, for the extension of the franchise, and for the improvement of conditions in workhouses.[11] The interest he took in naval surgeons and in the health of sailors thus united his professional and political interests.

At the end of 1839, when naval surgeons were placed on the same footing as other naval officers rather than non-commissioned officers, Wakley was among the first to celebrate. But several other grievances had still to be addressed. The Navy's unfavourable position relative to the Army was particularly evident in the position of assistant-surgeons – the lowest grade of the medical service. As Codrington pointed out, assistant-surgeons in the Navy possessed many disadvantages as regards pay and promotion,[12] but what really rankled was the fact that they were kept separate from commissioned officers. When making a passage on board ship,

5   'A Navy Surgeon', 20 December 1837, The Lancet (1837–8), i, p. 530.
6   'A Naval Surgeon of the Last Century', 8 January 1838, The Lancet (1837–8), i, p. 634.
7   'A Naval Surgeon of the Present Century', 29 January 1838, The Lancet (1837–8), i, p. 712.
8   'A Naval Surgeon', undated, March 1838, The Lancet (1837–8), ii, pp. 189–92.
9   'Naval Surgeons', The Lancet (1838–9), ii, p. 27.
10 'Letter from A Naval Surgeon', 8 July 1837, The Lancet (1837–8), i, p. 592; J.K. Laughton, 'Edward Codrington (1770–1851), Oxford Dictionary of National Biography (Oxford, 2004), hereafter ODNB. A former commander of the Channel Squadron, Codrington sat as Liberal MP for Devonport from 1832 to 1839. In the latter year, he was appointed Commander-in-Chief at Portsmouth.
11 W.F. Bynum, 'Thomas Wakley (1795–1862)', ODNB.
12 As reported in The Lancet (1839–40), ii, pp. 31–2.

assistant-surgeons in the Army were allowed to mess with lieutenants and other ward-room officers and had cabins or screened berths. Assistant-surgeons in the Navy, by contrast, were not permitted entry to the officers' mess, and they had to berth with young midshipmen who were notoriously rowdy and comparatively poorly educated. It was not an environment conducive to professional study, nor one in keeping with the gentlemanly status to which all medical practitioners aspired.[13] Within the Navy itself, the position of assistant-surgeons compared very unfavourably with that of young officers of the marines, who were received as gentlemen in the mess despite being raw youths with little liberal or professional education.[14] To make matters worse, the children of assistant-surgeons were not permitted to enter the Royal Navy Schools at Richmond and Camberwell at a nominal charge, as children of officers of ward-room rank were permitted to do, and all attempts to end this discrimination were blocked.[15]

The lack of respect given to assistant-surgeons in the Navy helps to explain the poor morale of the medical service and the fact that many young surgeons apparently preferred the Army. Denied the status of 'gentleman', and with recent cuts to rates of half pay for those not on active service, the naval surgeon was not simply in an unfavourable situation in relation to counterparts in the Army: he was an embarrassment to an entire class of practitioners who were seeking parity with the physician elite. For this reason, it is easy to understand why a journal such as *The Lancet* should have championed his cause. However, it stopped short of advising young men not to enter the Navy, as some of its correspondents did. Some of the most vehement critics of the Navy claimed that its emoluments were insufficient compensation for the indignities and dangers of a career at sea. But *The Lancet* appears to have taken the view that it was better to press for reform, and it would entertain seriously only those complainants who had constructive proposals.[16] Presumably, the journal was afraid of appearing to be irresponsible when it came to matters of national importance. Indeed, some its correspondents thought that the more extreme claims made about the life of assistant-surgeons were 'twaddle', while others protested that their exclusion from the officers' mess was actually a good thing, as most could ill afford to maintain themselves in the style to which most naval officers (often younger sons of aristocrats and landed gentry) were accustomed.[17]

[13] Ian Inkster, 'Marginal Men: Aspects of the Social Role of the Medical Community in Sheffield, 1790–1850', in D. Richards and J. Woodward (eds), *Health Care and Popular Medicine in Nineteenth Century England* (London, 1977); J.M. Peterson, 'Gentlemen and Medical Men: The Problem of Professional Recruitment', *Bulletin of the History of Medicine*, 29 (1985), pp. 138–68.
[14] 'A Late Naval Surgeon', undated, May 1841, *The Lancet* (1840–1), ii, p. 283.
[15] Dr J. Tweeddale, 25 May 1841, *The Lancet* (1840–1), ii, p. 444, and 8 July 1841, ibid., p. 638.
[16] 'One of the Robbed', undated June 1841, and reply of editor, *The Lancet* (1840–1), ii, pp. 552–4, and July 1841 and reply of editor, ibid., p. 703; 'A Surgeon of the New School', September 1841, ibid., pp. 933–7.
[17] 'A Naval Surgeon of the Old School', undated, *The Lancet*, 3 July 1841 (1841–2), i, pp. 525–6; Robert Hancome, August 1841, ibid., pp. 767–8.

In campaigning for better conditions, naval surgeons were well aware that their opponents could portray them as self-serving and that they would face considerable opposition to some of their demands. It was therefore necessary for them to emphasize that improvement of their professional conditions would be of advantage to the service and to the country as a whole. The lack of suitable berths for assistant-surgeons, for example, was blamed for the lack of professional distinction attained by the majority of naval surgeons. How could they study and keep up with the latest developments in surgery and medicine in an atmosphere that was positively hostile to intellectual endeavour?[18]

But the most persistent theme was the importance of surgeons in maintaining the health of naval vessels. This assertion was supported by *The Lancet*, which pointed out in 1838: 'It appears to us, that the case of the naval surgeons cannot be separated from the health of the Navy, or the services that the medical officers render.' As it reminded its readers, 'No question is of greater national importance than the health of the Navy', as this had an obvious bearing upon naval efficiency.'[19] To emphasize this point, the journal thought it necessary to shake the complacency that had grown around the issue following the achievements of the French Wars. Crucially, it pointed out that the mortality statistics which Blane had used to illustrate the great improvement of naval health following his appointment to the Naval Medical Board were misleading. Blane had claimed that there had been a marked reduction in deaths and in the numbers of sick sent to hospital. In 1779, at the time of the American War of Independence, 40,815 men had been sent to hospital and 2,654 had died. By 1804, the number sent to hospital had apparently declined to 11,978 and the number of deaths to 1,606; and in 1813 this had fallen further to 9,336 and 698, respectively. Although the journal did not deny that the health of the Navy had greatly improved over that time, largely as a result of the decline of scurvy and certain fevers, it showed that Blane had recorded only those casualties sent to the shore. In a 'strange misstatement', he had deliberately excluded deaths on board ships and admissions to their sick berths.[20]

Correspondents to the journal continued in similar vein, one alluding to what he regarded as 'that important and truly national subject, viz., the health of seamen'. In his view, there was no higher object than to protect the lives of men who were indispensable to 'our prosperity and superiority as a people'. But, he continued, the service had been badly neglected at the expense of what he termed 'the landed interest'.[21] This was presumably a slight against landowning politicians with links to the Army. Others, including *The Lancet*, pointed the finger at corruption in the Admiralty.[22] By the early 1840s, however, there were signs that naval health was beginning to receive the attention it deserved. During the 1830s Dr John Wilson had embarked on the collection of naval health statistics, and for the first time the

[18] F. N***s, 14 November 1844, *The Lancet* (1844), ii, p. 302.
[19] Editorial, 21 April 1838, *The Lancet* (1837–8), ii, p. 121.
[20] Ibid., pp. 124–5.
[21] Ninian Hill, 20 July 1838, *The Lancet* (1837–8), pp. 865–8.
[22] Editorial, 5 May 1838, *The Lancet* (1837–8), ii, p. 193.

Navy had a set of aggregated data. The first series covered the period 1830 to 1836, and by the 1840s these statistics, based upon the surgeons' journals which were submitted annually to the Admiralty, were yielding valuable comparative data on the health of different squadrons.[23]

The initiative mirrored a similar exercise in the Army, set in train in 1835 by Henry Marshall and Alexander Tulloch. As *The Lancet* noted, these moves were part of a more general trend towards government involvement in the field of public health. In part, this had been a consequence of the first visitation of Asiatic cholera to Britain in 1831–2, but the stimuli to sanitary reform were more diverse, arising from deep-rooted concerns about 'fever nests' in crowded cities and the confined spaces of factories and prisons. The hopeful signs remarked upon by *The Lancet* included the gathering of vital statistics under the General Register Office (created in 1837) and the passage of the Vaccination-Extension Act of 1840 and the Factory Act of 1833.[24] The fact that the health of sailors was now being considered alongside the health of workers is significant for reasons which will become clear later in this chapter, as is *The Lancet's* criticism of the protectionist Corn Laws and their effects on health in the same editorial. It argued that medical men ought not to be party to any law which placed an adequate supply of bread beyond the reach of the bulk of consumers. As we shall see, this was the first indication of a conjunction of several reforming interests – including free-traders, philanthropists and medical officers – which placed the issue of naval medical reform firmly on the agenda.

The Niger Expedition and the Perils of West Africa

Although there is evidence of increasing interest in naval health from the late 1830s, the subject was impressed most clearly on the minds of the public by the dangers of service in the Royal Navy's West Africa Squadron, which was engaged predominantly in operations against slaving vessels following the abolition of the slave trade and then the institution of slavery in British territories.[25] The dangers of the West Africa Service were emphasized time and again from the 1830s by medical officers when making their case for reform. Between 1837 and 1843 the mortality rate in the West Africa Squadron was 33 per cent, whereas that for the Navy as a whole was 14 per cent.[26] Even if they survived the 'white man's

---

[23] C. Lloyd and J.L.S. Coulter, *Medicine and the Navy, 1200–1900. Vol. IV, 1815–1900* (Edinburgh and London, 1963), p. 4.

[24] Editorial, 26 June 1841, *The Lancet* (1840–1), ii, pp. 482–3.

[25] On the Navy's role in the suppression of the slave trade, see Christopher Lloyd, *The Navy and the Slave Trade* (London, 1949); E.P. Leveen, *British Slave Trade Suppression Policies* (New York, 1977); Raymond Howell, *The Royal Navy and the Slave Trade* (London, 1987).

[26] James Watt, 'The Health of Seamen in Anti-Slavery Squadrons', *The Mariner's Mirror*, 88 (2002), pp. 69–78. Over an eighteen-month period in 1837–8, some 336 out of a thousand men engaged on anti-slavery operations in the West Africa Service died, almost all as a result of disease. Mortality rates per vessel ranged from 3 per cent to 71 per cent. See Sotherton-Estcourt Papers, F.529, Gloucestershire County Record Office (hereafter GCRO).

grave', sailors were likely to return prematurely aged and with a basket of chronic ailments.[27] The sickness rate of the West Africa Squadron was 1,797 per thousand men per year in 1837–43, while that for the Navy as a whole was 1,365 per thousand. In other words, men on the West Africa Service were likely to be admitted to hospital more than once a year. Much of this sickness was due to dysentery, diarrhoea, malaria and yellow fever, but rates of almost all diseases were higher, including chronic ailments such as rheumatism.[28] As one correspondent to *The Lancet* remarked, 'three and a half years upon the coast of Africa, or in the West Indies, are equivalent to an age in many of our military stations.'[29] Although the West Africa Service represented an extreme in naval mortality and morbidity, the loss of life experienced year-in, year-out on anti-slavery operations brought home the sacrifices sailors made in what some continued to regard as a just and noble cause. But as medical officers pointed out, few sailors shared these sentiments. The commanders of ships were entitled to nearly one-eighth of the money allotted to any vessel which captured a slaving ship and they often went to great lengths, ascending 'pestiferous rivers' and losing many of their crew in the reckless pursuit of prizes. But medical officers also blamed the Admiralty for the loss of life in West Africa. Most of the vessels used for anti-slavery operations were poorly ventilated ten-gun brigs which proved stifling in the tropical heat; they were proverbially known as coffins. It was manifestly unfair, critics claimed, to

> send Europeans *up their rivers* for that purpose, consigning numbers of our countrymen to a certain death, in a cause in which few of them are interested, except as a source of prize money – most unfair to treat those as dogs, who would willingly risk their lives where the honour or welfare of their country demand them.[30]

The Admiralty was criticized not simply for its indifference but for acting in a manner which positively invited heavy mortality.[31]

While there was mounting concern within the Navy and in some parts of the medical profession about deaths on the West Africa Service, it was not yet a matter of major public concern. But the dangers of the West Africa Service were soon to come under the spotlight as never before. The reason was the publicity given to the Niger Expedition of 1841–2. As Philip D. Curtin remarked many years ago, the expedition was significant because it marked the end of a humanitarian era in British foreign policy and growing criticism of anti-slavery operations

---

[27] Lloyd and Coulter, *Medicine and the Navy*, pp. 155–64; Philip D. Curtin, '"The White Man's Grave": Image and Reality, 1750–1850', *Journal of British Studies*, 1 (1961), pp. 94–110; Philip D. Curtin, *Death by Migration: Europe's Encounter with the Tropical World in the Nineteenth Century* (Cambridge, 1989).
[28] Watt, 'Health of Seamen', pp. 71–4.
[29] 'A Navy Surgeon', 20 December 1837, *The Lancet* (1837–8), i, p. 530.
[30] 'A Surgeon of the New School', September 1841, *The Lancet* (1840–1), ii, pp. 933–4.
[31] 'Mortality in the Navy and Army', *The Lancet* (1845), ii, p. 251.

in particular.[32] Curtin also concluded that the expedition had important implications for British medicine.[33] This chapter agrees with this assessment, although for rather different reasons.

The Niger Expedition of 1841–2 was the largest of a series of exploratory expeditions made in West Africa since the 1790s. In the 1820s and 1830s interest in the Niger intensified as West Africa rose in economic importance, with increasing demand in Britain for commodities such as palm oil. The expedition planned for 1841 was intended as the beginning of a more ambitious policy towards West Africa, which reversed the earlier doctrine of 'minimum commitment' to the region. Its aims were to conclude treaties with African chiefs in order to prohibit the slave trade; to purchase African commodities on terms favourable to African producers; and to establish British factories and a 'model farm' up-river to teach Africans elements of modern agriculture and 'innocent trade'.[34]

In April 1841 three steam ships – the *Albert*, the *Wilberforce* and the *Soudan* – set out for the Niger delta. All reached their destination: treaties were signed with local rulers and a model farm was established.[35] By August, however, fever started to appear among the crews.[36] There were just a few cases at first but in September the number increased sharply and it was reported that sickness prevailed to 'a considerable extent'. To be exact, by 18 September there had been eighty cases of fever and eight deaths. On the advice of the head surgeon, Dr James O. McWilliam, the expedition's commander, Captain H.D. Trotter, dispatched the *Soudan* down river to Fernando Po with such sick and convalescent cases as it could carry.[37] On 25 October, Trotter, who had joined McWilliam at Fernando Po, wrote to Lord John Russell, solemnly informing him that 'the steam-vessels of the Niger Expedition have been obliged to return from the Niger, owing to a most calamitous fever having broken out'. He continued, 'Only nine persons have escaped the fever, out of about 150 … and it is Dr. M' William's opinion that the nature of the fever has been such as to make it inadvisable in general for those who have had the disease to return to the coast of Africa.'[38] The casualties from fever were such that there were scarcely enough men to steer the vessels down river. The *Albert*, for example, came down under the command of Dr McWilliam, as its captain was too sick to pilot the vessel and its engineer had died. Once at

[32] Philip D. Curtin, *The Image of Africa: British Ideas and Action 1780–1850* (Madison, 1964), vol. 2, pp. 282–317.

[33] Ibid., pp. 343–62.

[34] Lord John Russell to the Lords Commissioners of H.M. Treasury, 26 December 1839, *Papers relative to the Expedition to the River Niger* (London, 1843), pp. 1–2.

[35] William Allen and T.R.H. Thomson, *A Narrative of the Expedition sent by Her Majesty's Government to the River Niger in 1841 under the Command of Captain H.D. Trotter* (London, 1968 [1848]).

[36] Dispatch from H.M. Commissioners of the Expedition to the Niger, to Lord John Russell, 18 August 1841, ibid., p. 43.

[37] H.M. Commissioners to Russell, 18 September 1841, ibid., p. 43.

[38] Trotter to Russell, 25 October 1841, ibid., p. 44.

Fernando Po, McWilliam also contracted 'river fever', but recovered to be praised by his captain for his strength and judgement.[39]

Taking stock of McWilliam's medical assessment, the government – now that of Sir Robert Peel – ordered what was left of the crew of the three steam vessels to return to Britain. However, one ship did re-enter the Niger in 1842 because a tender vessel had been left at the confluence of the Niger and Chadda rivers.[40] After the vessels arrived in Britain the Colonial Office's former disenchantment with West Africa returned, along with a more wary attitude to humanitarian ventures. But the high death rate did focus attention on the health of sailors and the problems of service in tropical stations. According to Curtin, in the decade after the Niger Expedition, 'tropical medicine passed through the most important series of practical reforms of the entire nineteenth century' – reforms which reduced the death rate for European newcomers in West Africa by half.[41] The term 'tropical medicine' is rather anachronistic as it did not come into general use until the 1890s following the establishment of schools of tropical medicine at London and Liverpool.[42] But whatever we choose to call it, the branch of medicine dealing with the health of Europeans overseas underwent a series of important reforms – reforms which may have had their origin in events on the Niger.

In Curtin's view, the medical significance of the Niger Expedition was fourfold. First, the expedition led to more and better intelligence about the medical topography of West Africa, which, in time, led to the selection of healthier garrison sites and settlements for Europeans. Secondly, the expedition re-opened debates over the causes and identity of African fevers, specifically the question of 'yellow fever'. Thirdly, the development of quinine prophylaxis against fever was a direct result of experiments made by medical officers on the expedition. And fourthly, the 1840s saw the abandonment of some of the more dangerous forms of treatment used in cases of tropical fever, such as bloodletting and, to a lesser extent, mercurial drugs.

While it may have contributed to a reduction in the mortality of Europeans, the last of these factors had no obvious connection to the Niger Expedition, and Curtin does not seriously attempt to establish one. The other three specific claims about the Niger Expedition warrant more scrutiny. With regard to medical intelligence, Curtin is certainly correct in arguing that efforts intensified. The government did circulate questionnaires to those who had recently travelled to Africa, and it consulted medical authorities in England and sent out Dr Richard Robert Madden (1798–1886) to the western portion of the Guinea Coast with a medical and political commission. The Niger Expedition itself also spent more time

---

[39] Trotter to Russell, 25 October 1841, ibid., p. 44.
[40] Trotter to Russell, 25 October 1841, ibid., p. 44.
[41] Curtin, *The Image of Africa*, vol. 2, p. 344.
[42] See for example Michael Worboys, 'The Emergence of Tropical Medicine: A Study in the Establishment of a Scientific Speciality', in G. Lemaine *et al.* (eds), *Perspectives on the Emergence of Scientific Disciplines* (The Hague, 1977), pp. 76–98; David Arnold (ed.), *Warm Climates and Western Medicine* (Amsterdam and Atlanta, 1996).

studying the medical topography of the region than any other scientific problem. But the significance of this data was probably no greater than that of the more systematic surveys conducted by military surgeons on the West African coast in the 1830s, or the later work of Dr Alexander Bryson, which was based on a detailed analysis of the health of the British naval squadron operating in West Africa and which offered concrete recommendations.[43] With the exception of the mortality and morbidity figures relating to the crew of the expedition, much of the information generated prior to and during it was anecdotal. In this respect, the significance of the Niger Expedition is far from obvious, and even Curtin does not consider it at length. In relation to this one specific claim, it is reasonable to conclude that the Niger Expedition did not generate any data that were particularly important, or any significant theoretical or practical insights. The statistical surveys of the 1830s and later 1840s were more important in all these respects.

Where Curtin is on firmer ground, and where the significance of the expedition is indisputable, is in regard to quinine prophylaxis as a measure against fever, or, more specifically, against what was generally known as the endemic or common coast fever of West Africa. The Navy ordered the medical officers on the three vessels to maintain the usual precautions against fever, which entailed giving the crew a mixture of Peruvian bark (the bark of the cinchona tree) in wine. This was a practice that went back to the previous century. But on the Niger Expedition, medical officers were permitted to substitute quinine for bark powder if they preferred. Quinine – which had been isolated from the bark in the 1820s – had already been subjected to therapeutic trials in a range of fevers, but it was in the treatment of malarial fevers that it had distinguished itself. It was not, however, yet in general use as a prophylactic, and there had been no systematic examination of its efficacy in that capacity. One of the Niger Expedition's medical officers – Dr T.R.H. Thomson – saw it as an opportunity to do just that and continued his experiments after the expedition left the Niger. Using himself as an experimental subject, he administered a higher dose than had previously been recommended (six to ten grains per day rather than two or three) and was entirely free from symptoms of fever while in Africa. Only after he returned to England, and stopped taking quinine, did the symptoms of fever begin to appear.[44] McWilliam also believed that taking quinine daily was among the most useful precautions that could be taken against fever on the West African coast, although he warned that there was no certain method of prevention.[45]

This episode has been well documented by Curtin and by historians such as Daniel Headrick, who see quinine as enabling European expansion even in the

[43] Alexander Bryson, *Report on the Climate and Principal Diseases of the African Station* (London, 1847).
[44] Curtin, *Image of Africa*, vol. 2, pp. 355–6; T.R.H. Thomson, 'On the Value of Quinine in African Remittent Fever', *The Lancet* (1846), i, pp. 244–5.
[45] James O. M'William, *Medical History of the Expedition to the Niger during the Years 1841–2, comprising an Account of the Fever which led to its abrupt Termination* (London, 1843), p. 188.

most malarious areas of Africa.[46] Studies such as those made by Bryson in 1847 appeared to confirm the findings of Thomson and, in 1848, the Director-General of the Army Medical Service sent a circular to West African governors, advising that quinine prophylaxis be instituted on a general basis.[47] In this case, there was clearly a direct link between the observations made on the Niger Expedition and subsequent developments which may have contributed to the prevention of sickness and mortality among Europeans. However, it is important to stress that the value of quinine prophylaxis has often been overstated. While it was a valuable treatment, its limitations as a prophylactic became increasingly evident and were fully exposed by the time of the First World War.[48] This helps to explain the disparity between falling mortality rates from the middle of the nineteenth century and the high morbidity which persisted in most tropical locations until the early 1900s.

The link between the Niger Expedition and debates over the identity and causes of fever is less clear-cut. It did place the spotlight on tropical fevers, but subsequent events were more important, especially in regard to the vexed question of yellow fever. Even then, it is not clear from Curtin's account how these inconclusive debates had a practical impact. But there is perhaps another reason – not considered by Curtin – why the Niger Expedition may be regarded as significant for medical reform in the Royal Navy. It is important because it marked the beginnings of a fusion between hitherto disparate interest groups: the humanitarian lobby (anti-slavery activists, factory reformers and so forth); those campaigning for the welfare of sailors (mostly former naval officers); sections of the medical profession (especially surgeon-apothecaries); and, less obviously, the proponents of free trade.

The heated debates over fevers that occurred in the 1840s and 1850s would have mattered little had they been confined largely to the medical profession, as they had been previously. Hitherto, the government had taken an interest in yellow fever only when it appeared in the Mediterranean, as it did occasionally between 1800 and 1820. The government sometimes sought the advice of medical practitioners but, in the absence of consensus, it did nothing to alter its existing quarantine regulations.[49] It remained anxious about the disease being introduced into Britain by merchant vessels or returning troops, particularly invalids from

---

[46] D.R. Headrick, *The Tools of Empire: Technology and European Imperialism in the Nineteenth Century* (Oxford and New York, 1981).

[47] Curtin, *Image of Africa*, vol. 2, p. 356.

[48] Mark Harrison, 'Medicine and the Culture of Command: The Case of Malaria Control in the British Army during the Two World Wars', *Medical History*, 40 (1996), pp. 437–52.

[49] Some medical practitioners believed the fever to be contagious: see for example William Pym, *Observations on the Bulam Fever, which has of late Years prevailed in the West Indies, on the Coast of South America, at Gibraltar, Cadiz, and other parts of Spain: with a Collection of Facts proving it to be a highly Contagious Disease* (London, 1815). But the majority of those who had served in the Caribbean or in Spain during the French Wars believed that yellow fever was merely a more serious form of common remittent fever, which arose from miasma: see for example Edward N. Bancroft, *An Essay on the Disease called Yellow Fever* (London, 1811);

the West Indies.[50] For the most part, the government was more concerned with cholera and plague than with yellow fever. Cholera had wreaked havoc during the epidemic of 1831–2 and posed a continuing threat to trade and public health. Although plague remained confined to the Mediterranean, quarantine was regularly imposed against vessels sailing to Britain from the Levant and Egypt, disrupting the supply of cotton to Britain's mills. The government was therefore asked by merchants to repeal or reform its quarantine legislation, but it was reluctant to do so for a host of reasons, not least because this would invite retaliation from other nations.

It was in such circumstances that the free-trade lobby began to form an association with medical practitioners, who were opposed to quarantine on the grounds that diseases such as cholera, plague and yellow fever were non-contagious.[51] But until the 1840s, only a few of the more radical practitioners were closely linked with merchants and their parliamentary supporters. Even merchants themselves were divided on the utility or otherwise of quarantine.[52] The humanitarian lobby also took little interest in these matters, although it occasionally denounced the abuses committed in lazarettos.[53] Nor was it particularly concerned with the welfare of soldiers and sailors – their champions were to be found largely within the forces themselves, or among those who had retired. Indeed, the public was largely indifferent to the welfare of servicemen and regarded losses from disease rather fatalistically.

In the decade after the Niger Expedition this situation began to change. Both quarantine reform and the welfare of sailors ceased to be sectional issues and came to be identified closely with the national interest. The well-publicized venture on the Niger directed attention towards the humanitarian role played by the Navy, and some of its participants – notably McWilliam – became public figures. This attracted sympathy towards the plight of sailors, particularly those on the West Africa Service. Other interest groups also became involved, the most important of which was the free-trade lobby. Merchants and manufacturers began to couch their

Thomas O'Halloran, *Remarks on the Yellow Fever of the South and East Coasts of Spain* (London, 1823).

50 John Booker, *Maritime Quarantine: The British Experience, c.1650–1900* (Aldershot, 2007), esp. ch. 10.

51 See Erwin H. Ackerknecht, 'Anticontagionism between 1821 and 1867', *Bulletin of the History of Medicine*, 22 (1948), pp. 562–93; Roger Cooter, 'Anticontagionism and History's Medical Record', in P. Wright and A. Treacher (eds), *The Problem of Medical Knowledge: Examining the Social Construction of Medicine* (Edinburgh, 1982), pp. 87–108; Margaret Pelling, *Cholera, Fever and English Medicine 1825–1865* (Oxford, 1978).

52 Peter Baldwin, *Contagion and the State in Europe 1830–1930* (Cambridge, 1999), pp. 97–8, 201–9; Mark Harrison, 'Disease, Diplomacy and International Commerce: The Origins of International Sanitary Regulation in the Nineteenth Century', *Journal of Global History*, 1 (2006), pp. 197–217; Booker, *Maritime Quarantine*, ch. 12.

53 See for example John Howard, *An Account of the Principal Lazarettos in Europe; with various Papers relative to the Plague: Together with further Observations on some Foreign Prisons and Hospitals; and additional Remarks on the present State of those in Great Britain and Ireland* (Warrington, 1789).

demands for quarantine reform in humanitarian language, drawing attention, for example, to the sufferings of returning sailors who were subjected to detention on vessels stricken with fever. In so doing, they joined forces with medical officers of the Navy, who denied that quarantine was medically valid, seeing environmental improvements as the only effective means of prevention.

Although the West Africa Squadron had long endured high mortality, the high-profile Niger Expedition brought the matter before the public in a way that earlier operations had not. It also came at a time when criticism was beginning to be voiced about 'philanthropy at a distance', exemplified by the character of Mrs Jellyby in Charles Dickens's *Bleak House* (1852–3). Public sentiment was increasingly turning to charity at home: to the plight of factory workers and the poor.[54] Some reform-minded naval officers sensed this and saw an opportunity to present their case to the public, making much of the neglect of sailors by comparison with African slaves. Writing to *The Times*, a naval officer sought to draw readers' attention to what he saw as:

> The evils of our present system of the prevention of the slave-trade, and to direct the public sympathy, which has so long raged in favour of the African blacks, towards their countrymen employed in the prevention of the slave-trade on the coast of Africa, whose sufferings ... pass by unknown and unnoticed. Dozens of vessels have been similarly desolated by fever on that station, but the records of them are buried at the Admiralty, and rarely meet the public eye; but many hundreds of bereaved families have to bewail their sorrows unheard.[55]

The perils of the West Africa Service – which Bryson was later to describe as 'the most disagreeable, arduous and unhealthy service that falls to the lot of British officers and seamen' – highlighted in extreme form the conditions endured by British sailors generally.[56] There was an undercurrent of racism, too: a sense that British lives ought not to be sacrificed for 'a foreign race, sunk in the lowest barbarism, having little in common with humanity save some similarity in form'.[57] It was easy to see why the Navy was suffering from low morale, poor recruitment and high rates of desertion.[58]

Of particular concern were conditions in the small steam-sloops used in antislavery operations and in the expedition up the Niger. The heat generated by the engines compounded the discomfort created by tropical heat and, in the opinion of some naval officers, contributed materially to the incidence of fever. Another anonymous correspondent to *The Times*, who claimed to have suffered from fever, remarked that:

[54] Boyd Hilton, *The Age of Atonement: The Influence of Evangelism on Social and Economic Thought, 1785–1865* (Oxford, 1988).
[55] 'A Naval Officer', *The Times*, undated cutting (mid 1840s), F.529, GCRO.
[56] Bryson, *Report*, p. 161.
[57] 'A Naval Officer', undated cutting (mid 1840s), F.529, GCRO.
[58] E.L. Rasor, *Reform in the Royal Navy: A Social History of the Lower Deck 1850 to 1880* (Hamden, Conn., 1976), pp. 9–10.

To cram, jam and compress 300 or 400 horse steam power, and 300 or 400 tons of coals into an engine room ... 58 feet long, 33 feet wide, and 21 feet deep, is to deny space and ventilation for the two engineers, three firemen, and one coal-man, who must form the watch there, roasting, stewing; and to send such a steamer to the West Coast of Africa, where the very coals in store support and team with vegetable life to be carried on board, stewed, and decomposed, forming malaria by natural heat, and generating fever more rapidly by the befitting influence of artificial heat, is abominably wrong.[59]

These opinions echoed medical concerns that conditions below decks in steam vessels resembled those of a tropical climate, even when they were not in tropical waters. Indeed, fears were expressed in some quarters that steam vessels might act as a kind of hot-house, incubating diseases that were normally confined to tropical regions. Thus preserved, the seeds of disease, if brought back to Britain at the right season, might even germinate there. Tropical metaphors were also becoming more common in descriptions of factories and other environments in Britain in which machinery generated heat. Friedrich Engels's *Condition of the English Working Class*, published in 1844 – just three years after the Niger Expedition – is a case in point.[60] This emphasis upon steam and artificial heat sets the language of hygienic reform in the Victorian Navy apart from earlier periods. Although Georgian naval reformers such as James Lind had stressed the importance of good ventilation and cleanliness in the prevention of so-called 'putrid' diseases such as scurvy and typhus, their reference points tended to be prisons and hospitals rather than factories. By the 1840s, concern over the health of sailors was inseparable from more general unease over the advent of a new, steam-powered industrial society.

The health of sailors in steam vessels was also brought to the fore by an old controversy which had been re-awakened by the Niger Expedition: the nature and causes of yellow fever. Dr McWilliam insisted that the fever which had claimed the lives of so many of his fellow crew members was not the dreaded yellow fever, but merely a form of the common remittent fever of the African coast. This fever was not contagious and was generated by tropical heat acting upon decaying vegetable matter; humidity accelerated the process of decay, producing founts of putrefaction in areas of lush tropical vegetation. Men worn down by fatigue and heat exhaustion, particularly in the cramped and over-heated conditions of steam vessels, were particularly liable to its effects.[61] This opinion was shared by the other surgeons engaged on the expedition, and was communicated to the Secretary of State for the Colonies, Lord Stanley.[62]

[59] 'One who has Suffered from Fever', *The Times*, undated cutting (mid 1840s), F.529, GCRO.
[60] Alan Bewell, *Romanticism and Colonial Disease* (Baltimore and London, 1999), pp. 272–4.
[61] M'William, *Medical History*, pp. 179–80.
[62] *Papers Relative to the Expedition to the River Niger*, PP 1843 [472] XLVIII: for example, Report from W. Cook, Surgeon of the Wilberforce, to Lord Stanley, Secretary of State for the Colonies, 11 March 1843.

The *Éclair* and Boa Vista Incidents

In the wake of the Niger Expedition, McWilliam's reputation was immense and, when another public scandal erupted over fever and the West Africa Service in 1845–6, he was called upon to make an official report. The scandal was caused by the fate of one particular vessel, the *Éclair*, which limped back to Britain in September 1845 with most of its original crew, and a number of volunteers who had boarded the vessel, dead or dying.[63] While the mortality rate was higher than normal – around two-thirds of the original crew – it was by no means unprecedented for vessels on the West Africa Service. The plight of the *Éclair* came to public attention for other reasons. Its commander – Walter Estcourt – was from a prominent landed family; his father was MP for Oxford University and his brother-in-law, A.H. Addington, was parliamentary under-secretary for the colonies.[64] Estcourt's death *en route* to Britain was bound to be noted by the press. Another reason why this particular vessel received attention was that it had stopped at the Portuguese island of Boa Vista – one of the Cape Verde Islands – on its return, where it took on volunteers. Some also boarded the *Éclair* at Madeira, although the crew were not allowed to land there as they had at Boa Vista. The Boa Vista landing was notable partly because of the embarkation of volunteers who helped to steer the stricken vessel back to Britain. Their bravery was widely praised, especially as some of them, such as the naval surgeon Sidney Bernard, later died from a fever they had contracted on the ship. More importantly, after the vessel had left Boa Vista, the island was devastated by an epidemic of fever, which many thought had been brought there by the *Éclair*. Claims for compensation and the imposition of quarantine against British vessels created a major diplomatic incident.

The epidemic on Boa Vista – which killed around a tenth of the population – was not common knowledge when the *Éclair* returned to Britain. However, the quarantine office of the Privy Council suspected that the disease might be yellow fever and – in keeping with the statutes – placed the vessel in quarantine. The crew were confined to their ship rather than in a lazaretto, which produced howls of fury in the press.[65] Naval officers protested against the inhumanity of the action, which continued to expose the crew to infection.[66] The bravery of the crew made their detention all the more unbearable, and editorials in the national and local press condemned the Privy Council for its actions. Naval men wrote that the

---

[63] Papers and newspaper cuttings relating to the *Eclair*, Sotherton-Estcourt Papers, F.533 and F.546, GCRO.

[64] Obituary of Commander Walter Grimston Bucknall Estcourt, *The Nautical Magazine and Naval Chronicle*, 12 and 14 December 1845, pp. 686–8.

[65] Editorial, *The Times*, undated cutting (mid 1840s), Sotherton-Estcourt Papers, F.529, GCRO; *Gloucester Journal*, 'The Plague on board the Eclair', 4 October 1845, p. 2, and 11 October 1845, p. 2.

[66] Undated cutting from the *Naval Intelligencer*, Sotherton-Estcourt Papers, F.529, GCRO.

action was symptomatic of the government's disregard for sailors, and they used the high mortality to highlight the perils of African service.

The furore over the treatment of the *Éclair*'s crew was also the occasion for another potent ingredient to enter the mixture. Advocates of free trade used the 'imprisonment' of the sailors on board their vessel as evidence of the inhumanity of quarantine, which they also regarded as a useless impediment to free trade. With repeal of the Corn Laws in the offing, the tide of public opinion was running in their favour and there were numerous calls for the reform, if not always for the repeal of the quarantine statutes. For the first time, too, the majority of medical practitioners were behind them, led by journals such as *The Lancet*.[67] As well as condemning the inhumanity of quarantine – and its vexatious restrictions upon trade and the movement of people around the empire – many practitioners believed that quarantine against yellow fever was unjustified on medical grounds. Following the lead taken by medical officers of the Army and Navy, they argued that the fever was primarily a disease of tropical conditions, generated by putrefaction.[68]

These issues became particularly important at the end of 1845, when some of the Mediterranean states imposed quarantine against all British shipping on the grounds that the fever might have taken root in Britain itself.[69] This proved damaging to Britain, as was the prospect of paying reparations to Portugal.[70] It was alleged that the commander of the vessel had misled the authorities on Boa Vista as to the true nature of the fever, and had been allowed to disembark under false pretences. The controversy prompted the Privy Council to dispatch McWilliam to the island to conduct an inquiry into the epidemic. His report made uncomfortable reading. After a searching investigation, McWilliam concluded that the fever was contagious and that it had probably been imported by the *Éclair*. But it was not, in his opinion, yellow fever – if it were, he reasoned, it would have afflicted the islands far more often.[71]

It seems likely that McWilliam was mistaken about the nature of the fever and that it was really yellow fever as understood today; however, the identity of the disease cannot be proved with certainty. Moreover, for the purposes of this discussion, its true nature is less relevant than the controversy and its ramifications. McWilliam's conclusion was an embarrassment to the British government, except in so far as it appeared to justify the decision to place the *Éclair* in quarantine.

[67] Editorial, 11 October 1845, *The Lancet* (1845), ii, pp. 402–3.
[68] Sir William Burnett, Director General of the Naval Medical Service, report to the Admiralty, 21 November 1845; Burnett to Admiralty, 11 December 1845, Sotherton-Estcourt Papers, F.546, GCRO.
[69] Capt. Gallway, H.M. Consul, Naples, to Earl of Aberdeen, 17 October 1845; Addington to Hon. W.L. Bathurst, Foreign Office, 10 November 1845; Aberdeen to the Hon. William Temple, 24 November 1845, Sotherton-Estcourt Papers, F.546, GCRO.
[70] The British government eventually agreed to pay compensation of 1,000 guineas to the inhabitants of Boa Vista. See General Board of Health, *Second Report on Quarantine: Yellow Fever*, PP 1852, XX, p. 101.
[71] James O. McWilliam, *Report on the Fever at Boa Vista* (London, 1847).

It certainly embarrassed the Admiralty, which sent another naval medical officer – Dr Gilbert King – to the island to conduct its own investigation. As might be expected, he concluded that the epidemic had not been imported, and had been produced by unusual meteorological conditions.[72] The whole affair also threw the spotlight once again on conditions in steam vessels and the possibility that some form of infectious miasma might be sustained within their engine rooms. At any rate, this was the opinion of the General Board of Health – created by the Public Health Act of 1848 – when it came to consider the matter a few years later. Under the presiding influence of the sanitarian Edwin Chadwick the Board deliberately excluded evidence of the disease having been spread by importation, and emphasised hygienic and meteorological factors instead.[73] Both the health of naval vessels and the health of the country therefore appeared to rest on the avoidance or removal of those conditions which gave rise to fever, rather than upon measures such as quarantine, which were deemed medically useless and damaging to trade.[74]

In the late 1840s and in the following decade, the health of sailors continued to be intertwined with the status of naval medical officers, particularly that of assistant-surgeons. The heroism of McWilliam on the Niger and of Sidney Bernard on the *Éclair* was frequently invoked to garner public support for their cause and to draw attention to the perils of tropical service.[75] McWilliam also made weighty interventions in his own right, becoming an ardent champion of medical officers and maritime health in the merchant marine as well as in the Navy.[76] By the late 1840s the status of assistant-surgeons and the related issue of naval health were being extensively discussed in the national and local press. Newspapers such as *The Times*, *The Morning Herald* and *The Morning Chronicle* threw their weight behind the campaign, as did popular periodicals such as the *Spectator* and *Punch*.[77] The matter was finally settled in the House of Commons in 1850, after young graduates had been warned off the Navy by the royal colleges.[78] After that, conditions of service for assistant-surgeons began to improve, although the surgeons and their supporters continued to vent their frustration at the slow pace of reform.[79] But the leisurely pace of change ensured that the broader issue

[72] 'Report of Dr King on the Fever at Boa Vista, addressed to Sir William Burnett, 10 October, 1847', Sotherton-Estcourt Papers, F.550, GCRO.

[73] See Christopher Hamlin, *Public Health and Social Justice in the Age of Chadwick: Britain, 1800–1854* (Cambridge, 1998).

[74] *Report of the General Board of Health on Quarantine*, PP 1849, XXIV; *Second Report on Quarantine: Yellow Fever*, PP 1852, XX, p. 101.

[75] Editorial, *The Lancet*, 26 June 1847 (1847), i, p. 680.

[76] Editorial, *The Lancet*, 17 June 1848 (1848), i, pp. 670–1; J.O. McWilliam, *An Exposition of the Case of the Assistant Surgeons of the Royal Navy* (London, 1849); W.A. Greenhill, rev. Lynn Milne, 'James Ormiston McWilliam (1808–1862)', ODNB.

[77] J.O. McWilliam letters and newspaper cuttings, MS.6830, WMS, Wellcome Library, London.

[78] See for example *The Lancet* (1849), i, pp. 216, 297, 436, 566; (1850), i, p. 449.

[79] See for example *The Lancet* (1850), i, p. 738; (1850), ii, pp. 538–9; (1853), ii, p. 84; (1855), i, p. 324; (1859), p. 248.

of naval health remained on the political agenda. Time and again, supporters of medical reform in the Royal Navy emphasised that the health of sailors was vital to the service's efficiency and ought to be the first consideration of the Admiralty.[80] The poorly ventilated and overcrowded conditions endured by sailors continued to be likened to those suffered by slaves in Africa or pauper children crammed into workhouses at home.[81]

Ventilation had been recognised as a problem since the mid eighteenth century and various devices had been introduced to improve it. The problem, however, seemed to be magnified on steam vessels – especially for those who worked in the engine room – and particularly in hot climates. During the Niger Expedition, for example, even the most modern devices had been found wanting. The vessels all had a tube system of ventilation which pumped fresh air into each compartment of the ship and which allowed 'vitiated' or respired air to escape. In calm weather, this could be powered by the vessel's paddle-wheel. Air was also 'medicated' with various substances such as chlorine in an attempt to purify or disinfect it. But McWilliam later reported that the medication process had proved useless because there was no way of knowing in advance which type of poison a crew would encounter. More importantly, the ventilation system had failed to render sufficient air fit for respiration to the lower deck.[82] In the coming years, many more experimental devices were tried out in an attempt to alleviate the problem. The practice of regularly washing decks – which had in any case been declining since the early 1800s – also gave way to greater emphasis upon dryness, in the belief that humidity was conducive to fevers, rheumatism, and consumption (tuberculosis).[83] In tropical stations and among squadrons like the one in West Africa, a number of special measures began to be taken from the 1840s which similarly contributed to the decline in mortality. These included more care over the location of hospitals, improvements in the purity of water supplies, and the standardization of prophylaxis with quinine. But it is important not to exaggerate the impact of these reforms. Indeed, some fundamental problems such as overcrowding had yet to be addressed. Surgeons complained that sailors had less breathing space in their quarters than 'felons condemned to imprisonment'.[84]

The decline in mortality among sailors was accordingly fitful. In 1834 the annual death rate in the Navy as a whole was 20.4 per thousand men, but after falling in the early 1850s it rose in the years after the Crimean War to a high of 25.8 per thousand in 1858. After that year there was a sustained reduction in mortality which was probably due to improvements in hygiene and diet prompted

---

[80] Editorial, 3 June 1848, *The Lancet* (1848), i, pp. 615–16; 'Parliamentary Intelligence', 22 February 1862, *The Lancet* (1862), i, p. 239.

[81] Editorial, 27 January 1849, *The Lancet* (1849), i, p.103.

[82] M'William, *Medical History*, pp. 253–4, 267.

[83] Rasor, *Reform*, pp. 100–1; Michael Lewis, *The Navy in Transition: A Social History 1814–1864* (London, 1965), pp. 252–3.

[84] Surgeon of HMS *Modeste*, quoted in Lloyd and Coulter, *Medicine and the Navy*, pp. 54–5.

by problems encountered during the Crimean War. In 1859, for example, the food allowance given to sailors was increased and its quality improved. However, conditions below decks improved more slowly. In 1862, the First Lord of the Admiralty, Sir John Pakington, asked the respected doctor and former mail packet surgeon Gavin Milroy to write a report on the health of the Navy. A convinced sanitarian and colleague of Chadwick, Milroy attributed most of the worst outbreaks of disease on naval vessels to defective ventilation, overcrowding, and accumulations of filth in the hold. One outcome of the inquiry was that the Admiralty issued an order for the improvement of ventilation on all steam vessels. Together with other improvements, such as less overcrowding below decks, these initiatives may have contributed to the rapid and persistent decline in mortality that occurred among sailors from the mid 1860s.[85] By 1868 the death rate in the Navy had fallen to 8.9 per thousand and by 1895 it had been reduced further to only 6.6 per thousand men.[86] While it is difficult to separate the effects of these reforms from improved nutrition and sanitary conditions in civilian life, the fall in mortality certainly coincided with major initiatives within the service and, in this respect, mirrored similar trends within the Army.[87]

Conclusion

This chapter has argued that the reform of naval medicine and health from the 1840s was a direct result of widespread public concern created by public awareness of the plight of sailors in the West Africa Squadron. The issue of naval health became increasingly prominent during the 1830s, as surgeons gathered support for their demands for better pay and conditions. But it was not until the 1840s that their professional campaign – and the related issue of naval health – began to attract support outside the Royal Navy and the medical profession. The response to the *Éclair* and Boa Vista incidents shows that several reformist interests became intertwined during the 1840s. Those who sought the improvement of conditions for sailors found allies in free-trade opponents of quarantine, and in a large and increasingly influential section of the medical profession which denied or minimized the contagious nature of tropical fevers. This new coalition of interests began to shape the course of public health in Britain during the 1850s, but it also spurred practical measures designed to protect the health of seamen. The opponents of contagion proposed an alternative to quarantine in the form of practical sanitary action. Moreover, with the spotlight of the humanitarian lobby now fixed upon the Navy, it became harder to justify inaction. These are the main reasons why the 1840s and early 1850s may be regarded as a turning point in the

---

[85] 'Health of the Navy', *The Lancet* (1862), i, pp. 440–1.
[86] Rasor, *Reform*, pp. 101, 103.
[87] See Curtin, *Death by Migration*, and Alan R. Skelley, *The Victorian Army at Home: The Recruitment and Terms and Conditions of the British Regular* (London, 1977).

history of British naval medicine. From then on, the public was no longer prepared to countenance what it regarded as needless deaths from disease. Once a matter of indifference, there was now a sense that sanitary measures, like those beginning to be implemented in civilian life, could and should be used to protect the lives of servicemen.

6

Mortality and Migration: A Survey

Hamish Maxwell-Stewart and Ralph Shlomowitz

When the convict John Popjoy was disembarked from the transport vessel *Larkins* in 1817 he was found to be tattooed on his right arm with the verse 'Rocks, hills and sands, and barren lands, kind fortune set me free, from roaring guns and women's tongues, O Lord deliver me.'[1] There is much evidence to suggest that the emphasis of this talismanic tattoo was misplaced, for shipwrecks were comparatively rare events: of 337 convict voyages to the colony of Van Diemen's Land in the fifty years between 1803 and 1853, only two were wrecked. Nevertheless, in the age of sail, a trans-oceanic voyage was a dangerous undertaking – but the vast majority of deaths on the long run to Australia were caused by disease.

During the past few decades, a number of scholars have attempted to quantify the mortality suffered by seaborne populations in the age of sail. Most of these studies have related to the bulk shipping of what can be termed 'institutional' populations in steerage. These include African slaves transported to the Americas (and the crews on board these slave vessels); British convicts transported to North America and Australia; various streams of Asian, Pacific Islander and African indentured labour shipped to various destinations around the world; and British emigrants whose passage was paid by the receiving colonies in Australia, New Zealand and South Africa.[2]

It is well recognized in this literature that seaborne migrant populations were at risk of sickness and death during four distinct stages in the process of migration: on the route to the port of embarkation; at the port while awaiting departure; during the sea voyage; and after arrival at their destination. It is also recognized that diseases acquired in one stage could result in death in a subsequent stage. Furthermore, the accumulated insults of harsh treatment, poor and insanitary living arrangements and malnutrition experienced by some migrant

---

[1] Tasmanian Archives and Heritage Office, CSO1/416/9354.

[2] For recent surveys of this literature, see R.L. Cohn, 'Maritime Mortality in the Eighteenth and Nineteenth Centuries: A Survey', *International Journal of Maritime History*, 1 (1989), pp. 159–91; R. Haines, R. Shlomowitz and L. Brennan, 'Maritime Mortality Revisited', *International Journal of Maritime History*, 8 (1996), pp. 133–72; R. Haines and R. Shlomowitz, 'Explaining the Modern Mortality Decline: What Can We Learn from Sea Voyages?', *Social History of Medicine*, 11 (1998), pp. 15–48; H.S. Klein, S.L. Engerman, R. Haines and R. Shlomowitz, 'Transoceanic Mortality: The Slave Trade in Comparative Perspective', *William and Mary Quarterly*, 58 (2001), pp. 93–117.

groups would have had long-term consequences for their health. The privations suffered by slaves, for example, on the march to the coast and when confined in crowded and insanitary conditions at coastal forts, would have made them much more vulnerable to sickness and death both during the Middle Passage and after arrival in the Americas.

This survey, accordingly, will bring together not only studies of mortality suffered during the sea voyage (for which quantitative evidence is most readily available), but also the information available on the mortality suffered by slaves, convicts, indentured labourers and free migrants before departure and after arrival at their destination. The voyages that we examine span the period from the mid seventeenth century to the early twentieth century, although the vast bulk of the pre-1800 data relates to the Atlantic slave trade. The chapter will commence with an examination of the existing literature highlighting the various explanations put forward by historians to explain this mortality. It then proceeds to introduce new data on the mortality suffered by convicts after arrival in Van Diemen's Land (Tasmania) in the period 1830 to 1853.

Pre-embarkation Mortality

Information does not appear to be available on the mortality suffered by migrants on their journey to the port of embarkation, but for some groups we have quantitative estimates of mortality at the port while awaiting embarkation. These include male convicts who were housed in hulks in England, and Indian indentured workers who were kept in depots in Calcutta while awaiting departure. For both these migrant groups, the decline in hulk or depot mortality was mirrored by a decline in mortality on board vessels departing from those ports. This could have been due to similar forces being at work – such as improved sanitation – bringing about lower mortality.[3] The decline in mortality at sea was also due, in part, to improved screening practices reducing the number of sick passengers being permitted to embark on the sea voyage.

Information is also available on the deaths suffered by slaves during what is called the 'coasting period' or 'loading period' in which slaves were bought along the coast of Africa, a period which was usually much longer than the Middle Passage itself. Voyages that experienced more deaths during the coasting period were also usually associated with more deaths during the Middle Passage.[4]

---

3   J. McDonald and R. Shlomowitz, 'Mortality on Convict Voyages to Australia, 1788–1868', *Social Science History*, 13 (1989), pp. 285–313 (see, in particular, appendix A); R. Shlomowitz and J. McDonald, 'Mortality of Indian Labour on Ocean Voyages, 1843–1917', *Studies in History*, 6 (1990), pp. 35–65; R. Shlomowitz and L. Brennan, 'Mortality and Migrant Labour en route to Assam, 1863–1924', *Indian Economic and Social History Review*, 27 (1990), pp. 313–30 (see, in particular, table 3 and discussion on pp. 325–7).
4   Klein *et al.*, 'Transoceanic Mortality', tables 1 and 9. See also S.J. Hogerzeil and D. Richardson, 'Slave Purchasing Strategies and Shipboard Mortality: Day-to-Day Evidence from the Dutch African Trade, 1751–1797', Chapter 7 in this volume.

Table 6.1 Mortality on ocean voyages

Nature of voyage	Period	Number of voyages	Average length (days)	Crude death rate per month per 1,000
African slaves to Americas	1664–1864	2,429	64	59.6
British and Irish convicts to Australia	1788–1814	68	174	11.3
	1815–1868	693	122	2.4
British and Irish emigrants to New York	1836–1853	1,077	45	10.0
British and Irish emigrants to Australia	1838–1853	258	109	7.4
	1854–1892	934	92	3.4
African indentured labour to the West Indies	1848–1850	54	29	48.7
	1851–1865	54	29	12.3
Indian indentured labour to Mauritius, Natal, West Indies and Fiji, departing from Calcutta	1850–1872	382	88	19.9
	1873–1917	876	65	7.1
Chinese indentured labour to Americas	1847–1874	343	116	25.5
Pacific Island indentured labour to: Queensland	1873–1894	558	111	3.0
Fiji	1882–1911	112	117	3.6

Note: The data are restricted to completed voyages, exclusive of shipwrecks. The mortality statistic used standardises voyage mortality for voyages of different length. While there is evidence of falling mortality on British slave vessels in the late eighteenth and early nineteenth centuries, other trends are more difficult to discern. For this reason the data for the 200-year period of the slave trade represented in this table have not been desegregated.

Sources: For slave voyages, R. Haines, J. McDonald and R. Shlomowitz, 'Mortality and Voyage Length in the Middle Passage Revisited', *Explorations in Economic History*, 38 (2001), pp. 503–33, table 1; for non-slave voyages, R. Haines, R. Shlomowitz and L. Brennan, 'Maritime Mortality Revisited', *International Journal of Maritime History*, 8 (1996), pp. 133–72, table 1.

Mortality during the Sea Voyage

Table 6.1 brings together information on the crude death rate (that is, the overall death rate presented over a constant period of time) suffered by a number of migrant populations on the sea voyage from the seventeenth to the early twentieth century. For a subset of these voyages, information is available to estimate age-specific death rates for three age groups: infants, children and adults; these estimates are presented in Table 6.2. For some slave voyages, information is also available on the age-specific death rate of two groups – children and adults – but

Table 6.2 Mortality on ocean voyages by age classes

Nature of voyage	Period	Number of voyages	Death rate per month per 1,000		
			Adult	Child	Infant
British and Irish emigrant voyages to New York	1836–1853	118	4.5	13.7	97.7
British and Irish emigrant voyages to Australia	1838–1853	364	2.4	18.2	66.1
	1854–1892	1,036	1.0	7.9	40.1
Indian labour voyages to:					
Fiji	1879–1916	87	4.0	17.8	54.7
Mauritius	1860–1872	280	12.6	40.4	90.4
Natal	1884–1900	141	2.7	7.0	21.3
British Guiana	1874–1901	175	3.7	24.1	80.9
Trinidad	1859–1899	140	4.8	16.3	67.2
Jamaica	1874–1895	12	3.6	6.1	52.8

Source: R. Haines, R. Shlomowitz and L. Brennan, 'Maritime Mortality Revisited', *International Journal of Maritime History*, 8 (1996), pp. 133–72, table 2.

as the age distribution within the group 'children' is not known, it is difficult to evaluate these data.[5]

The main findings that can be read from these tables are: slaves suffered much higher death rates than non-slave populations; infants were at much greater risk of death at sea, as on land; and the death rate of adult British emigrants to Australia by the mid nineteenth century had declined to roughly that of the land-based population (about ten per thousand per annum), but infants and children remained at increased risk. Babies born at sea were at the most risk: the neo-natal mortality rate (the ratio of deaths of babies aged less than 28 days to the number of live births) on voyages to the colony of South Australia between 1847 and 1872, at 172.5 per thousand, was more than four times that on land.[6]

When standardised for differing voyage lengths, the death rates on British and Irish emigrant ships to Australia were much lower than on similar voyages to New York, reflecting the greater attention to sanitation and hygienic measures on board ships bound for Australia. It is difficult to explain the variability in death rates on Indian voyages other than to suggest that the higher death rates on board ships to

---

5 Klein *et al.*, 'Transoceanic Mortality', table 7; Hogerzeil and Richardson, 'Slave Purchasing Strategies', table 7.3.

6 R. Haines and R. Shlomowitz, 'Deaths of Babies Born on Government-Assisted Emigrant Voyages to South Australia in the Nineteenth Century', *Health and History*, 6 (2004), pp. 113–24 (see, in particular, pp. 117, 119). For age-specific death rates for adult males in England and Wales in 1861, see S.H. Preston, N. Keyfitz and R. Schoen, *Causes of Death: Life Tables for National Populations* (New York, 1972), p. 224.

Mauritius were mostly earlier. Hence it seems possible that measures to improve sanitation and hygiene were less developed than in later voyages to other colonies.

A major gap in our knowledge relates to the specific diseases to which migrants succumbed. Surgeons' reports that included the ascribed causes of death are available for some British slave vessels in the late eighteenth century, and for British convict and emigrant ships bound for Australia.[7] But these were atypical voyages, as their mortality, as will be discussed below, had already declined to a relatively low level. The surgeons' reports also give the date of each death over the length of the passage. For slave voyages in the late eighteenth century and British emigrant voyages to South Australia in the nineteenth century, most deaths occurred in the middle of the voyage, so the distribution of deaths had a humped shape on a graph.[8] Tracing individual deaths by cause of death over the course of the sea journey yielded an unexpected finding for the voyages of British emigrants to South Australia: epidemics of diseases, such as measles, did not burn out before the end of the three- or four-month passage.[9]

Mortality after Arrival

We also have quantitative estimates of the mortality suffered by slaves after arrival in the Americas during the 'selling period', which could be a protracted period lasting many weeks. It has been found that more deaths during the Middle Passage were associated with more deaths during the selling period, presumably because epidemics on the Middle Passage continued into the selling period.[10] Furthermore, it is well recognised in the literature that slaves encountered 'new' diseases in the Americas, such as tuberculosis and pneumonia, in the so-called 'seasoning period' of the first few years after arrival.[11]

Some of the best evidence we have of post-disembarkation mortality is for indentured Pacific Island and Indian labourers, both while housed in depots after arrival and during successive years of their contracts. Table 6.3 presents death rates for the initial two weeks spent in depots before allocation to employers, and for

---

[7] R.H. Steckel and R.A. Jensen, 'New Evidence on the Causes of Slave and Crew Mortality in the Atlantic Slave Trade', *Journal of Economic History*, 46 (1986), pp. 57–77; M. Staniforth, 'Diet, Disease and Death at Sea on the Voyage to Australia, 1837–1839', *International Journal of Maritime History*, 8 (1996), pp. 119–56; R. Haines and R. Shlomowitz, 'Causes of Death of British Emigrants on Voyages to South Australia, 1848–1885', *Social History of Medicine*, 16 (2003), pp. 193–208.

[8] Steckel and Jensen, 'New Evidence'; Haines and Shlomowitz, 'Causes of Death', p. 201. This humped-shaped distribution of deaths, however, is not confirmed for voyages of a Dutch company which also kept records of deaths for each day of the voyage; see Chapter 7.

[9] Haines and Shlomowitz, 'Causes of Death', pp. 201–2.

[10] Klein *et al.*, 'Transoceanic Mortality', tables 2, 10. See also Chapter 7, Table 7.2.

[11] P.D. Curtin, 'Epidemiology and the Slave Trade', *Political Science Quarterly*, 83 (1968), pp. 190–216. See also R. Shlomowitz, 'Introduction', in his *Mortality and Migration in the Modern World* (Aldershot, 1996).

Table 6.3 Mortality of Indian and Pacific Island migrant workers in Fiji

	Indians	Pacific Islanders
During residence in depots after arrival (rate per 1,000 per fortnight)[a]	2.4	25.3
During each year of the indenture (rate per 1,000 per year)[b]		
First	41.9	144.2
Second	34.9	52.5
Third	22.8	27.2
Fourth	20.6	
Fifth	19.6	

[a] For Indians, 1879–1916; for Pacific Islanders, 1878–1909.
[b] For Indians, 1885–1894; for Pacific Islanders, 1878–1881.

Source: R. Shlomowitz, 'Mortality and the Pacific Labour Trade', *Journal of Pacific History*, 22 (1987), pp. 34–55, see, in particular, pp. 44–5.

each year of their indenture in Fiji for Pacific Island workers (who were recruited from Vanuatu, the Solomon Islands, Papua New Guinea and Kiribati) and for Indian workers. Excess mortality (that is, deaths in excess of what would have been suffered if they had not migrated) during the first year of the indenture also occurred among Pacific Island migrants in Queensland, Papua New Guinea and the Solomon Islands.[12] The same mortality pattern also held for Indian migrants in diverse regions, including Assam and Malaya.[13] The explanation for the trend for mortality to be higher in the first year than subsequent years of the indenture will be discussed below.

This is a trend that is also evident in post-voyage death rates for convicts landed in Van Diemen's Land. Table 6.4 provides data for death rates at sea and during the first twelve months of colonial servitude for male prisoners arriving in the period 1830 to 1853.[14] While overall convict death rates in Australia were low

[12] R. Shlomowitz, 'Mortality and the Pacific Labour Trade', *Journal of Pacific History*, 22 (1987), pp. 34–55 (in particular, see pp. 47, 49); R. Shlomowitz, 'Epidemiology and the Pacific Labor Trade', *Journal of Interdisciplinary History*, 19 (1989), pp. 585–610 (in particular, see p. 596).
[13] R. Shlomowitz and L. Brennan, 'Mortality and Migrant Labour in Assam, 1865–1921', *Indian Economic and Social History Review*, 27 (1990), pp. 85–110 (see, in particular, pp. 95–100); R. Shlomowitz and L. Brennan, 'Mortality and Indian Labour in Malaya, 1877–1913', *Indian Economic and Social History Review*, 29 (1992), pp. 57–75 (see, in particular, p. 64). See also R. Shlomowitz and L. Brennan, 'Epidemiology and Indian Labour Migration at Home and Abroad', *Journal of World History*, 5 (1994), pp. 47–67.
[14] Tables 6.4, 6.5 and 6.6 employ data drawn from a wider Australian Research Council-funded project, 'Founders and Survivors: Australian Lifecourses in Historical Context', which we are conducting in conjunction with Janet McCalman, Gavan McCarthy, James Bradley and Shyamali Dharmarge from the University of Melbourne, Rebecca Kippen from the Australian National University and Alison Venn from the University of Tasmania. The aim of this work

Table 6.4 Monthly mortality of convicts in Van Diemen's Land 1830–53

Period	Rate per 1,000 per month
During voyage	2.3
During each month of the first year of servitude in the colony	
1	3.6
2	3.4
3	2.1
4	2.0
5	1.8
6	1.6
7	1.1
8	1.2
9	0.9
10	0.9
11	1.2
12	1.1

Source: Tables 6.4, 6.5 and 6.6 employ data drawn from a wider Australian Research Council-funded project, 'Founders and Survivors: Australian Lifecourses in Historical Context', examining the impact of convict transportation on the health and well-being of convicts and their descendants. The data used in these tables are drawn from 184 voyages which carried a total of 44,589 male convicts to Van Diemen's Land in the period 1830–53. Data on the length of passage, and the voyage and post-voyage death rates, have been obtained from C. Bateson, *The Convict Ships, 1787–1868* (Sydney, 2004), the Tasmanian Archives and Heritage Office description registers (CON 31, 32, 33) and death registers (CON 63 and 64), and the National Archives (Kew) musters for convicts in Van Diemen's Land (HO 10/38 and 10/47–52). See note 14 for more details.

relative to a similar-aged cohort in the British Isles, the death rate in the first two months after landing was higher than that suffered during the voyage.[15] Thereafter

is to examine the impact of convict transportation on the health and well-being of convicts and their descendants. The data used in these tables are drawn from 184 voyages which carried a total of 44,589 male convicts to Van Diemen's Land in the period 1830–53. Data on the length of passage, and the voyage and post-voyage death rates, have been obtained from C. Bateson, *The Convict Ships, 1787–1868* (Sydney 2004), the Tasmanian Archives and Heritage Office description registers (CON 31, 32, 33) and death registers (CON 63 and 64), and the National Archives (Kew) musters for convicts in Van Diemen's Land (HO 10/38 and 10/47–52). It should be noted that the death registers only cover the post-1840 period. A check against annual returns for the number of convicts dying while under sentence from 1830 to 1838 suggests that 10 per cent of all deaths were not recorded in shipping registers and musters (Tasmanian Archives, CSO1/700/15332). No such returns have been located for the post-1840 period, but better record-keeping and the high correspondence between death annotations added to description registers and the death registers suggest that the post-1840 data are more complete.

[15] The death rate for 20–24-year-old males in England and Wales in 1861 was 8.2 per thousand per year, rising to 8.4 for 25–29-year-olds and 10.1 for 30–34-year-olds. As can be seen from

the rate steadily declined until it stabilised after six months. In contrast to slave voyages to the Americas, encounters with 'new' diseases are unlikely to have been responsible for this elevation in the post-arrival death rate. There is no evidence that nineteenth-century Van Diemen's Land possessed a disease environment that was particularly lethal for Europeans. On the contrary, the evidence suggests that, like New Zealand, death rates for resident Europeans were actually lower than they were for the equivalent age groups in the British Isles.[16]

The particularly detailed records for convicts landed in Australia can be used to explore the factors that contributed to post-arrival death rates. These are the only data in the age of sail where it is has proved possible to study the link between mortality and migration at the individual level in order to measure the knock-on effects of excess mortality at sea. While these data provide no evidence that the length of a passage had an impact on post-arrival mortality, the level of morbidity encountered *en route* to Australia does appear to have had an effect on death rates post-arrival. As Table 6.5 demonstrates, convicts on those voyages that experienced at least one death were at greater risk of dying in the first year in the colony than those who arrived on mortality-free passages. Furthermore, those who arrived on the thirty-three voyages on which four or more deaths occurred experienced a 50 per cent higher death rate in the first year. Even on mortality-free voyages, however, there is evidence that the effects of a long passage at sea impacted upon post-arrival survival rates – suggesting the landing of some sick convicts from otherwise death-free voyages. Convicts landed from these voyages experienced twice the risk of death in the first two months that they did in the first year in the colony as a whole. Nevertheless, their risk of death in that first year was no greater than for troops stationed in barracks in the British Isles, a population recruited from a similar socioeconomic stratum of British and Irish society. Thereafter, the convict risk of mortality declined still further.

The comparison with death rates amongst soldiers is revealing for other reasons. Even ignoring losses on active service, soldiers experienced greater levels of mortality than civilian populations. Thus, the mean annual death rate for troops stationed in the British Isles in the period 1830–53 was 14.3 per thousand. This was approximately 40 per cent higher than civilian rates.[17] Troops stationed in Australia in the same period experienced a very similar death rate, of 14.5 per thousand. This is significantly higher than the death rate for the male convict population which, according to official returns, averaged just 10.6 per thousand in the period 1824–38 (excluding executions).[18] While it may seem anomalous that

---

Table 6.6, these rates are similar to those experienced by convicts in Australia after the effects of the voyage had diminished. The mean age of male convicts upon arrival in Australia was 26. See Preston *et al.*, *Causes of Death*, p. 224.

[16] Philip Curtin, *Death by Migration: Europe's Encounter with the Tropical World in the Nineteenth Century* (Cambridge, 1989), p. 7.

[17] Curtin, *Death by Migration*, p. 194.

[18] Tasmanian Archives CSO5/1/130/3087, CSO1/746/61110, CSO1/741/16030 and CSO49/7; and M. Austen, *The Army in Australia, 1840–50* (Canberra, 1979), pp. 209–46.

Table 6.5 Mortality during voyage and first year of arrival – male convicts landed in Van Diemen's Land 1830–53

Number of deaths at sea	Number of voyages	Number of convicts landed	Death rate in Van Diemen's Land (per 1,000 per year)		
			First 60 days	First 180 days	First year
None	45	9,475	34.4	21.8	15.6
One	45	10,573	36.9	22.7	17.2
Two or three	61	15,896	40.3	28.8	20.2
> three	33	8,253	57.9	38.1	24.2

Note: The number of deaths during the first 60 days after arrival and first 180 days after arrival have been expressed as a death rate per year.

Source: See Table 6.4 above.

convicts sentenced to penal servitude should die at a lesser rate than those sent out to guard them, the difference can probably be explained by the way that the two populations were distributed. Although upon arrival convicts were housed in barrack-style accommodation, most of them were quickly dispersed to private settlers for whom they worked as 'assigned servants'. Soldiers, on the other hand, were concentrated in military barracks and were therefore at greater risk of exposure to infectious diseases.

As it is likely that crowded accommodation elevated death rates, this makes it difficult to isolate the extent to which hard labour regimes were responsible for excess mortality. This is because convicts undergoing hard labour were routinely accommodated in barracks. The death rate at Macquarie Harbour penal station for example – a place of punishment notorious for its level of coercion – was thirty-three per thousand per year, or more than treble the death rate for the colony as a whole.[19] The extent to which this excess mortality was due to accommodation practices, diet, the harsh climate, labour regimes, or a combination of the above, is difficult to determine. The burial register for the penal settlement at Port Arthur, however, recorded the category of labour the convict was deployed in prior to death. This revealed that there was a huge disparity in mortality between those engaged in ganged and non-ganged labour, the former dying at a rate of forty-eight per thousand per year and the latter at just thirteen per thousand per year.[20] Since both groups were accommodated in the same settlement (the majority were housed in the principal barracks) these findings would suggest that

[19] Hamish Maxwell-Stewart, Closing Hell's Gates: The Death of a Convict Station (Sydney, 2008), p. 253.
[20] Hamish Maxwell-Stewart, 'The Rise and Fall of John Longworth: Work and Punishment in Early Port Arthur', Tasmanian Historical Studies, 6:2 (1999), p. 105.

Table 6.6 Annual mortality of convicts landed in Van Diemen's Land and Norfolk Island

Death rate	Assignment period 1830–9	Probation period 1840–53	Norfolk Island[2] 1843–6
During voyage (rate per 1,000 per month)	2.4	2.2	2.0
During each year of servitude (rate per 1,000 per year)			
First	17.5	20.3	33.0
Second	9.1	9.8	13.4
Third	8.7	9.0	15.4
Fourth	9.4	6.3	8.2
Fifth	9.4	6.8	8.9
Sixth	8.0	6.2	13.4

Note: Norfolk Island was primarily a place of secondary punishment for convicts who had been reconvicted in the Australian colonies. Between 1843 and 1846, however, a total of 1,697 male convicts were landed there from eight vessels arriving direct from the British Isles. These prisoners underwent probation on Norfolk Island before being transferred to Van Diemen's Land.

Source: Tasmanian Archives and Heritage Office: CON 31, 32, 33, 63 and 64. The National Archives (Kew): HO 10/38 and 10/47–52.

levels of labour and punishment, as well as the quality of rations received, played a role in influencing different mortality outcomes.

In 1840 a new system of convict management was introduced for male prisoners. Rather than being 'assigned' to private settlers, convicts instead had to undergo a stint of probationary hard labour on the roads. As Table 6.6 reveals, under this hard labour regime death rates in the first year in the colony rose. While the overall rate of increase was slight (and could possibly be attributed to the undercounting of deaths amongst the pre-1840 arrivals), the trend was particularly marked amongst those prisoners unfortunate enough to be landed on Norfolk Island. This was a place notorious for its hard labour regime. What is intriguing about these returns is that mortality rates on voyages to Norfolk Island were lower than those for voyages as a whole. While the effects of a long sea voyage were sufficient to elevate post-arrival mortality rates, the type of conditions and the levels of work convicts were subjected to after arrival may have had an impact too. Further study might help to throw fresh light on this issue. Surgeons' journals for convict voyages to Australia contain detailed information on morbidity.[21] These records will provide an opportunity to explore the link between sickness (as opposed to death) at sea and mortality on land. Since the individual returns

[21] TNA, ADM, 101 series.

for convicts disembarked in Van Diemen's Land provide information on rationing, accommodation, work and punishment, it should also be possible to assess the manner in which the consequences of a long sea passage may have worked in combination with local conditions to influence death rates.

Discussion

Two questions, in particular, have engendered much debate on the link between mortality and migration. What factors explain the excess mortality of slaves in the Middle Passage? And what explains the excess mortality suffered by indentured workers, particularly Pacific Island migrant workers, during their contracts of indenture?

One answer to both these questions is that migrants were exposed to new diseases to which they had not acquired immunity in their childhood disease environment. This explanation has most applicability to Pacific Islanders who were 'virgin soil' populations (that is, populations free of the infectious diseases that afflicted Europe, Asia and to a lesser extent Africa) before European intrusion into the Pacific. This explanation also has some applicability to slaves who had not been exposed to many European diseases in their childhood disease environment in Africa. An alternative answer is that migrants were exposed to harsh treatment, poor food, and crowded and insanitary living conditions. Both slaves and indentured workers, in addition, were exposed to a harsh work regime. It is inferred that improvements in these conditions would have reduced mortality. The blame for the excess mortality, according to this view, resides with Europeans in various roles such as ship captains and employers of labour.

Some of these arguments can be traced back to the anti-slavery campaigns of the late eighteenth and early nineteenth centuries. Those opposed to the slave trade argued that high mortality rates during the Middle Passage could be attributed to the greed of slavers who deliberately overcrowded their vessels in search of higher profits. The pro-slavery lobby emphasized that it was in the slavers' interests to land as many live slaves as possible – arguing instead that the problem of excess mortality was caused by the poor condition of the slaves at point of purchase on the African coast. This effectively shifted the blame for high mortality rates from European to African slaving practices.[22] We will attempt to show the various arguments historians have put forward to distinguish these explanations.

---

[22] Steckel and Jensen, 'New Evidence', p. 57.

The Middle Passage

A number of arguments have been put forward in the literature in support of the epidemiological explanation (that is, that slaves became exposed to 'new' diseases to which they lacked immunity), and the subsequent evaluation of these arguments illustrates how historians have debated this issue.

First, the marked variability in death rates of slave voyages from different African regions of departure has allowed some historians to infer that some African regions were more epidemiologically hostile than others.[23] Yet as the average death rate of slave voyages from each African region of departure was much higher than on voyages made by convicts, indentured servants and free migrants, this type of evidence alone cannot explain why slaves were at such greater risk of mortality.

A second type of evidence employed in support of the epidemiological argument relies on the results of statistical tests of association between death rates and a measure of crowding: the 'passenger-per-ton' ratio. Using this ratio, it has been argued that statistical tests indicate that decreased crowding would not have reduced mortality – hence indirectly supporting the view that it was slaves' lack of immunity to disease that caused mortality, rather than crowding. However, we would argue that this is an incorrect extrapolation from the statistical findings: those employing these arguments are extrapolating a narrow range of passenger-per-ton ratios on slave voyages to non-slave voyages, which is statistically irregular as the passenger-per-ton ratio was much higher on slave than on non-slave vessels. We would therefore argue that there is no convincing evidence that mortality was not influenced by crowding, rather than lack of immunity.

Thirdly, it has been argued that as most slave deaths occurred early in the Middle Passage, they could be attributed to pre-embarkation conditions.[24] More recent research, however, shows that most deaths did not occur early in the voyage.[25] A fourth argument has suggested that a comparison of slave mortality with the mortality suffered by related seaborne populations who were subject to less severe mistreatment can yield insights into why slaves were at such increased risk of death. The European crews of slave vessels are one such group: it has been found that their death rates were comparable to those of slaves, and when mortality was high for slaves on particular vessels, the crews were also at increased risk.[26] It is not clear, however, why the crews were also at such increased risk, since their immunities and susceptibilities (to malaria and yellow fever, in particular) differed from those of the slaves on board their vessels. The mortality suffered

[23] Klein et al., 'Transoceanic Mortality', table 6.

[24] J.C. Miller, 'Mortality in the Slave Trade: Statistical Evidence on Causality', Journal of Interdisciplinary History, 11 (1980), pp. 385–434.

[25] Steckel and Jensen, 'New Evidence', p. 62; Chapter 7, this volume, Figure 7.3; Robin Haines, J. McDonald and Ralph Shlomowitz, 'Mortality and Voyage Length in the Middle Passage Revisited', Explorations in Economic History, 38 (2001), pp. 503–33.

[26] Klein et al., 'Transoceanic Mortality', table 11. See also S.D. Behrendt, 'Crew Mortality in the Transatlantic Slave Trade in the Eighteenth Century', Slavery and Abolition, 18 (1997), pp. 49–71.

by another group, the so-called 'liberated Africans', has also attracted attention in this literature. Liberated Africans were ex-slaves who had been captured by the Royal Navy as part of Britain's anti-slavery campaign and escorted to Sierra Leone and other places where British Admiralty and International Mixed Commission courts met. Many of these ex-slaves were trans-shipped to the West Indies as indentured servants. Initially, their death rates were comparable to those suffered in the transatlantic slave trade, but after 1850 their death rates declined markedly (see Table 6.1).[27]

A corollary of the epidemiological hypothesis is that it was not possible to significantly reduce the death rate of slaves in the Middle Passage. Using the new W.E.B. Du Bois Institute database on the transatlantic slave trade, however, it has been shown that from the mid eighteenth century the British were able to significantly reduce death rates during the Middle Passage by setting in place a series of administrative reforms to reduce the exposure of slaves to infectious diseases.[28] These measures included a reduction in overcrowding, isolation of the sick, clean water, an improved diet, and paying much more attention to sanitation and private hygiene. The continued decline in death rates on the voyages of convicts, emigrants and indentured labour over the following century was, accordingly, due to a progressive tightening of these administrative reforms. (And it is notable that a similar decline in mortality had been seen on board Royal Naval vessels.) Together these various arguments cast doubt on the suggestion that the extraordinarily high death rate suffered by African slaves in the Middle Passage was *mainly* due to their exposure to new diseases to which they lacked immunity.

The Colonial Plantation

There was, unfortunately, a lag in the introduction of public health measures to reduce mortality on colonial plantations, until the twentieth century. Although little could be done to ameliorate airborne diseases given the crowded conditions of plantation life, a reduction in the incidence of bacillary dysentery required the construction of latrines, and education in their use. Whereas ship populations were under close surveillance, reforms were more difficult to implement on plantations. Planters were usually reluctant to incur the expenditure necessary to maintain the health of their workers; they lacked the authority to implement many of these measures (such as making workers use latrines or designated defecation

---

[27] R. Shlomowitz, 'Mortality and Voyages of Liberated Africans to the West Indies, 1841–1867', *Slavery and Abolition*, 11 (1990), pp. 30–41.

[28] D. Eltis, S.D. Behrendt, D. Richardson and H.S. Klein (eds), *The Trans-Atlantic Slave Trade: A Database on CD-ROM* (Cambridge, 1999); Robin Haines and Ralph Shlomowitz, 'Explaining the Decline in Mortality in the Eighteenth-Century British Slave Trade', *Economic History Review*, 53 (2000), pp. 262–83. See also N. van Manen, 'Preventive Medicine in the Dutch Slave Trade, 1747–1797', *International Journal of Maritime History*, 18 (2006), pp. 129–85.

areas while working in the fields, and insisting that they only drink from protected wells, streams, and pools); and such measures were difficult to enforce due to the dispersed nature of the agricultural labour force.

The health problems of workers on colonial plantations were magnified when indentured workers were recruited from 'virgin soil' populations in the Pacific. That the excess mortality suffered by migrant Pacific Island workers can be attributed to their exposure to exotic diseases is shown in their much higher death rates as compared to Indian migrant labourers who worked on the same plantations in Fiji, so facing identical work and environmental conditions (see Table 6.3). It is also shown in the pattern of mortality: the highest death rates occurred immediately after the arrival of Pacific Island migrant workers in Fiji, before planter coercion or poor work and living conditions had time to destroy their health (see Table 6.3). A further telling piece of evidence is that whereas tuberculosis usually took a chronic course among Europeans, it usually appeared as an acute rapidly progressive disease, with a high fatality rate, among migrant Pacific Islanders, reflecting their lack of previous exposure to the disease.[29]

Conclusion

This survey has attempted to bring together estimates of the mortality suffered by various migrant populations before embarking on their sea voyage, during this voyage, and shortly after their arrival. It has highlighted the various hypotheses that historians have advanced to explain why slaves were so much more at risk than non-slave populations, and the eventual decline in mortality on both slave and non-slave voyages, and the arguments historians have used to distinguish among these hypotheses. The survey has also highlighted the debate over the causes of the excess mortality of indentured Pacific Island workers soon after their arrival at their place of work. It has also indicated how work on the relationship between on-board morbidity and post-disembarkation labour management and punishment regimes in convict Australia may help to throw further light on these issues. The link between mortality and migration remains an exciting area for future research.[30]

Of course in any survey there is always a danger of losing sight of the individual. It is important to remind ourselves that the trans-oceanic migrations that played such a prominent role in shaping the modern world came at a price. The deaths that occurred on the journey to the coast, at the point of embarkation, at sea and after arrival were individual tragedies, the details of which will only be known for the vast majority in the aggregate. There are exceptions, however, and

---

[29] Shlomowitz, 'Epidemiology', table 12.
[30] One such area is morbidity. See, for example, R.V. Jackson, 'Sickness and Health on Australia's Female Convict Ships, 1821–1840', *International Journal of Maritime History*, 18 (2006), pp. 65–84.

we will end by relating just one. John Popjoy not only survived the voyage in a convict vessel to Australia, but succeeded in gaining a free pardon and a voyage back home to the British Isles. Tattoo not withstanding, he met his end when the vessel he was working was blown onto a sandbank off Boulogne and wrecked.[31]

7

Slave Purchasing Strategies and Shipboard Mortality: Day-to-Day Evidence from the Dutch African Trade, 1751–1797

Simon J. Hogerzeil and David Richardson

Ever since British abolitionists first highlighted the issue in the 1780s, the mortality of enslaved Africans in the Middle Passage from Africa to America has been a preoccupation of scholars studying the Atlantic slave trade. Following Curtin's pioneering work on the epidemiology of the slave trade in the late 1960s, discoveries of new shipping data have allowed major strides to be made in tracking long-run trends in slave mortality.[1] Such data have also been used to evaluate possible causes of shipboard mortality of slaves. Historians now tend to give less credence to the impact of crowding of slaves on board ship, intensive though that was by most historic standards, and prefer instead to place greater weight on the place of embarkation of captives in Africa and on declining levels of shipboard epidemics as factors in shaping mortality trends.[2] In this respect, the trends in mortality are seen as reflective of broader changes in public health and disease prevention in the Atlantic world.[3] Despite the tendency of shipboard mortality of slaves to fall, notably in the eighteenth century, the loss of slaves in transit

---

[1]   See, for example, Herbert S. Klein, *The Middle Passage* (Princeton, 1978); Raymond L. Cohn and Richard A. Jensen, 'The Determinants of Slave Mortality Rates on the Middle Passage', *Explorations in Economic History*, 19 (1982), pp. 269–82; David Eltis, 'Mortality and Voyage Length in the Middle Passage: New Evidence from the Nineteenth Century', *Journal of Economic History*, 44 (1984), pp. 301–18; Raymond L. Cohn, 'Deaths of Slaves in the Middle Passage', *Journal of Economic History*, 45 (1985), pp. 685–92; Richard H. Steckel and Richard A. Jensen, 'New Evidence on the Causes of Slave and Crew Mortality in the Atlantic Slave Trade', *Journal of Economic History*, 46 (1986), pp. 57–77; Herbert S. Klein and Stanley L. Engerman, 'Slave Mortality on British Ships 1791–1797', in Roger Anstey and P.E.H. Hair (eds), *Liverpool, the African Slave Trade and Abolition* (Liverpool, 1976), pp. 113–26; Herbert S. Klein, Stanley L. Engerman, Robin Haines and Ralph Shlomowitz, 'Transoceanic Mortality: The Slave Trade in Comparative Perspective', *William and Mary Quarterly*, 58 (2001), pp. 93–117.
[2]   Klein and Engerman, 'Slave Mortality'.
[3]   Robin Haines and Ralph Shlomowitz, 'Explaining the Decline in Mortality in the Eighteenth Century British Slave Trade', *Economic History Review*, 53 (2000), pp. 262–83.

remained an inevitable part of the slave trade, a fact reflected in the insurance policies for slave voyages. Until now, however, the relationship between slave mortality and purchasing strategies of traders on the African coast has been only vaguely understood. A critical constraint to understanding the relationship is the lack of data relating to patterns of slave purchases in Africa by shipmasters and the actual time spent on board ship by slaves. This essay sheds light on both these issues.

Slave mortality has been pivotal to discussions of the 'Middle Passage' from Africa to the Americas. Historians typically define it as starting when ships left the coast. For each slave, however, it actually began as soon as he or she boarded ship. This might be weeks, if not months, before the ship began its voyage to the Americas. Moreover, a considerable number of enslaved Africans died before the Atlantic crossing. Understanding how shippers adapted their purchasing strategies to the risks of slave mortality in transit, and how this affected survival rates, requires redefining the Middle Passage to embrace the whole time spent by slaves on board ship. In other words, we have to shift attention from the merchant's point of view to the slave experience. Only then will we be able further to advance understanding of slave mortality or survival in transit and the factors that helped to shape mortality and survival.

This chapter focuses on day-to-day slave purchasing strategies pursued by masters of thirty-nine Dutch voyages to 'Guinea' (or West Africa) for slaves in 1751 to 1797, when the slave trade in general and the Dutch slave trade in particular were at their height. It also examines day-to-day slave mortality between the first purchase and final sale of slaves for the same voyages and the factors associated with it. The chapter falls into four sections. The first discusses the sources used and the methodology adopted to analyse them. The second describes the slave purchasing strategies followed by shipmasters and explores some of the reasons underlying them. The third examines the relationship between purchasing strategies and shipboard mortality of slaves. The final section outlines the implications of our findings for understanding the Middle Passage and slave mortality on board ship.

Sources and Methodology

The Middelburgsche Commercie Compagnie (hereafter MCC) was a Dutch company that dispatched some 118 slaving voyages to Africa between the 1730s and 1790s. Its records are among the most detailed of all slave-trading groups. They have long attracted the attention of students of the slave trade, but to our knowledge they have not previously been used to reconstruct the day-by-day slave purchase and slave mortality patterns that the high survival rate of logs, journals and other papers for MCC ships makes possible. Records of this sort exist for seventy MCC slaving voyages (60 per cent of known voyages); of these thirty-nine are for voyages destined for West Africa or 'Guinea', and thirty-one for West Central Africa, principally the Loango Coast. We shall focus here on the Guinea voyages. 'Guinea' in this context is defined as the coastal area between the River

Senegal in the north and Cape Lopez in the south and comprises Senegambia, Sierra Leone, the Windward Coast, the Gold Coast, the Bight of Benin (or Slave Coast), and the Bight of Biafra.[4]

Appendix I summarises the data on the names of the ships, masters and surgeons as well as on ships' tonnages and voyage schedules for the thirty-nine voyages included in this study. Thirty-six of the thirty-nine voyages were dispatched before 1780, the remaining three in 1788–94. All but one ship returned home to Middelburg after journeying to Africa and thence to America with slaves. Even the one ship that failed to complete its triangular voyage – the *Zang Godin*, which sailed in 1773 – delivered slaves to America before being abandoned as unseaworthy. Fourteen different ships made these thirty-nine voyages, with just over half the voyages (twenty out of thirty-nine) being made by just four ships – the *Willem V*, *Philadelphia*, *Johanna Cores*, and *Nieuwe Hoop*. Concentration of management of voyages was much lower, however, for no less than twenty different captains were involved in the voyages. Only two made more than two voyages in this capacity. Of the twenty-nine surgeons involved, only one made more than two voyages. Such patterns of management do not appear unusual in the eighteenth-century slave trade.[5] By contrast, the mean time taken to complete the MCC voyages in our sample group – 572 days (ranging from 357 to 1,370 days) – was seemingly longer than that of contemporary British and French traders.[6] One important factor determining this was time spent at the African coast, a point to which we return later.

In common with other ships logs, those of the MCC provide daily reports on ship location, wind strength and direction, and rainfall from the start until the conclusion of voyages. What distinguishes the MCC records from those of other traders is that logs are often accompanied by trade books that provide daily

---

[4] All the primary materials used in this paper are from the MCC records at Zeeuws Archief in Middelburg, Netherlands. The document numbers for the thirty-nine voyages studied are 391–97, 511–17, 537–41, 542–45, 748–51, 775–80, 781–86, 830–36, 837–41, 842–47, 853–57, 858–62, 896–902, 903–09, 910–15, 916–21, 922–28, 968–72, 973–77, 994–98, 999–1003, 1004–12, 1103–10, 1125–29, 1153–59, 1189–92, 1193–97, 1217–21, 1234–38, 1239–45, 1246–51, 1252–56, 1302–06, 1312–17, 1385–90, 1391–96, 1397–1401, 1405–10, and 1411–18.

[5] Most captains had made earlier voyages in a lower rank or to a different region. In a sub-analysis, muster rolls for all the MCC voyages with complete documents (70 out of 118, including the 39 voyages in our study) were studied to estimate the work experience of captain and surgeon. These rolls list the full name, rank, date of entry on board ship, date of death or departure from service, salary and advance payments for each crew enlisted. In our sample, captains were generally more experienced than surgeons. With median experience the captain would be on his fourth slaving venture (second time as a captain) for the MCC, but the surgeon would have no previous experience at all. We can discount that captains may have acquired earlier experience with other companies. Our MCC findings are, nevertheless, consistent with claims that most slave captains had earlier worked as junior officers in other trades (see Stephen D. Behrendt, 'The Captains in the British Slave Trade from 1785 to 1807', *Transactions of the Historic Society of Lancashire and Cheshire*, 140 (1991), pp. 79–140) and returned several times to the same area; see David Eltis, *The Rise of African Slavery in the Americas* (Cambridge, 2000), p. 135.

[6] David Eltis and David Richardson, 'Productivity in the Transatlantic Slave Trade', *Explorations in Economic History*, 32 (1995), pp. 465–84.

accounts of slave purchases, deaths and sales. In almost every case the age and sex of the slaves concerned is noted. Interspersed with these data are accounts of coastal purchases of water, food, wood and other consumables, as well as periodic inventories of slaves on board, purchased and dead. The last provide useful cross-references for our own calculations of the same. For the most part, the causes of the slaves' deaths are not reported, but there are anecdotal reports of accidental deaths, suicides, uprisings and epidemics, notably of smallpox, scurvy and diarrhoea. Reports relating to the crew paralleled those relating to slaves.[7]

Combined into one dataset, the MCC records permit a day-to-day reconstruction of life and death on thirty-nine slaving voyages to Guinea in the second half of the eighteenth century. The total number of enslaved Africans involved in these voyages was 9,880. To facilitate analysis of their experience, we divided voyages into five phases: (1) the journey from Middelburg to the first place of purchase of slaves; (2) the purchase or trading period in Africa (hereafter the 'loading phase'); (3) the sailing time from last place of purchase in Africa to the principal place of slave sale in the Americas (conventionally known as the 'Middle Passage', but hereafter the 'crossing phase'); (4) the time spent in the Americas selling slaves and obtaining a return cargo (or 'selling phase'); and (5) the homeward voyage. In this essay we concentrate on phases (2) to (4) when slaves were on board ship.

Following Curtin's pioneering census of the slave trade published in 1969, historians have typically divided trading locations in Atlantic Africa into seven regions – Senegambia, Sierra Leone, Windward Coast, Gold Coast, Bight of Benin, Bight of Biafra and West Central Africa.[8] We have followed the same procedure in analysing the data of our thirty-nine MCC voyages, one of which, though initially destined for Guinea, completed its loading in West Central Africa. Where the specific location of any slave purchase was not given, we assumed this was the same as those for immediately adjacent days of slave purchase. The key variables used to track daily events through time were location (or port); number of slaves traded and number of slaves who died, each by age and sex; number of crew entering or leaving the ship; and number of crew deaths. Data describing location were cross-matched between the logbooks and trade journals. Where there was conflict between sources, preference was given to data from trade journals. Cross-matching slave purchase data with muster rolls and ship specifications allowed us to calculate packing levels of slaves through time and to assess the experience of particular shipmasters and surgeons in handling slaves.

---

[7]   One of the authors (SJH) was surprised to read in one of the captain's logs (MCC 844; 17 June 1771) that thirteen checks worth 26,626 Dutch guilders had been entrusted to a certain captain Martynus Bruijne Hoogerzeyl of the ship *De Meermin*, for transport from Paramaribo to Middelburg. The Hogerzeil genealogy revealed that Martynus's father, whaling commander Bruin Okkerse Hoogerzeyl, was the brother of the author's seventh-generation grandfather, commander Michiel Okkers Hoogerzeyl (1696–1779). Mixed feelings about this family link were confirmed when another log book (MCC 1239; 24 February 1765) identified Martynus as captain of *De Meermin*, arriving in Paramaribo with 328 slaves from Angola.

[8]   For the original classification see Philip D. Curtin, *The Atlantic Slave Trade: A Census* (Madison, 1969).

For the reconstruction of patterns of slave mortality on board ship one ideally requires data allowing one to construct 'life tables' describing the number of days on board ship from initial purchase to sale or death of each individual slave in the sample. Such information is available for only one voyage in our sample.[9] The next best option is to calculate daily hazards and exposure-based death rates of slaves. Daily hazard is defined as the number of slave deaths per day relative to the total number on board on that particular day. It can be calculated for both slaves and crew and in the case of slaves disaggregated for both age and sex. Exposure is the sum of the days spent on board ship by a group of people expressed in person-years (or py). This provides the denominator for a calculation of the true death rate on board ship, reported as the number of deaths per thousand person-years exposure (or d/py). The use of true death rates in captivity allows for a standardized comparison of slave and crew mortality across different groups and periods. It is also to be distinguished from the percentage loss in transit, which relates to the total number of slave deaths as a proportion of slave purchases irrespective of the length of the voyage or the time spent on board ship, and which has been the primary measure of slave mortality used in most studies of shipboard mortality since the late 1960s.

Slave Purchasing Strategy

We begin our analysis by looking at the time spent on board ship by slaves and at the underlying slave purchasing strategies of MCC shipmasters. In investigating these issues we use pooled data for 9,880 slaves purchased across the thirty-nine voyages (mean purchase 253 slaves, ranging from 71 to 390). As a group, these 9,880 slaves were actually on board ship for 61.3 per cent (or 13,646 days) of the 22,238 days taken to complete the voyages. Put another way, the typical MCC slaving voyage to Guinea in 1751 to 1797 lasted some 570 days (or nineteen months) (95 per cent confidence interval (hereafter CI) 513–627 days), during which the ship would have some slaves on board for 350 days (95 per cent CI 316–383 days), or just under a year. The last figure includes 223 days (95 per cent CI 199–247 days) in the loading phase, seventy-one days (95 per cent CI 65–77 days) in the crossing phase, and fifty-six days (95 per cent CI 42–70 days) in the selling phase. The mean length of time spent by MCC ships in the crossing does not appear exceptional in the period 1750–75, but the Company's ships do seem to have spent much longer than those of other carriers acquiring slaves in Africa.[10] To our knowledge,

[9] This was the voyage of the *Philadelphia* which left Middelburg in 1754 (Zeeuws Archief, 903–09) and is listed as voyage 6 in Appendix I.

[10] Evidence in the revised edition of the Atlantic slave trade database, first published in 1999 and now available at www.slavevoyages.com, shows that the mean time between first purchase of slaves and departure from last place of purchase for ships trading in West Africa in 1754 to 1797 was 138.56 days (N = 1245; StD = 98.79), or some 85 days less than we compute for the thirty-nine MCC voyages in our sample (David Eltis, Stephen D. Behrendt, David Richardson

however, there are no data currently available on the ratio of days with slaves on board to total voyage days. This ratio – roughly six out of ten days in these thirty-nine MCC voyages and, when allowance is made for longer loading times by MCC ships, perhaps five out of ten days on most other voyages – underlines the need for historians to re-consider the concept of the 'Middle Passage' to include the time spent by slaves on board ship before departing the shores of their homeland. More specifically, the fact that MCC ships typically took up to six or even eight months in 1751–97 to acquire a shipload of slaves requires us to take account of the pace at which slaves were acquired in Africa when seeking to assess life and death on board slave ships.[11]

It is possible to ascertain the African coastal place of purchase of over 99 per cent of the slaves acquired by the thirty-nine MCC voyages in our sample. All but one of the ships began their purchase of slaves at Upper Guinea, which comprised the sub-regions of Senegambia, Sierra Leone and the Windward Coast west of the Gold Coast; the Windward Coast was by far the most common initial trading destination. However, Upper Guinea was not the only source of slaves for these MCC ships, for while typically starting trade there, most went on to complete their purchase of slaves further south, with the Gold Coast being the preferred destination for the great majority. This pattern is underlined by the data shown in Table 7.1, which shows that of the 9,880 slaves bought by MCC ships, 6,718 (or 68.0 per cent) were taken at the Windward Coast and 2,224 (or 22.5 per cent) at the Gold Coast. The remaining 938 slaves (or 9.5 per cent) were taken at various places north of the Windward Coast or east and south of the Gold Coast. This pattern of trade differentiated that of the MCC ships from that of British, British colonial and French traders. They sometimes purchased whole complements of slaves at the Windward Coast. In other cases they collected a few slaves, *troque au vol* (in chance or casual barter), as they sailed along the Sierra Leone coast and Windward Coast to places further south.[12] Rarely, however, do they seem to have acquired two-thirds of their slaves *troque au vol* and the remainder at markets

and Manolo Florentino, *The Transatlantic Slave Trade, 1527–1867: A Revised and On-line Data-base* [www.slavevoyages.com]). On crossing times, data for all carriers suggest that the mean time for crossing was 81 days in 1751–75 (N = 785 voyages). For ships leaving the Gold Coast, it was 84 days (N = 144) (Eltis *et al.*, *Slave Trade Database*). The annual total number of slaves purchased by ships in our sample decreased over the period studied, from ± 450 per year in the 1750s to ± 100 in the 1790s (r^2=0.235, p=0.013). Over the same period the mean crowding during the Middle Passage halved from 2.1 to 0.9 slaves per ton (r^2=0.43, p<0.001). This is in line with earlier studies (Haines and Shlomowitz, 'Explaining the Decline in Mortality'). The finding of Steckel and Jensen ('New Evidence') that the loading phase and Middle Passage became shorter over the years was not confirmed in our study. Yearly slave death rates did not decrease for the loading phase and the crossing, despite less crowding.

[11] James C. Riley, 'Mortality in Long-Distance Voyages in the Eighteenth Century', *Journal of Economic History*, 41 (1981), pp. 651–6, p. 653.

[12] Examples of such trade can be found in the diaries of the the slave-trader-turned-abolitionist, John Newton, who took in slaves at Sierra Leone and the Windward Coast in three voyages he commanded in 1750 to 1753: see Bernard Martin and Mark Spurrell (eds), *The Journal of a Slave Trader (John Newton), 1750–1754* (London, 1962), pp. 27, 50, 75, 90.

Table 7.1 Numbers of slaves purchased per region
during the loading phase

	N	Days (%)	Traded (%)	Men (%)	Women (%)	Boys (%)	Girls (%)
Senegambia	1	10 (0.1)	33 (0.3)	13 (0.3)	19 (0.5)	1 (0.1)	0 (0.0)
Sierra Leone	5	18 (0.2)	25 (0.3)	6 (0.1)	14 (0.4)	3 (0.3)	2 (0.2)
Windward Coast	36	5,507 (63.3)	6,718 (68.0)	2,709 (62.9)	2,568 (69.9)	811 (74.9)	630 (77.2)
Gold Coast	34	1,650 (19.0)	2,224 (22.5)	1,189 (27.6)	819 (22.3)	148 (13.7)	68 (8.3)
Bight of Benin	3	130 (1.5)	211 (2.1)	102 (2.4)	71 (1.9)	12 (1.1)	26 (3.2)
Bight of Biafra	5	578 (6.6)	190 (1.9)	44 (1.0)	63 (1.7)	38 (3.5)	45 (5.5)
W. C. Africa	1	129 (1.5)	387 (3.9)	186 (4.3)	93 (2.5)	64 (5.9)	44 (5.4)
Unknown	35	680 (7.8)	88 (0.9)	56 (1.3)	25 (0.7)	6 (0.6)	1 (0.1)
Total sample	**39**	**8,702**	**9,880**	**4,305**	**3,672**	**1,083**	**816**

Note: As noted in the text, in this essay Guinea is defined as comprising Senegambia, Sierra Leone, the Windward Coast, the Gold Coast, the Bight of Benin and the Bight of Biafra. Slaves with an unknown place of purchase were very largely if not wholly bought within the boundaries of Guinea as defined here. 'N' represents the number of ships having spent one day or more in a specific region; 'Days' the number of days spent in a specific region; 'Traded' the net number of slaves purchased in a specific region.

Source: Middelburgsche Commercie Compagnie 1751–97.

further south. The unusual sequential regional pattern of slave purchases by MCC ships probably helps to explain their slow turnaround times in West Africa in 1751–97, noted earlier. It also needs to be taken into account when exploring not only the levels and patterns of shipboard slave mortality on MCC ships but also how far they were representative of the trade more generally.

At the Windward Coast, MCC ships spent about 153 days (95 per cent CI 132–174 days) acquiring slaves, whereas at the Gold Coast purchases took about forty-nine days (95 per cent CI 38–59 days). Slaves were acquired at the Windward Coast at various places, with no single location predominating. Some spreading of purchases across trading venues was also evident at the Gold Coast, but 44 per cent of slaves taken there were bought at Elmina and a similar percentage at Anomabu, Apam and Axim combined. Widening the perspective to the regional level again, the implication of the regionally sequential patterns of purchase was that two-thirds of the slaves in our sample – mostly those purchased at the Windward Coast – spent up to six months longer (or 48–200 days) on board ship than the rest.

As Elmina was a major trading venue for Dutch slave ships from the late seventeenth century onwards, it is unsurprising that MCC ships purchased over 40 per cent of their Gold Coast slaves there.[13] More surprising is the fact that up to two-thirds of the slaves acquired by MCC ships trading to Guinea came from the Windward Coast. Dutch traders certainly visited this region from the late seven-

---

[13] On Dutch trading patterns before 1750, see Johannes M. Postma, *The Dutch in the Atlantic Slave Trade, 1600–1815* (Cambridge, 1990).

Figure 7.1 Mean numbers of slaves purchased per week during the loading phase

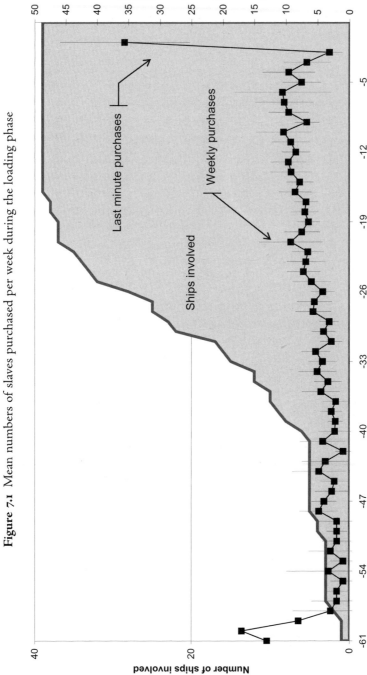

Note: Time-units are expressed as the number of weeks before departure. The numbers of slaves purchased are defined as mean numbers purchased per week for the number of ships involved, and are plotted with 95 per cent confidence intervals.

Source: Middelburgsche Commercie Compagnie 1751–97.

teenth century, but the second West India Company, which dominated Dutch slaving before its demise in 1730, seems largely to have neglected it as a source of slaves.[14] The trading pattern of the MCC probably represented, therefore, an innovation in Dutch slaving activity, which, when combined with simultaneous moves by British traders and British colonial traders, contributed to a remarkable upsurge in slave exports from the Windward Coast in the third quarter of the eighteenth century.[15] This, in turn, seems to have been a response to more general pressures on slave supply in other regions of West Africa in the face of growing international slave exports after 1750.[16] In the case of MCC ships, concentration of slave purchase at the Windward Coast may also have reflected a decline of Dutch competitiveness relative to the British and French in the larger Gold Coast, Slave Coast and Bight of Biafra slave markets after the demise of the second West India Company. In the MCC period, the French dominated the Slave Coast and the British the Bight of Biafra and to a lesser extent the Gold Coast.

During their stay in Africa, MCC ships trading at Guinea (defined as rows 1–6 of Table 7.1) acquired some 1.19 slaves per day on average. This was lower than loading rates achieved by British ships trading to Sierra Leone and the Gold Coast in 1791 to 1797, but broadly similar to daily loading rates of Liverpool ships trading at the Windward Coast and Gold Coast in 1750 to 1775 computed by other means.[17] Unlike earlier estimations, however, rates derived from MCC accounts allow us to quantify and visualize short-term fluctuations in the rate and sex and age distribution of slave purchases across the whole loading phase, thereby exposing previously unknown features of the process. Purchasing strategies typically involved buying a few slaves every few days, with ships actually taking on board small clusters of slaves less than twice per week during their stay in Africa. During most of the purchase period, this pattern of acquisition was fairly homogeneous or constant, as is shown in Figure 7.1, with slaves being acquired at the rate of up to five a week up to twenty weeks before departure from Africa, and rising to about eight a week (95 per cent CI 7.3–8.8 slaves) between twenty and six weeks before departure. But during the last four weeks of loading, acquisition patterns changed for all ships, but particularly for those finishing off their purchase at the Gold Coast. The records for the thirty-two

---

[14] Ibid.
[15] On the broader picture of the shift towards the Windward Coast, see David Richardson, 'Slave Exports from West and West-Central Africa, 1700–1810: New Estimates of Volume and Distribution', *Journal of African History*, 30 (1989), pp. 1–22; David Eltis, 'The Volume and Structure of the Atlantic Slave Trade: A Reassessment', *William and Mary Quarterly*, 58 (2001), pp. 17–46.
[16] On lengthening loading times between 1725 and 1775, see Eltis and Richardson, 'Productivity in the Transatlantic Slave Trade'.
[17] For the 1791–7 estimates, see B.K. Drake, 'The Liverpool–African Voyage, c.1790–1807: Commercial Problems', in Roger Anstey and P.E.H. Hair (eds), *Liverpool, the African Slave Trade, and Abolition* (Liverpool, 1976), p. 155; for those for 1750–5, see Paul E. Lovejoy and David Richardson, '"This horrid hole": Royal Authority, Commerce and Credit at Bonny, 1690–1840', *Journal of African History*, 45 (2004), p. 379.

Figure 7.2 An illustration of age- and sex-specific purchasing strategies: voyage no. 10

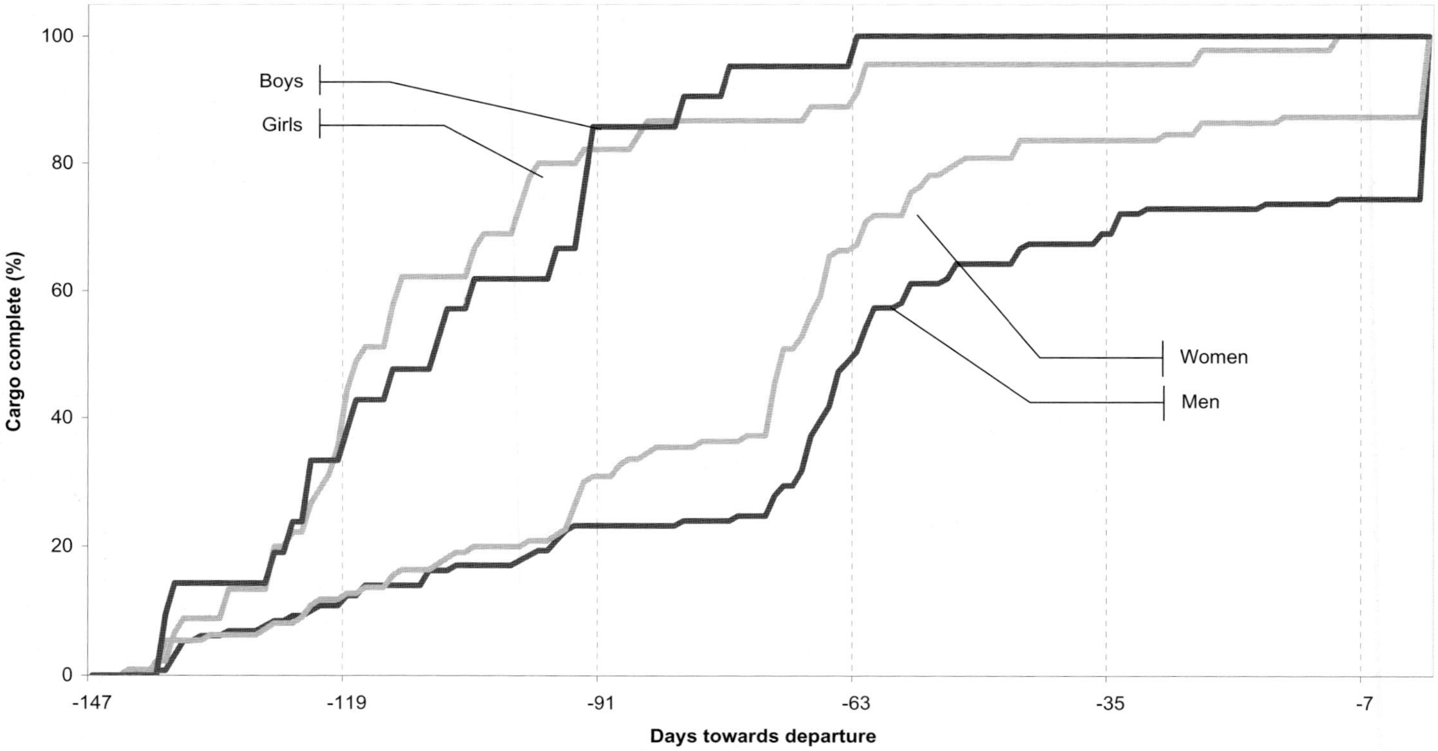

Note: Numbers on board by age and sex are expressed as a percentage of the final cargo, and should not be confused with absolute numbers. Time-units are expressed as the number of days before departure; vertical gridlines indicate one-month intervals.

Source: Middelburgsche Commercie Compagnie 1751–97: an illustration of purchasing strategy on the *Philadelphia* sailing between 1756 and 1758.

ships in the last category show that most placed an order for a large number of slaves about a month before departure. An easing of loading rates to about three slaves a week then ensued, to be followed by a surge of acquisitions to close to forty slaves a week just before departure. Indeed, of the 2,023 slaves acquired at Elmina, Anomabu, Apam and Axim on the Gold Coast, some 1,350 (or two-thirds) embarked during the last week of purchase. This pattern of loading is less evident for the remaining five ships in our sample.[18] Taking all ships in our sample, it appears that while the loading phase typically lasted eight months, over 78 per cent of the slaves were on board a month before the ship left the coast, and 21.8 per cent (or 2,151) of the 9,880 slaves embarked during the last month and 14.7 per cent (or 1,390) during the final week before sailing.

MCC accounts also provide day-to-day information on the age and sex of the slaves purchased. We do not know the age at which MCC shippers distinguished children from adults, but it was likely to have been around 14 years. Of the 9,880 slaves purchased in our sample, some 81 per cent were described as adult. Sex ratios were 55 per cent male, 45 per cent female. These proportions varied little by age or between voyages. Such age and sex distributions of slave purchases were broadly similar to those achieved by other carriers of slaves from the same regions and at the same time.[19] In this respect, at least, MCC voyages may be seen as representative of all voyages to the Windward Coast and Gold Coast after 1750. Further investigation of MCC accounts shows, however, that age and sex ratios of slave acquisitions commonly varied during the course of individual ship purchases, as illustrated for one typical voyage in Figure 7.2.

From the beginning, masters bought mixtures of slaves and, overall, bought more adults, including men, on the Windward Coast than in other parts of West Africa. Typically, however, they also tended to buy proportionately more girls and boys early in their purchase than throughout the whole purchase. Thus, half the final purchase of girls and boys was normally completed in less than 45 per cent of the total loading phase of ships. This contrasts with the purchase pattern for women and men, where half the purchase of slaves in these two categories was achieved only after 60 per cent and 69 per cent, respectively, of the loading phase. The implication of this is that the last-minute surge in purchases, described earlier, centred disproportionately on adults, especially men. This is underlined by the fact that whereas the typical voyage embarked between 6 per cent and 9 per cent of the total purchase of girls and boys during the final week on the coast, the

---

[18] A minority of five ships traded in the Bight of Biafra or Gabon during the final month. Numbers traded increase slightly towards the end (from four to six per week per ship), but show no peak during the final week (r=0.08, p=0.38). Interestingly, both groups show an unexpected decrease (p>0.34) in slave exposure during the final week, which could only be explained for the Gabon group in which one ship lost twenty-one slaves in a revolt two weeks before departure.

[19] The sex ratio for ships leaving Sierra Leone (which included the Windward Coast) in 1751–75 was 58.3 per cent male and 41.7 per cent female (N = 26 voyages). For the Gold Coast the ratio was 62.1 per cent male and 37.9 per cent female (N = 68) (Eltis et al., Slave Trade Database). Interestingly, the percentage of children on voyages from the Gold Coast in the same period was 21.4 per cent (N = 42 voyages) and from Sierra Leone was 34.7 per cent (N = 25).

same figures were 17 per cent and 12 per cent for men and women respectively. In short, the loading of adult slaves and especially men by MCC ships proceeded at a more uneven rate than that of children.

The combination of sequential sex-specific purchasing preferences and selective last-minute purchases had other important implications. It meant that, as most ships started trading at the Windward Coast, this region contributed proportionately more children to the final slave purchase than regions visited later. The reverse was true of the Gold Coast, which contributed proportionately more adults, especially men. Overall, seven times more children were taken from the Windward Coast than from the Gold Coast on our thirty-nine MCC voyages (1,441 compared to 216). For adults this ratio was just 2.5 (5,777 compared to 2,008). These ratios contrast with an overall ratio of slaves embarked in the two regions of three to one. Similar calculations show that the Gold Coast contributed a disproportionate share of the adult slaves taken by MCC ships from the two regions.

These age and sex patterns of slave purchase meant that, *ceteris paribus*, children would have been expected to spend more time on board ship than adults before MCC ships left the coast. Indeed, the MCC accounts show that on the day before they left Africa girls and boys had typically spent 132 days (95 per cent CI 115–150 days) and 124 days (109–139), respectively, on board ship whereas women had spent 101 days (86–116) and men just 91 days (70–113). In other words, children were typically exposed to on-board conditions for forty-one days longer on average than adults before the crossing started, and often much longer. Widening the perspective to include the crossing and selling phases of voyages, it appears that, while children comprised only 19 per cent of the slaves purchased by our MCC ships, they accounted for 23 per cent of the total exposure time lived by the 9,880 deportees on board ship. In other words, the slave purchasing strategies of MCC shippers put children at risk for longer periods of time than adults, particularly men.[20] This has important implications for interpreting the age- and sex-related shipboard slave mortality rates described later.

Explaining age- and sex-related slave purchasing strategies by MCC shippers is more difficult than documenting them. We have found no evidence in instructions to shipmasters from the MCC bearing on such matters, but evidence from other accounts reveals that masters trading to the Windward Coast were sometimes instructed to be selective in terms of the quality of, and price paid for, slaves early

---

[20] Aggregated for all voyages, ships spent more than three times as many days at the Windward Coast as at the Gold Coast (a ratio of 3.34), and bought three times (3.02) as many slaves accordingly. Naturally, given that numbers on board were much larger in later stages of the voyage, this translates to a smaller ratio in terms of slave exposure (1.53). But the fact that adults, and especially men, were purchased later is reflected in a relatively stronger shift for male and female exposure (to ratios of 1.36 and 1.46 respectively), and a somewhat weaker shift for boys and girls (1.96 and 1.95). This implies that, in terms of exposure to risk, the Windward Coast was relatively less important to adults than children.

in their transactions.[21] The precise strategy adopted by MCC shipmasters was likely to have been a response to several factors. The most obvious was that adult slaves, particularly males, were more expensive to buy than children. Premiums on prices of adult males varied widely over time and place, but rates for adult males of 20 per cent above the mean price for slaves were not uncommon, and the mark-up on adult males was even higher relative to children.[22] Price data found in MCC records confirm these impressions. As time spent on board ship was widely considered a health hazard for slaves, a deferral in purchasing high-value adult males was perhaps to be expected. In other words, it reflected a policy adjustment by MCC shippers to coastal price differentials among categories of slaves, largely dictated, it seems, by planter preferences for adult males in the Americas.[23]

It would be misleading, however, to attribute slave purchasing strategies by MCC shipmasters purely to coastal relative prices for slaves or to demand-side factors. Such strategies were conceivably shaped, too, by African-centred factors as well as perceptions of the shipboard survival capacity of different categories of slaves. The intensity of MCC activity at the Windward Coast after 1750 almost certainly reflected pressures on slave supply capacity as well as the strength of competition for slaves in other regions of Atlantic Africa at that time.[24] It brought MCC shippers, too, into contact with emergent slave supply systems that were perhaps less efficient than the well-established systems of the Gold Coast in satisfying shippers' preferences for slaves. This might explain the higher ratios of children and females taken by MCC ships from the Windward Coast relative to the Gold Coast. Differences in regional patterns of slave exports may also have been linked to a higher propensity of slaves shipped from the Windward Coast to rebel on board ship. This rebelliousness has been increasingly well documented by historians. It was attributed by some contemporaries not just to Windward Coast

[21] In 1768 David Tuohy, bound for the Windward Coast in a Liverpool ship, was told to 'Be very carefull in the beginning of your Purchase that the Slaves be Choice, and such as will stand, for you know, they will be considerably longer on Board, and are to stand the whole Purchase, this requires a particular nicity both in regard to the Quality of the Slaves, and in the Price, and not so Necessary to be Observed, at, or near the close of your Purchase when you are then lying at great Expence and Risk.' Folliott Powell, Hen[ry] Hardwar, Ja[me]s Clemens and Mat[thew] Stronge to Capt. David Tuohy, 9 July 1768, Liverpool Record Office, 380 TUO 4/3.
[22] On general price ratios, see Richard N. Bean, *The British Trans-Atlantic Slave Trade 1650–1750* (New York, 1975); David Eltis and David Richardson, 'Prices of African Slaves Newly Arrived in the Americas, 1673–1865: New Evidence on Long-Run Trends and Regional Differentials', in David Eltis, Frank Lewis and Kenneth Sokoloff (eds), *Slavery in the Development of the Americas: Essays in Honor of Stanley L. Engerman* (Cambridge, 2004), pp. 181–218.
[23] The premium of adult males at the coast contrasted sharply with the contemporary premium on females in the interior of West Africa, where demand for female labour was high; Paul E. Lovejoy and David Richardson, 'Competing Markets for Male and Female Slaves: Slave Prices in the Interior of West Africa, 1780–1850', *International Journal of African Historical Studies*, 28 (1995), pp. 261–93.
[24] On the general lengthening of loading times after 1750, see Eltis and Richardson 'Productivity in the Transatlantic Slave Trade'; Klein *et al.*, 'Transoceanic Mortality', p. 111. On coastal price trends see David Richardson, 'Prices of Slaves in West and West-Central Africa: Toward an Annual Series, 1698–1807', *Bulletin of Economic Research*, 43 (1991), pp. 21–46.

slaves but to adult males generally and those from the Gold Coast in particular.[25] The relative lateness in finalising the loading of adult males may therefore have been just as much an adjustment to fears of slave rebellion as to the price premium on adult male slaves. Whatever weight one attaches to particular factors, however, the slave purchasing strategies followed by MCC shippers were likely the rational outcome of a complex set of demand- and supply-side factors. We turn now to explore their relationship to shipboard mortality of slaves.

Shipboard Mortality

It is widely recognised that there was a large spread and skewed distribution of slave mortality on board ship from voyage to voyage and that this presents problems for establishing a meaningful measure of mortality levels.[26] The slave mortality experience on MCC ships was no exception.[27] The pooling of data relating to 9,980 slaves, however, enables us to discern some fairly clear and robust macroscopic trends in shipboard mortality on thirty-nine MCC voyages to Guinea between 1751 and 1797.[28] Our focus on such trends limits our capacity to interpret

---

[25] David Richardson, 'Shipboard Revolts, African Authority, and the Atlantic Slave Trade', *William and Mary Quarterly*, 58 (2001), pp. 69–92. There is evidence that outside Upper Guinea, which includes the Windward Coast, higher ratios of women were correlated to the incidence of slave ship revolts; Stephen D. Behrendt, David Eltis and David Richardson, 'The Costs of Coercion: African Agency in the Pre-Modern Atlantic World', *Economic History Review*, 54 (2001), pp. 454–76.

[26] Herbert S. Klein, *The Atlantic Slave Trade* (Cambridge, 2002), p. 136.

[27] In total, 1,290/9,880 (13 per cent) of the slaves purchased on our thirty-nine MCC voyages were lost in transit. This corresponds to a pooled death rate of 273 d/py for a total slave exposure of 4,724 person-years. If we restrict ourselves to the loading phase alone, the pooled death rate of the total sample was 203.66 d/py. However, the range of the rates for each of the thirty-nine voyages varied from 0 to 1235.49 with a mean of 198.96 (95 per cent CI 126.3–271.6) and a median of 129.39. Which of these values to report? The mean is not very reliable here because of the wide confidence interval. The 5 per cent trimmed-mean, which disregards high and low extremes, is 167.56. Still more sophisticated estimations of the centre (Huber's M-estimator, Tukey's Biweight, Hampel's M-estimator and Andrews' Wave) range from 260.30 to 262.68. Such wide differences in mortality between the voyages make it difficult to express that in one meaningful figure.

[28] Descriptions of trends in average mortality over two-week periods for the thirty-nine voyages in our sample yielded unworkable confidence intervals. Very wide short-term variations obscured any longer-term trend in mortality. Methodologically, pooling the daily mortality records per week or per month reduces the effect of extreme values and increases the statistical significance. This can be illustrated by correlating the death rates of the thirty-nine voyages with time from the start of loading in weekly (r=0.35) or monthly (r=0.417) periods. By pooling all voyages together, the correlations further increase over daily (r=0.170), weekly (r=0.604) or monthly (r=0.768) periods. The correlations seem stronger but the variance between voyages or details of time patterns disappear. By experimenting with shorter time spans and subsets for each sex and age group, various other (non-significant, non-linear) fluctuations can be visualised. They offer tempting hypotheses pertaining, amongst others, to differences in sex- and age-specific timing of mortality, but these cannot be verified as yet.

Table 7.2 Summary data for thirty-nine voyages

	Loading	Crossing	Selling	Total
Duration (days)				
Mean (95% CI)	223 (199–247)	70.97 (65–77)	55.79 (42–70)	349.89 (316–383)[e]
Median (range)	208 (112–427)	67 (45–130)	42 (3–222)	334 (207–728)
Trade deficit (slaves)				
Mean (95% CI)	253 (234–273)	0.00	-220.66 (201–240)	32.66 (22–43)[a]
Median (range)	260 (71–390)	0.00	-223 (45–349)	23 (2–71)
Exposure (person-years)				
Mean (95% CI)	65.95 (55–71)	45.22 (40–51)	12.94 (9–17)	121.12 (110–132)
Median (range)	60.42 (17–144)	45.72 (12–90)	8.58 (0–74)	118.13 (30–189)
Number of deaths (slaves)				
Mean (95% CI)	12.82 (9–17)	17.76 (10–26)	2.48 (1–4)	33.08 (22–44)[a]
Median (range)	8 (0–50)	10 (0–137)	1 (0–19)	22 (2–174)
Lost-in-transit (%)				
Mean (95% CI)	n/a	7.07[b] (4–10)	n/a	12.96 (9–17)[c]
Median (range)	n/a	4.05 (0–58)	n/a	9.00 (1–65)
Death rate (d/py)[d]				
Mean (95% CI)	199.0 (126–271)[f]	379.0 (195–564)[f]	342.3 (83–601)	259.86 (193–327)
Median (range)	129.4 (0–1235)	213.6 (0–3476)	85.3 (0–4263)	181.28 (29–922)

Notes: (a) Differences between the mean 'trade deficit' and 'number of deaths' are due to human error in the historical trade records; (b) Lost-in-transit during middle passage alone = deaths during the Middle Passage/number on board at the onset of the Middle Passage *100; (c) lost-in-transit = total number of death/total number of slaves purchased*100; (d) Death rate = number of deaths per 1,000 person-years; (e) Total number of trade days (travel to Africa, and return to NL excluded), the numbers for the entire voyage are: mean (95 per cent CI) 570.21 (513–627) and median (range) 521 (357–1370); (f) The difference in death rates between the loading and crossing phases is significant (p=0.02).

Source: Middelburgsche Commercie Compagnie 1751–97.

the short-term fluctuations in slave mortality that other historians have heroically attempted to describe, but it does reveal previously unnoticed differences in slave mortality experience as well as some persistent time trends in mortality over voyages.[29] It also sheds new light on the impact of shipboard and African conditions on such mortality.

We begin by providing in Table 7.2 some basic mean and median values of voyage duration as well as slave purchases, exposure, loss in transit and death rates for the thirty-nine voyages in our sample. To give a very general impression: the typical MCC voyage to Guinea in 1751 to 1797 purchased 253 slaves (range 71–390), lost 33 slaves (range 2–174) during the course of its voyage, and sold 220 slaves (range 45–349) in the Americas. The loss in transit, defined in this case to include the loading, crossing and selling phases, averaged 13 per cent (range 1–65

---

[29] On short-term fluctuations, the trend of the rate of loss during voyages, and its interpretation, see Miller, 'Statistical Evidence'.

Figure 7.3 Centred moving average slave death rates during loading and sailing for thirty-nine MCC ships (1751–1791)

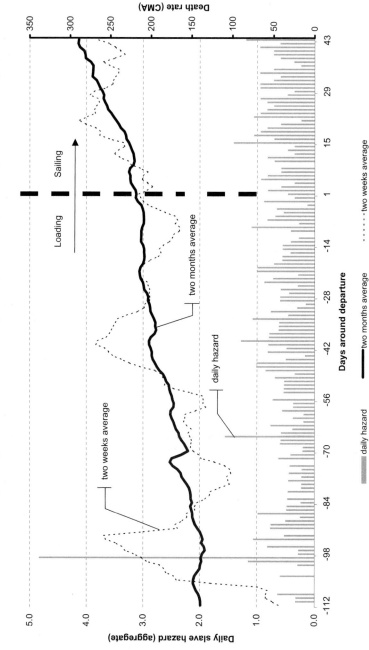

Note: Data are scaled on two vertical axes. The left axis expresses daily hazards, the right axis expresses centred moving average death rates. Daily hazard is the number of deaths on a given day, divided by the number of slaves on board (aggregated for all thirty-nine voyages); death rate is the number of deaths per thousand person-years at risk (d/py), aggregated for all thirty-nine voyages, expressed as centred moving averages over periods of two weeks and two months.

Source: Middelburgsche Commercie Compagnie 1751–97.

per cent). Though problems exist in making comparisons, this seems not to have been untypical at this time.[30] When account is taken of the actual time spent by slaves on board ship, the data reveal a mean slave death rate for the thirty-nine voyages of 259 deaths per 1,000 person-years (range 29–922 d/py). Given the age structure of the populations involved, this was an extraordinary rate by any standard.[31] It is witness to the enormous human costs of the Atlantic slave trade.[32]

Our methodology allows us to go beyond these crude measures of mortality, and to investigate the impact on mortality of risk factors such as length of time on board ship, geographical location of trade, and the age and sex of slaves. Table 7.2 provides information relating to the first of these. It shows that the loading phase accounted for almost 66 (or 54.5 per cent) of the 121 person-years spent on average by slaves on board ship. It also accounted for 41 per cent of slave deaths. This amounts to a much higher proportion of total slave deaths on board ship at the coast than has sometimes been estimated.[33] Nevertheless, though ships spent more days loading slaves than sailing to the Americas, death rates were lowest during loading (199 d/py). Thereafter, they averaged 379 d/py during the crossing, and 342 d/py during the selling phase for all thirty-nine voyages in our

---

[30] If mortality is expressed as percentage 'lost-in-transit', it is important to state explicitly which time period is described, and how the denominator is defined. If lost-in-transit is defined as percentage of the total number of slaves purchased, the mean percentage lost-in-transit in our sample was 12.96 per cent (95 per cent CI 9–17). But this definition becomes ambiguous if applied to a single phase of the voyage. As a percentage of the total number of slaves purchased, the number of deaths during the crossing alone was 6.59 per cent. Using the number of survivors on the first day of the crossing as the denominator, the percentage increases slightly to 7.07 per cent. As previous studies often do not state if they consider the total voyage (from first purchase to last sale) or only the crossing, and whether they use the total number purchased or the number of survivors at the start of the crossing as denominator, it is difficult to compare our MCC phase-specific loss-in-transit figures with the available literature. Having said that, the mean loss rate of slaves on all ships in 1750–1800 is estimated to have been 11.2 per cent (Klein et al., 'Transoceanic Mortality', p. 114), and for the quarter-century from 1751 to 1775, in which the bulk of the thirty-nine MCC voyages in our sample were concentrated, it was 14.2 per cent (N = 809; StD 14.5) in general and 13.7 per cent (N = 184; StD 12.7) if only voyages to the Windward Coast and Gold Coast are included (Eltis et al., Slave Trade Database).

[31] Eltis et al., Slave Trade Database. The point is further emphasised when one takes account of slave deaths during the enslavement process and forced journey to the African coast. One of the few losses in transit of Europeans that comes close to that of slaves on MCC vessels is that of Dutch passengers travelling to the Cape of Good Hope in the 1730s when losses were estimated at 23.07 per 1,000 per month (Riley, 'Mortality in Long-Distance Voyages', p. 652) or 276.84 d/py.

[32] To illustrate: a death rate of 259 d/py equates to a loss of 5.4 persons (2.1 per cent) in the first month for a shipload of 250 slaves. In our sample, death rates regularly hit >2,000 d/py over very short periods. At such a rate of loss, a ship with 250 slaves would have lost 42 slaves (17 per cent) in the first month, and half its purchase within four months.

[33] For estimates of deaths at the coast, see Klein and Engerman, 'Slave Mortality'; Klein et al., 'Transoceanic Mortality'; Klein, Atlantic Slave Trade, p. 157. Data for the eighteenth century, most of it relating to British ships in the 1790s, suggests deaths during coasting averaged less than 10 per cent of slaves purchased or 18–30 per cent of total slave deaths on board ship.

Table 7.3 Slave death rates during loading, by region at the time of death

| | N | Deaths (%) | Exposure (%) | Death rates | | | | |
				All	Men	Women	Boys	Girls
Senegambia	1	0 (0.0)	0.71 (0.0)	0.00	0.00	0.00	0.00	0.00
Sierra Leone	5	0 (0.0)	1.55 (0.0)	0.00	0.00	0.00	0.00	0.00
Windward Coast	36	206 (41.2)	1231.51 (50.2)	167.27	280.49	145.19	40.25	92.82
Gold Coast	38	152 (30.4)	802.71 (32.7)	189.36	223.84	187.24	98.81	181.22
Bight of Benin	3	35 (7.0)	46.50 (1.9)	752.62	1316.21	261.98	557.68	0.00
Bight of Biafra	5	13 (2.6)	82.93 (3.4)	156.75	141.45	62.23	324.73	231.64
W. C. Africa	1	25 (5.0)	58.33 (2.4)	428.60	417.62	562.08	0.00	687.38
Unknown	39	69 (13.8)	230.84 (9.4)	298.90	352.67	254.59	418.00	130.40
Total sample	39	500 (100.0)	2455.08 (100.0)	203.66	295.33	175.17	97.69	142.19

Note: 'N' represents the number of ships trading in a specific region; 'Exposure' numbers of person-years at risk; 'Deaths' the absolute number of slave deaths; 'Death rates' number of deaths per 1,000 person-years (d/py).

Source: Middelburgsche Commercie Compagnie 1751–97.

sample.[34] Four of the thirty-nine voyages, however, experienced slave losses in transit of over 30 per cent. Discounting these produces the result in Figure 7.3.[35] This reveals that, even in the case of the thirty-five voyages where losses in transit were under 30 per cent, slave mortality rates doubled in more or less linear fashion from 146 d/py four months before ships sailed from Africa, to 290 d/py six weeks after sailing from the continent. These findings confirm the suggestion of Steckel and Jensen, based on British data, that slave mortality rates were normally lower during the stay of ships in Africa than during the Atlantic crossing.[36] But they also indicate that on MCC ships mortality rates rose systematically the longer slaves

[34] The death rates in the crossing on our MCC voyages were seemingly lower than the mean rate for most slave ships in 1751–75 and 1776–1800, when annualised rates were 626.4 per 1,000 (N = 450) and 552 per 1,000 (N = 650), respectively (Klein *et al.*, 'Transoceanic Mortaltiy', p. 113). There is no clear explanation of the lower mortality rate on MCC ships in the crossing, but it may in part have been linked to the geographical distribution of trade in Africa. Few slaves taken by our MCC ships came from Senegambia, the Bight of Benin and Bight of Biafra, but ships from these regions comprised over a third of the ship records in 1751–1800, on which general estimates of Middle Passage mortality have been calculated. Ships from these regions typically had higher mortality rates in the crossing than those leaving other regions, including the Windward Coast and Gold Coast (Klein *et al.*, 'Transoceanic Mortality', p. 114).

[35] Removal of the four voyages in question lowers the mean death rate for the remaining thirty-five ships from 259.86 to 204.95 d/py. The average number of days on board before departure decreases marginally from 99 to 95 days, and mean exposure remains the same. Then, the daily death rates for the thirty-five ships were aggregated. Centred moving average daily death rates were then computed, with spans of fourteen and fifty-six days, and plotted from sixteen weeks before departure to six weeks of crossing. For this period of twenty-two weeks, data were available for all thirty-five voyages and inform Figure 7.3.

[36] Steckel and Jensen, 'New Evidence'. Our findings are also consistent with those of Klein *et al.*, 'Transoceanic Mortality', pp. 111–13, which show a sharp rise in mortality between the coasting and crossing phases of voyages in 1751–1800.

Table 7.4 Mean numbers of slaves purchased and death rates by age and sex

Adults			
	Men	Women	Subtotal
Slaves purchased	110 (100–122)	94 (85–103)	205 (185–223)
Exposure	47.61 (42–54)	45.57 (41–50)	93.19 (83–103)
Death rate	402.46 (242–562)	214.03 (158–271)	295.85 (217–374)
Children			
	Boys	Girls	Subtotal
Slaves purchased	28 (24–32)	21 (18–24)	49 (42–55)
Exposure	15.65 (13–18)	12.27 (10–14)	27.92 (24–32)
Death rate	149.45 (89–212)	145.17 (100–194)	146.25 (105–187)
All slaves			
	Males	Females	Total
Slaves purchased	132 (126–151)	115 (106–124)	253 (234–273)
Exposure	63.27 (56–70)	57.84 (52–63)	121.12 (110–132)
Death rate	329.81 (220–439)	196.01 (145–247)	259.86 (193–327)

Note: Mean numbers purchased and deaths by age and sex for thirty-nine voyages for all days with slaves on board (phases 2–4). 'Death rate' represents number of deaths per 1,000 person-years of exposure; 'Exposure' number of person-years at risk. Numbers in parenthesis are 95 per cent CIs.

Source: Middelburgsche Commercie Compagnie 1751–97.

were on board ship, whether ships were at the coast or at sea. Only landfall and sale of slaves in the Americas seems to have tempered such trends; but as Table 7.2 reminds us, even in the selling phase mean mortality rates remained higher than at the African coast. The imperative for MCC traders to sell slaves as quickly as possible after reaching the Americas was evident.

Our data allow us to investigate risk factors for slaves other than time. Table 7.3 refers to the loading period (or phase 2) and provides data on the coastal location of ships at the time of slave deaths. These show that while trading on the Windward Coast ships experienced slave mortality rates of 167 d/py. Rates rose to 189 d/py during trading on the Gold Coast. It is likely that this rise in mortality rates between the Windward Coast and Gold Coast was in part a result of time factors, with sick or exhausted slaves bought on the Windward Coast dying while ships completed their slave purchase further south. But one cannot rule out the possibility that it may also have been caused by unhealthy Gold Coast slaves dying soon after purchase.

The data offer a rather clearer picture when it comes to looking at age and sex as risk factors for slaves. Table 7.4 refers to the entire period when slaves were on board (phases 2–4) and offers disaggregated data on slave mortality by age and sex. Some caution in interpreting the data on mortality by age is needed when relying on only two categories – adults and children – and when the boundaries between the two are blurred and the precise age distributions within them unknown. The data suggest, however, that mortality rates for adults were system-

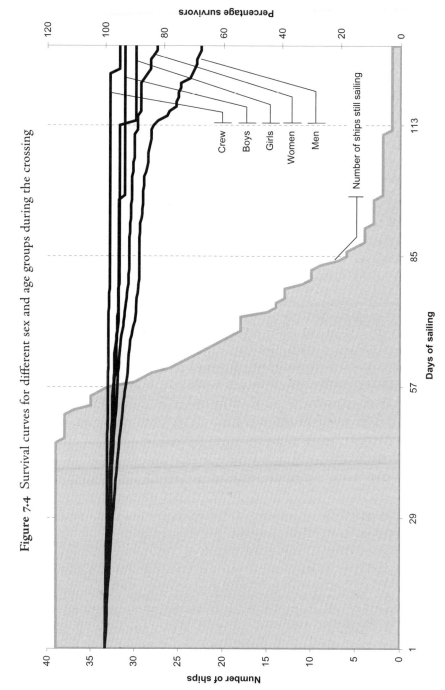

Figure 7.4 Survival curves for different sex and age groups during the crossing

Note: Survival is expressed as the percentage remaining of the slaves and crew departing from Africa. Time-units are expressed in days of sailing; vertical gridlines indicate one-month intervals.

Source: Middelburgsche Commercie Compagnie 1751–97.

atically higher than for children. Moreover, among adults, they were much higher for males than for females. Thus, at 296 d/py, the mortality rate for adults was more than double that of children, while at 402 d/py, the mortality rate of men was some 88 per cent higher than the 214 d/py for women. Such findings inform Figure 7.4, which reveals survival rates for groups of slaves by age and sex during the crossing. It shows a steeper decrease in surviving adult males compared to other groups. On MCC ships, at least, it appears that being an adult male slave was a risk in itself.[37]

Multivariate analysis allows us to assess the relative contribution of these and other risk factors to shipboard slave mortality. Our analysis uses all daily records for all thirty-nine voyages during the loading, crossing and selling phases in a non-linear multivariate model, with separate regressions for loading and crossing phases. The results are expressed as relative risks and refer to the odds of dying on any given day.[38] The constant for each regression is the adult male on the first day, located on the Windward Coast, for the loading phase, and departing from the Windward Coast for the crossing phase. Table 7.5 presents the results for the loading phase, Table 7.6 for the crossing.

During the loading phase (Table 7.5), the odds of dying for an adult male on the first day of loading were equivalent to a death rate of 54.76 d/py. For adult women, the odds were 0.59 of those for men (32.30 d/py); for girls 0.54 (29.57 d/py); and for boys 0.40 (21.90 d/py). These baseline odds worsened with every month the ship took to load (x 1.21), during the rainy season from June to August (x 1.47) or during the following trimester to November (x 1.40).[39] They were maybe better on the Gold Coast (x 0.77), and certainly better in the Bight of Biafra (x 0.17), but worse in West Central Africa (x 2.64) and much worse still in the Bight of Benin (x 5.61).[40] No other significant risk factors were found during

---

[37] This stands in sharp contrast with some recent findings which suggest that in 1776–1800, when the data are most abundant, mean loss rates of slaves did not vary much by age or sex (Klein *et al.*, 'Transoceanic Mortality', p. 116). These findings are based on a much larger sample of voyages than we use here but the calculations upon which they are based relate to percentage losses in transit and, unlike our findings, make no allowance for differentials in time spent on board ship by different categories of slaves.

[38] Relative risks (hazard ratios) were obtained assuming a proportional hazards model. Estimation was done using methods for discrete survival data. The likelihood was rewritten as relating to a binary regression model (D.W. Hosmer and S. Lemeshow, *Applied Survival Analysis* (Chichester, 1999), p. 258), and logistic regression with a random ship effect was used to obtain estimates of hazard ratios.

[39] The rainy season varied between Upper Guinea and the Bight of Biafra. August and September were, however, the months with the lowest levels of slave deliveries at Sierra Leone and the Windward Coast, a pattern linked, it seems, to the harvest cycle as well as rainfall patterns. See Stephen D. Behrendt, 'Markets, Transaction Cycles, and Profits: Merchant Decision Making in the British Slave Trade', *William and Mary Quarterly*, 58 (2001), pp. 184–5.

[40] The sample sizes of deaths for the Bight of Benin and Bight of Biafra are very small.

Table 7.5 Relative hazards for slaves during loading
for thirty-nine MCC voyages

Risk factor	Univariate		Multivariate		
	Relative hazard	p=	Relative hazard	p=	
Constant[a]	145.53	<0.0001	54.76	<0.0001	***
	(109.71–193.02)		(25.60–116.93)		
Age and sex categories					
Man, adult (reference)[b]	1.95 (1.62–2.35)	<0.0001	1.00 (n/a)	n/a	n/a
Woman, adult	0.74 (0.61–1.00)	<0.01	0.59 (0.48–0.73)	<0.0001	***
Boy, child	0.48 (0.34–0.69)	<0.001	0.40 (0.27–0.58)	<0.0001	***
Girl, child	0.71 (0.50–0.99)	0.04	0.54 (0.38–0.77)	<0.01	**
Time & exposure					
Duration of loading (months)	1.16 (1.11–1.22)	<0.0001	1.21 (1.12–1.32)	<0.0001	***
Exposure last week (days)	1.00 (1.00–1.00)	<0.0001	1.00 (1.00–1.00)	0.85	n.s.
Crowding (slave/ton)	1.79 (1.41–2.26)	<0.0001	1.08 (0.51–2.26)	0.84	n.s.
Rainy season					
Dry season (reference)	0.70 (0.56–0.88)	<0.01	1.00 (n/a)	n/a	n/a
June–August	1.02 (0.82–1.28)	0.85	1.47 (1.08–1.99)	0.02	*
September–November	1.36 (1.10–1.67)	<0.01	1.40 (1.06–1.83)	0.02	*
Crew experience					
Captain (voyages)	1.03 (0.91–1.16)	0.65	1.01 (0.87–1.16)	0.94	n.s.
Surgeon (voyages)	1.00 (0.78–1.30)	0.97	0.98 (0.74–1.30)	0.89	n.s.
Region of loading					
Windward Coast (reference)	0.74 (0.60–0.91)	<0.01	1.00 (n/a)	n/a	n/a
Gold Coast	1.15 (0.92–1.44)	0.20	0.77 (0.58–1.02)	0.07	*
Bight of Benin	2.92 (1.73–4.91)	<0.001	5.61 (3.08–10.20)	<0.0001	***
Bight of Biafra	0.14 (0.06–0.35)	<0.0001	0.17 (0.07–0.44)	<0.001	***
West Central Africa	3.11 (0.66–14.66)	0.15	2.64 (0.47–14.97)	0.26	n.s.
Unknown	1.27 (0.95–1.69)	0.11	1.17 (0.83–1.65)	0.36	n.s.
Random factor	1.79 (1.27–2.52)	<0.01	1.76 (1.24–2.52)	<0.01	^^

(a) The constant is expressed as a death rate (95 per cent CI), the unit is deaths/1,000 person-years; (b) The brackets refer to 95 per cent confidence intervals. * = significant at the 0.05 level; ** = significant at the 0.01 level; *** = significant at the 0.001 level.

Notes: Relative risks (hazard ratios) were obtained assuming a proportional hazards model. Estimation was done using methods for discrete survival data. The likelihood was rewritten as a likelihood for a binary regression model (see Hosmer and Lemeshow, *Applied Survival Analysis* (Chichester, 1999), p. 258), and logistic regression with a random ship effect was used to obtain estimates of hazard ratios. The constant for the regression is the adult male on the Windward Coast during the dry season, on an empty ship, on the first day of loading, with captains and surgeons on their first slaving voyage.

Source: Middelburgsche Commercie Compagnie 1751–97.

Table 7.6 Relative hazards for slaves during the crossing
for thirty-nine MCC voyages

Risk factor	Univariate		Multivariate		
	Relative hazard	p=	Relative hazard	p=	
Constant[a]	253.12 (190.10–337.03)	<0.0001	124.54 (15.30–1014.60)	<0.0001	***
Age and sex categories					
Male, adult (reference)[b]	1.83 (1.57–2.15)	<0.0001	1.00 (n/a)	n/a	n/a
Woman, adult	0.78 (0.66–0.92)	<0.01	0.60 (0.51–0.72)	<0.0001	***
Boy, child	0.51 (0.37–0.70)	<0.001	0.37 (0.27–0.52)	<0.0001	***
Girl, child	0.49 (0.34–0.72)	<0.001	0.36 (0.24–0.53)	<0.0001	***
Time & exposure					
Duration of crossing (months)	1.52 (1.38–1.67)	<0.0001	1.47 (1.30–1.67)	<0.0001	***
Crowding (slave/ton)	0.16 (0.16–0.29)	<0.0001	0.91 (0.53–1.58)	0.73	n.s.
Rainy season					
Dry season (reference)	0.60 (0.48–0.75)	<0.0001	1.00 (n/a)	n/a	n/a
June–August	2.23 (1.75–2.84)	<0.0001	1.64 (1.25–2.16)	<0.001	***
September–November	0.74 (0.52–1.04)	0.08	1.06 (0.75–1.51)	0.73	n.s.
Crew experience					
Captain (voyages)	1.11 (0.98–1.25)	0.10	1.16 (1.02–1.33)	0.03	*
Surgeon (voyages)	1.04 (0.80–1.35)	0.71	0.95 (0.69–1.30)	0.74	n.s.
Last region before departure					
Windward Coast (reference)	1.04 (0.29–3.69)	0.95	1.00 (n/a)	n/a	n/a
Gold Coast	0.81 (0.39–1.70)	0.56	1.14 (0.27–4.84)	0.85	n.s.
Bight of Biafra	0.97 (0.26–3.62)	0.96	1.31 (0.14–4.28)	0.75	n.s.
West Central Africa	1.47 (0.26–8.16)	0.65	2.46 (0.32–19.16)	0.38	n.s.
Unknown location	1.65 (n/a)[c]	n/a	2.18 (0.29–16.17)	0.44	n.s
Random factor	1.91 (1.35–2.69)	<0.001	1.58 (1.21–2.06)	<0.01	**

(a) The constant is expressed as a death rate (95 per cent CI), the unit is deaths/1,000 person-years; (b) The brackets refer to 95 per cent confidence intervals; (c) Region of departure is unknown for two voyages; the regression provided no confidence intervals. * = significant at the 0.05 level; ** = significant at the 0.01 level; *** = significant at the 0.001 level

Notes: Relative risks (hazard ratios) were obtained assuming a proportional hazards model. Estimation was done using methods for discrete survival data. The likelihood was rewritten as a likelihood for a binary regression model (see Hosmer and Lemeshow, *Applied Survival Analysis* (Chichester, 1999), p. 258), and logistic regression with a random ship effect was used to obtain estimates of hazard ratios. The constant for the regression is the adult male during the dry season, departing from the Windward Coast, on an empty ship, on the first day of sailing, with captains and surgeons on their first slaving voyage.

Source: Middelburgsche Commercie Compagnie 1751–97.

loading.[41] During the Atlantic crossing (Table 7.6), the odds of dying started at 124.54 d/py for men. They were lower for women (x 0.60), for boys (x 0.37) and for girls (x 0.36). They increased every month during the crossing (x 1.47) and during the rainy season (x 1.64). Strangely, mortality seems to have increased with the increased experience of the ship captain (x 1.16). It is important to note, however, that not all variations in slave mortality can be explained by the factors referred to above (random factors of x 1.76 and x 1.58 for loading and crossing). Nevertheless, these results suggest that, together with time-related variables and seasonality, age and sex were critical factors in shaping the survival chances of enslaved Africans deported on MCC ships from West Africa to the Americas between 1751 and 1797. On the basis of this MCC evidence, therefore, Africans plainly did not enter the trade with an equal probability of surviving.

Implications

The principal finding of this longitudinal study is that slave exposure and mortality patterns on board MCC ships trading to Guinea after 1750 were not homogeneous. Depending on the region of embarkation, large proportions of slaves spent much longer on board ship than others. Adult males tended to be purchased later than children. There was a slow but continuous rise in mortality throughout the loading and crossing phases of voyages, with a dramatic rise in mortality at the end of very long crossings. Adult males were at higher risk than other slaves, especially children. The overall slave mortality rates found on MCC ships between 1751 and 1797 were, at 199.0 d/py and 379.0 d/py, respectively, for the loading and crossing phases, much higher than those found by Steckel and Jensen for British ships in the period 1792 to 1796 in the only other study using standardized shipboard slave mortality rates known to us.[42] This is true whether we use mean or median values for mortality on MCC ships to compare with the British data. We cannot explain this discrepancy, but it is worth noting that Steckel and Jensen acknowledge that their estimates of mortality rates were low. Our study, nevertheless, endorses their finding that mortality rates during the crossing were much higher than during the loading phase of the voyage.

In some respects MCC voyages to West Africa were atypical of the slave trade in the second half of the eighteenth century. They had an unusual balance of trade between the Windward Coast and the Gold Coast. They typically took over 60 per cent longer to purchase slaves at the coast than their contemporary rivals, yet

---

[41] To give an example: an adult woman during the final weeks of loading on a typical ship in Elmina (based on six months loading, five months on board, 250 slaves at 2.0 slaves per ton, during the rainy season, the captain on his second voyage and the surgeon on his first, on the Gold Coast, random effects included), according to Table 7.5, would have seen her odds of dying multiplied by 4.3 from a death rate of 54.76 to approximately 235.15 d/py since her arrival on board (i.e. $54.76 \times 0.59 \times (1.21)^6 \times (1.00)^{150 \times 28} \times (1.08)^2 \times 1.47 \times (1.01)^2 \times 0.98 \times 0.77$).

[42] Steckel and Jensen, 'New Evidence'.

experienced relatively low mortality rates among slaves in the crossing from West Africa to the Americas. The juxtaposition of these last two factors may in part have reflected the concentration of MCC West African trade at the Windward Coast and Gold Coast. Ships leaving these two regions typically experienced lower mortality in the crossing than those leaving Senegambia, the Bight of Benin and Bight of Biafra – which are included in more general calculations of mortality. The apparently exceptional nature of some features of MCC voyages to West Africa suggests the need for similar micro-studies of slave mortality for other regions of trade in Atlantic Africa.

Even with these caveats, however, our investigation of shipboard experience of slaves on MCC vessels trading to West Africa encourages reflection on conceptual-isations of the Middle Passage; on the impact of age and gender on slave purchase and mortality patterns; and on the relative importance of African and shipboard conditions in determining mortality trends. These are inter-related issues. By way of conclusion we briefly examine each of them.

The image of the Atlantic slave trade as a triangular trade linking three conti-nents – Europe, Africa and the Americas – has been a powerful factor in shaping the historiography on the Middle Passage. Conventionally defined as the ocean voyage between Africa and the Americas – and thus the second of the three legs of the triangular trade – the Middle Passage has become a metaphor for the horrors of transatlantic slavery. Viewed as an ocean crossing, it has also become the principal focus of efforts to measure changes in shipboard slave mortality through time and across space, with the proportions of slaves leaving Africa lost in transit being the key measure of such mortality. Reconstruction of voyages by MCC ships reveals, however, that the Atlantic crossing occupied little more than one-fifth of the time that ships had 'human cargo' on board. This may have been a lower proportion than in most instances, simply because MCC ships typically spent longer acquiring slaves at the coast than other ships. Nevertheless, it remains the case that the Atlantic crossing typically took only a fraction of the time that most ships spent trading in Africa. This was especially true of the period 1751 to 1775 in which the MCC voyages included in this study were concentrated.[43] To better understand life and death on board slave ships, therefore, we need to adopt a broader definition of the Middle Passage. This should embrace all the time when slaves were on board ship, and needs to take account of differences in time spent on board ship by individual slaves or groups of slaves as a result of shippers' slave purchasing strategies. This study is a first step in redefining the Middle Passage in this more comprehensive fashion and in clarifying the differences in time spent on board by different groups of slaves.

Redefining the Middle Passage places the slave purchasing strategies of ship-pers at the heart of discussions of shipboard slave mortality. The reconstruction of MCC voyages reveals a bias towards purchasing children and females at the

---

[43] Coasting or loading times of all ships in 1751–75 were evidently longer than normal; Eltis and Richardson, 'Productivity in the Transatlantic Slave Trade'; Klein et al., 'Transoceanic Mortality', p. 111.

start of loading and towards purchasing men in the final weeks. In the case of MCC ships, this had regional implications as ships tended to begin trade at the Windward Coast and conclude it on the Gold Coast. In terms of mortality, an important finding is that, against a background of rising mortality throughout the loading and crossing phases for all slaves, death rates of children and women remained lower than those of men. This fact may have been appreciated by some MCC shipmasters, at least half of whom made multiple slaving voyages. It may thus have reinforced other factors, such as the higher price of adult males and fear of shipboard rebellion, to which we alluded earlier, in shaping the slave purchasing strategies of such masters in Africa.

The age- and sex-related differentials in mortality on MCC ships contrast sharply with the findings of other studies of mortality using loss-in-transit data, which, if anything, show higher losses of children than adults.[44] The MCC mortality findings need to be confirmed by other studies, but should they prove representative, they have potentially wider implications. Confirmation of our findings would underline the role of gender as well as economic factors in shaping shippers' preferences for adult male slaves. Such preferences typically resulted in substantial premiums on prices of adult males at the coast. It might also help to explain the well-documented increases in proportions of children entering the Atlantic slave trade between the late seventeenth and early nineteenth centuries – increases that to date have largely escaped convincing explanation.[45] Understanding why slaves on board MCC ships had differential rates of mortality by age and sex, and the typicality of these experiences, has, therefore, a significance that extends well beyond the voyages covered by this study.

Finally, patterns of mortality on board MCC ships help to inform the ongoing debate over the relative importance of shipboard and African conditions in influencing mortality rates of slaves in transit. Differential rates of loss of slaves by African region of embarkation – notably between the Bight of Biafra and other regions – and allegedly high incidences of mortality in the early stages of the Atlantic crossing have tended to be seen as indicative of African influences on slave mortality. The MCC records used here offer very little new direct evidence on either of these arguments. Only a tiny share of the slaves included in this study came from the Bight of Biafra. Extraordinary variations in mortality over short intervals also make it unwise to do more than track macroscopic time-related trends in voyage mortality. Nevertheless, differentials in mortality rates of slaves by age and sex raise questions about the effectiveness of developments in shipboard sanitation and hygiene in lowering shipboard mortality rates equally for all

---

[44] Evidence for loss in transit for 199 voyages in 1651–1825 shows a child loss of 7.9 per cent compared to 6.7 per cent for adults (Klein *et al.*, 'Transoceanic Mortality', p. 116). The densest data are for 1776–1800 (151 voyages), when losses were 4.8 per cent and 4.6 per cent respectively.
[45] David Eltis and Stanley L. Engerman, 'Fluctuations in Sex and Age Ratios in the Transatlantic Slave Trade, 1663–1864', *Economic History Review*, 46 (1993), pp. 308–23.

slaves,[46] and point, instead, to the condition of slaves at the time of embarkation as critically important in determining their survival rates. This was particularly the case with adult males, relatively high proportions of whom embarked late in the loading phase yet succumbed at higher rates than other slaves in the crossing. Precisely why this happened is uncertain. It could have been associated with pressures on captains to take adult males to satisfy owners' and buyers' expectations, thereby encouraging them to be less rigorous in slave selection, especially in the final stages of transactions at the coast, when risks to the slaves on board ship were rising. Equally, it may have been associated with differences in enslavement and slave marketing processes between the Windward Coast and Gold Coast which caused adult males to reach the coast in less healthy condition than others. Having said that, it is worth remembering that men were typically seen as the primary instigators of shipboard rebellions and suffered the highest casualties during such incidents. Rebellions were not unknown on MCC ships. Moreover, men were commonly incarcerated on board in rooms separate from women and children, and were often held in irons, particularly while ships were close to Africa. To our knowledge, the implications of differences in slave management strategies on shipboard mortality rates have until now escaped attention, principally because age and sex differentials in slave mortality have largely gone unnoticed. But the housing of children with women, some of whom may have been related, conceivably helped to nurture material and spiritual support systems among slaves lodged in the 'women's rooms' – support systems that were less easy to inculcate and sustain among isolated and shackled men.

Though our evidence may point towards the primacy of African influences on age- and sex-based differentials in slave mortality, it would clearly be premature to disregard slave resistance, shipboard management practices, and even mutual support systems among the enslaved as factors affecting differences in their survival rates on MCC ships. Patterns of shipboard slave mortality on MCC voyages to Guinea in the period 1751 to 1797 open up, therefore, new avenues of enquiry into the complex inter-relationship between African conditions, trading and management strategies, and life and death on board slave ships.

---

[46] Haines and Shlomowitz, 'Explaining the Decline in Mortality'. Haines and Shlomowitz relate their argument specifically to British trading activity but there are claims that innovations developed by one group of traders were commonly adopted by others: see Klein, *Atlantic Slave Trade*, p. 159.

Appendix I Summary data for the thirty-nine Middelburgsche Compagnie Commercie voyages to Guinea, 1751–95, included in this chapter

	Ship	Tons	Captain*	Surgeon*	Departure	Loading	Crossing	Selling	Return	Arrival
1	Willem V	143	Jacobse (1/1)	Schradij (1/1)	11–10–1751	15–02–1752	26–08–1752	06–10–1752	14–10–1752	27–04–1753
2	Mid. Welvaren II	133	Kerkhoven (1/1)	Hemmekam (1/1)	19–08–1752	12–10–1752	26–10–1753	10–01–1754	24–03–1754	03–06–1754
3	Philadelphia	120	Menkenveld (1/1)	Nolson (1/1)	18–10–1752	29–01–1753	28–10–1753	22–01–1754	24–02–1754	04–06–1754
4	Willem V	143	Jacobse (2/2)	Schradij (2/3)	11–08–1753	21–10–1753	16–03–1754	02–06–1754	02–09–1754	26–10–1754
5	Mercurius	97	Stam (1/1)	Everwijn (1/1)	13–09–1753	18–10–1753	11–07–1754	08–09–1754	17–10–1754	19–01–1755
6	Philadelphia	120	Menkenveld (2/2)	Hemmekam (2/2)	21–09–1754	12–10–1754	25–05–1755	21–07–1755	20–09–1755	21–12–1755
7	Mid. Welvaren II	133	Kerkhoven (2/2)	Voort (1/1)	20–10–1754	07–02–1755	23–09–1755	28–10–1755	08–01–1756	03–05–1756
8	Johanna Cores	119	Tuijneman (1/1)	Kervink (1/1)	12–02–1756	19–04–1756	20–10–1756	29–04–1757	02–06–1757	02–11–1757
9	Vliegende Faam	101	Moor (1/1)	Bertram (1/1)	05–03–1756	20–07–1756	09–04–1757	02–07–1757	30–08–1757	05–02–1758
10	Philadelphia	120	Menkenveld (3/3)	Pacouw (1/3)	06–09–1756	15–10–1756	08–04–1757	29–06–1757	10–08–1757	12–11–1757
11	Philadelphia	120	Menkenveld (4/4)	Pacouw (2/4)	24–06–1758	31–07–1758	20–01–1759	08–04–1759	18–05–1759	10–09–1759
12	Philadelphia	120	Menkenveld (5/5)	Couperus (1/1)	22–02–1760	09–05–1760	07–10–1760	26–01–1761	22–02–1761	08–07–1761
13	Willem V	143	Jacobse (6/6)	Wante (1/3)	09–03–1761	13–05–1761	01–10–1761	03–01–1762	09–01–1762	16–05–1762
14	Johanna Cores	119	Tuijneman (4/4)	Kervink (3/4)	16–03–1762	04–05–1762	19–10–1762	21–02–1763	11–06–1763	01–08–1763
15	Willem V	143	Jacobse (7/7)	Wante (2/4)	10–10–1762	26–01–1763	18–08–1763	22–10–1763	13–01–1764	14–04–1764
16	Eenigheid	178	Pruijmelaar (2/7)	Henkel (1/1)	14–08–1763	29–11–1763	30–10–1764	29–12–1764	18–01–1765	08–08–1765
17	Johanna Cores	119	Molder (1/4)	Sprungli (2/2)	14–10–1763	04–05–1764	31–10–1764	27–02–1765	28–03–1765	01–07–1765
18	H. u Langzaam	198	Menkenveld (3/7)	Couperus (3/3)	09–07–1764	01–11–1764	13–07–1765	06–09–1765	06–10–1765	12–03–1766
19	Willem V	143	Jacobse (8/8)	Wante (2/5)	24–10–1764	19–03–1765	20–10–1765	10–02–1766	25–03–1766	30–06–1766
20	Johanna Cores	119	Mulders (4/6)	Pieterse (2/2)	10–10–1766	29–04–1767	11–10–1767	02–02–1768	21–04–1768	14–06–1768
21	Nieuwe Hoop	163	Bouque (1/3)	Callenfels (1/1)	27–10–1766	13–02–1767	21–09–1767	27–10–1767	06–03–1768	30–05–1768
22	Nieuwe Hoop	163	Bouque (2/4)	Okke (2/2)	27–08–1768	25–10–1768	23–05–1769	18–07–1769	07–09–1769	16–12–1769

#	Ship									
23	Zang Godin	137	Sprang (1/2)	Rodrigo (1/1)	28-09-1768	31-03-1769	31-10-1769	26-01-1770	08-02-1770	12-06-1770
24	Johanna Cores	119	Sap (1/4)	Schillemans (1/1)	04-01-1769	21-03-1769	05-10-1769	05-01-1770	19-01-1770	12-06-1970
25	Welmeenende	140	Haijen (1/1)	Fusie (1/1)	04-07-1769	09-09-1769	16-02-1770	08-04-1770	08-05-1770	25-06-1970
26	Nieuwe Hoop	163	Wilton (1/4)	Rudersdorf (1/1)	30-04-1770	20-06-1770	15-01-1771	31-03-1771	01-06-1771	04-09-1771
27	Vliegende Faam	101	Kakom (1/4)	Feutsch (1/1)	14-08-1770	13-10-1770	10-04-1771	10-07-1771	13-07-1771	21-12-1771
28	Zang Godin	137	Sprang (2/3)	Plevier (1/1)	21-10-1770	04-03-1771	24-08-1771	04-10-1771	07-10-1771	13-04-1772
29	Vliegende Faam	101	Kakom (2/5)	Feutsch (2/2)	28-08-1772	31-10-1772	26-09-1773	25-10-1773	30-10-1773	05-06-1774
30	Zang Godin	137	Hoffman (1/3)	Rusche (1/1)	06-04-1773	12-08-1773	21-09-1774	03-10-1774	No return	N/A
31	Welmeenende	140	Haijen (3/3)	Kober (1/1)	21-07-1773	10-10-1773	30-01-1774	02-04-1774	05-05-1774	27-08-1774
32	H. u Langzaam	198	Kakom (3/6)	(unknown)	06-04-1775	12-05-1775	07-10-1775	02-02-1776	14-03-1776	17-06-1776
33	Nieuwe Hoop	163	Wilton (2/5)	Pieterse (3/3)	13-07-1775	06-10-1775	24-05-1776	31-07-1776	14-10-1776	02-06-1777
34	H. u Langzaam	198	Kakom (4/7)	Lebeke (1/1)	06-06-1777	08-08-1777	31-01-1778	29-03-1778	03-07-1778	20-09-1778
35	Vigilantie	194	Magielsen (1/2)	Verschuere (1/1)	09-08-1778	08-10-1778	07-02-1779	01-05-1779	28-05-1779	08-09-1779
36	Nieuwe Hoop	163	Goodwill (1/4)	Leeuwen (1/1)	19-02-1779	18-05-1779	06-10-1779	12-01-1780	17-03-1780	20-05-1780
37	Zeemercuur	219	Kakom (6/9)	Weber (1/1)	07-10-1787	18-02-1788	20-04-1789	08-07-1789	15-02-1790	28-04-1790
38	Zeemercuur	219	Zill (1/1)	Bal (1/2)	27-10-1791	08-03-1792	10-04-1793	21-06-1793	04-10-1793	22-01-1794
39	Vergenoegen	209	Breedau (2/2)	Nijs (1/2)	20-10-1793	18-06-1794	12-01-1795	05-03-1795	23-05-1795	19-09-1797

* Figures indicate the number of voyages (including the present one) in the capacity of captain/surgeon over the total number of voyages in any capacity, from a sample of seventy muster rolls studied.

8

Ships, Families and Surgeons: Migrant Voyages to Australia in the Age of Sail

Robin Haines

Introduction

In the first decades of the nineteenth century, the newly formed colonies of Australia eagerly sought immigrants to exploit their rich natural resources, and looked to the mother country for their recruits. The importation of labour from the northern hemisphere required considerable sums of money, however. From 1831, each of Australia's colonial governments funded immigration from the sale of land to well-off settlers, the proceeds of which were earmarked for recruiting suitably qualified emigrants from Scotland, Ireland, England and Wales. The occupations in greatest demand in Australia were shepherds, herdsmen, agricultural labourers, rural tradesmen such as fencers, ditchers, well-diggers, carpenters and stonemasons, farm and domestic servants, and so forth. Families with older children were preferred because the children represented future labour, and married couples were thought to be more stable entrants into the labour market. Between 1831 and 1900, 750,000 such emigrants, assisted by Australia's colonial governments, arrived on its shores.[1]

Safely conveying these emigrants to the Antipodes was a challenging undertaking. The distance by sea from Britain to Australia spans twelve to fourteen thousand miles, depending on the route – usually a non-stop passage that would take from three to five months in the nineteenth century. The average time spent at sea for the non-stop voyage was around a hundred days from the mid 1840s, although some record-breaking voyages spent as little as seventy-seven days at sea, using the extreme Great Circle route. In addition to the length of the journey were the terrifying seas of the Southern Ocean, and the dangers of the rapid spread of disease amongst passengers confined in very close quarters. Nevertheless, the relatively few voyages that suffered high mortality due to violent epidemics, as well as the surprisingly few shipwrecks that occurred, have arguably attracted dispropor-

---

[1] See Robin Haines, *Emigration and the Labouring Poor: Australian Recruitment in Britain and Ireland, 1831–1900* (London, 1997), for comprehensive tables on numbers emigrating by year, to each colony.

tionate attention, serving to characterize Australia's immigrants in the age of sail as victims of perilous voyages. In reality, the intervention of the state (following a small number of fatal voyages) – through careful regulation of migrant voyages, including the provision of surgeons on board – meant that emigrant families were given the best possible chance of a healthy, safe passage. Indeed, for children and adults travelling under the auspices of the state and housed in steerage – between decks – the chances of surviving the long ocean voyage to Australia were far greater than those of their peers who sailed the much shorter, unregulated Atlantic crossing to North America.[2]

This survey, therefore, will highlight the positive effects of such regulation – and the critical role of the surgeon – on health and mortality on board emigrant vessels to Australia in the nineteenth century. It will first examine the challenges of the emigrant voyage, including conditions on board ship, then turn to adult and child health and mortality, before evaluating the measures taken by the authorities and surgeons to improve health on board. This process is assisted by a rich seam of information that the regulation of migrant voyages has left for researchers to mine.[3] Owing to the survival of a large amount of official documentation we know far more about surgeons and emigrants travelling on government-assisted ships to Australia than we do of passengers and their doctors carried on private ships. Emigrants assisted by colonial governments were, like convicts, subjected to more official scrutiny than any other groups in history before the twentieth century. Application procedures were strict, as were the criteria governing eligibility for an assisted passage. Before departure, emigrants were screened by Emigration Commission officers; before disembarkation, colonial immigration agents at the ports of arrival interviewed the emigrants. These officials reported upon the state of health and behaviour of the emigrants, and on their merit as potential labourers in the colonies' agricultural economy. Reports also show emigrant complaints about aspects of the voyage, including the surgeon's superintendence. Alongside official records are the letters and diaries of emigrants such as Ellen Moger, who

---

[2]   Robin Haines and Ralph Shlomowitz, 'Explaining the Modern Mortality Decline: What Can We Learn from Sea Voyages?', *Social History of Medicine*, 11 (1998), pp. 15–48; Robin Haines and Ralph Shlomowitz, 'Maritime Mortality Revisited', *International Journal of Maritime History*, 8 (1996), pp. 133–72; Robin Haines, *Life and Death in the Age of Sail: The Passage to Australia* (London, 2006); Robin Haines, *Doctors at Sea: Emigrant Voyages to Colonial Australia* (London, 2005).

[3]   Manuscript sources (for example, official correspondence and reportage, and private letters, diaries and journals) and contemporary published sources, including specific colonial and imperial Parliamentary Papers, newspapers, pamphlets and books can be found in archives and libraries in the UK and Australia. Full details of these voluminous sources can be found in Robin Haines, *Emigration and the Labouring Poor*, pp. 367–73; Haines, *Doctors at Sea*, pp. 216–20; Haines, *Life and Death in the Age of Sail*, pp. 330–4. Journal articles by Haines, and Haines and Shlomowitz, cited below, offer further archival sources related to specific matters regarding health and death at sea in the eighteenth and nineteenth centuries.

sailed to Australia in 1840,[4] and Sarah Brunskill, who sailed with her husband George in 1838.[5]

The conduct and efficiency of the surgeons were also scrutinized and reported upon. Surgeons submitted their official logs and summary reports upon arrival in Australia. They kept formal records of births and deaths, and on the on-board supervision routines that had been adapted from highly successful health regimes first introduced on convict voyages in 1815, and embodied in the official 'Instructions to Surgeons'.[6] (These, in their turn, appear to have been influenced by the experience of Royal Navy surgeons in men-of-war vessels during the French Wars, and had helped to considerably reduce mortality at sea in the period 1779 to 1814.) In this way reports and correspondence ricocheted between London and the colonies – whose governments footed the bill and expected to receive value for the funds invested in their labour force. Colonial complaints were vociferous when emigrants failed to arrive in good health or on a clean and well-run ship. Hence, these prototypical 'ten pound poms' (representing half of Australia's nineteenth-century arrivals) left in their wake a vast archive of information concerning their ages, occupations, religious persuasion, literacy, origins, family status and health.[7]

Sickness and Mortality on the Voyage

Life on board emigrant vessels was never going to be easy. A voyage of such length went through several climatic zones where passengers suffered extremes of heat and cold. Moreover, as the letters and diaries of emigrants and the reports of surgeon superintendents attest, many emigrants experienced an occasionally terrifying passage. This was sometimes exacerbated by the practice of taking the extreme Circle Route, which led vessels into even heavier seas. Seasickness afflicted many. The problems of large populations of people living in such crowded quarters, and the resulting malodorous environment, made life miserable for many passengers.

Disease, however, was the main threat stalking such migrant vessels. Pathogens such as measles, scarlet fever, smallpox, typhus, typhoid fever or, less often,

4   Letter from Ellen Moger to her parents, dated Gouger Street, Adelaide, 18 January 1840, State Library of South Australia (SLSA) D6249(L). An account of her voyage on the *Moffatt* can be found in Haines, *Life and Death in the Age of Sail*, pp. 103–21.
5   'Letter written on the Voyage to South Australia [on the *Thomas Harrison*] by George and Sarah Brunskill to her parents in Ely, Cambridgeshire, 1838–39', 27 November 1838, SLSA, D5203(L), typed transcript.
6   South Australia is the best served of all states, where a long run of surgeons' reports, from 1848 to 1885, survives in State Records (SA). For all ships arriving between 1848 and 1885, including individual data on births and deaths, and details of the voyage, see Robin Haines, Judith Jeffery and Greg Slattery, *Bound for South Australia: Births and Deaths on Government-Assisted Immigrant Ships, 1848–1885*, CD-ROM (Adelaide, 2004). Very few individual surgeons' reports survive in the state archives of the other Australian states.
7   For an analysis of the attributes of the emigrants, including literacy, see Haines, *Emigration and the Labouring Poor*.

cholera, picked up at the port of departure, erupted far from shore, creating potentially horrendous epidemic conditions on board, especially for children.[8] In 1838, a fortnight into her voyage from Plymouth to the newly formed colony of South Australia, 26-year-old Sarah Brunskill wrote to her parents, 'At ten minutes past seven in the morning our dear boy breathed his last on my lap. Oh! how can I proceed! My heart is almost ready to burst. Soon after four his body was consigned to the deep about 90 miles from Oporto.'[9] Sarah's young son had died from convulsions and dehydration following a severe attack of diarrhoea. Later the very same day tragedy struck again, when her daughter died from an acute attack of measles:

> For her we prayed that she might be saved, but no, God in his good time thought fit to take her also to Himself, about ½ past twelve her dear spirit flew to that mansion from which no traveller returns, so you see in less than 24 hours our darlings were both in the bosom of God. Time, the soother of all things, will I hope reconcile us, but to say how we now feel I cannot [say that], away from all our friends, bereaved of our darlings, our cup is indeed full! 'Tis said all is for good, and that I hope we shall find, but the stroke is most severe. What great sin have we committed to be so severely punished? Did we think too much of our darlings to do our duty to our God, or what?[10]

She went on to write, 'Two little angels they looked, so beautiful in death ... The Union Jack was thrown over them, and the burial service performed.' Having witnessed a total of twenty burials at sea on their voyage, Sarah and her husband arrived safely, and went on to have a further eight children in the colony.[11]

Another emigrant who arrived in South Australia in 1839 recorded her family's four-month experience on a vessel carrying 318 migrants to the new colony. The grief-stricken Ellen Moger wrote to her parents:

> [At first], Edward and the children suffered but little from sickness. But as we entered on a warmer climate, the dear children [were] gradually getting weaker and, for want of proper nourishment, became at last sorrowful spectacles to behold ... Poor little Alfred was the first that died on the 30th of Oct., and on the 8th of Nov., dear Fanny went and three days after, on the 11th, the dear babe was taken from me. I scarcely know how I sustained the shock, though I was certain they could not recover, yet when poor Fanny went it over-powered me and from the weakness of my frame, reduced me to such a low nervous state that, for many weeks, I was not expected to survive.[12]

Death became a commonplace. Describing a sunset, Ellen observed,

---

[8] Haines, *Life and Death in the Age of Sail*; Haines, *Doctors at Sea*.
[9] George and Sarah Brunskill, 'Letter written on the Voyage'.
[10] Ibid.
[11] See Haines, *Life and Death in the Age of Sail*, pp. 85–95.
[12] Letter from Ellen Moger to her parents.

Whilst gazing on the beautiful scene you are, perhaps, interrupted by the sad tolling of a bell, informing you some poor victim to sickness and privation was about to be launched into a watery grave; such events are not uncommon, but the mind, I assure you, soon becomes hardened and callous on board a ship.[13]

Ellen witnessed the burial at sea of thirty passengers, predominantly children who had succumbed to disease. Indeed, children typically bore the brunt of disease on board ship. Of the assisted migrants who died at sea in the nineteenth century *en route* to Australia, three-quarters were under the age of 6. Ninety per cent of these victims were under the age of 3; half were under the age of 1.[14]

In reality, there was very little that a doctor could have done to save children suffering from an epidemic of measles, whooping cough or scarlet fever on board. It is surprising, rather, that more children – who often comprised one-third or more of those on board – did not die under the crowded conditions at sea. For infants and children under the age of 6, both on land and at sea, this was an era when the virulent infectious diseases of childhood – mainly measles, whooping cough, scarlet fever and diarrhoea – swept through the most vulnerable age groups.

Despite epidemics on some Australia-bound migrant ships, such disasters were rare after the mid nineteenth century and most voyages were, for adults, remarkably successful in terms of health and well-being. Countless south-bound emigrants enjoyed unremarkable passages, without rough seas or illness. Given the negative reputation of emigrant voyages, it is perhaps surprising to learn that over 98 per cent of government-assisted immigrants who boarded vessels at ports in the United Kingdom disembarked in Australia after their long voyage in reasonable health, ready to take on the challenges of working in the new colonies. Many declared that they had never felt fitter or fatter in their lives.[15] By the 1850s,

[13] Ellen Moger, quoted in Haines, *Life and Death in the Age of Sail*, p. 110.
[14] For comparative voyage loss rates (New South Wales, Victoria, South Australia, Queensland, according to contemporary official published data), see Haines, *Life and Death in the Age of Sail*, tables 1 and 2, pp. 29–30.
[15] The examples are too numerous to cite here, but, amongst the large volume of letters and diaries assayed in the books cited above, see, for example, the words of Ellen Moger cited below, and the diaries and letters of Julia Cross on the *James Fernie* from Southampton to Moreton Bay in 1885, who declared 'all my children look uncommon well considering the voyage … Many who boarded thin are fat now.' See 'Diary letter written by Julia Cross', Ely Museum, Ely, a copy of which is also housed in the Oxley Library, Brisbane, at M1550. Julia's voyage and settlement are discussed in Haines, *Life and Death in the Age of Sail*, p. 206. Most emigrants, including Edward Allchurch in 1866, mention the constant supply of puddings, pork and pastries (see 'The Voyage of the *Atalanta*, Plymouth to Adelaide, 1866: A Diary by Edward Allchurch', transcribed and edited by Adelaide McLean and Harold Baker, privately printed (n.d.). Surgeons, too, often reported children and adults growing fatter as the voyage progressed (see, for example, Surgeon Strutt's delight that the children in his charge looked 'well and fat', as they might well do given that he personally cooked for them, three times weekly, puddings of sago and other soft cereals so that they might avoid the suet that plagued the digestion of many adults). 'Journal of Dr Edward Strutt on board the *St Vincent* 1848', Freer Family Papers, MSS 8352, 8345, Box 913/5, La Trobe Collection, State Library of Victoria. All of the diaries mentioned here are discussed in detail in Haines, *Life and Death in the Age of Sail* or in *Doctors at Sea*.

adult mortality on government-assisted emigrant ships bound for Australia had enjoyed such a remarkable decline that it matched adult death rates in Britain; similarly, the mortality of older children was close to that of children at home. Two-thirds of all ships suffered five or fewer deaths, in spite of the large number of children on board. Ten per cent of ships suffered no deaths at all – a considerable feat of management given that a substantial proportion of their occupants were children.[16]

Regulation

How was it that Australia-bound emigrant ships were so successful in reducing mortality rates before the advent of modern medical science? The answer lies in the regulatory framework imposed by the authorities on state-assisted migrant vessels to Australia – as witnessed by their favourable comparison with survival on the much shorter, unregulated Atlantic crossing to North America.[17]

The Emigration Commission

To protect the immigrants, and to oversee the systematic scrutiny of procedures at sea (and on landing), colonial officials at the ports of arrival set up immigration departments. These officials managed procedures governing the reception and hiring of migrants, and they liaised first with the office of the Agent General for Emigration, a branch of the Colonial Office in London, and, from 1840, the Colonial Land and Emigration Commission, whose staff gradually expanded into a large unit of experts, many of whom remained in the department for decades. They oversaw the imposition of rules and regulations governing recruitment, selection, and the chartering and provisioning of suitable ships on behalf of the Australian colonies.[18]

Contrary to popular opinion, migrant ships bound for Australia in the nineteenth century were governed by strictly enforced regulations that went far beyond those of the Passenger Acts under which British merchant ships sailed. The Acts specified that every vessel carrying fifty or more passengers through the tropics, with an anticipated voyage time exceeding eighty days by sail or forty-five by steam, was required to carry a qualified surgeon. Though the Acts also regulated private ships, medical practitioners hired by private shipping companies were not required to keep official records, although they also gradually adopted the procedures that

---

[16] All figures mentioned in this chapter are derived from tables, data, and discussion included in those of my journal articles and books mentioned in footnotes above and below, resulting from a large project with my colleague Ralph Shlomowitz funded by the Australian Research Council on slave, convict and emigrant voyages in the eighteenth and nineteenth centuries.

[17] Haines and Shlomowitz, 'Explaining the Modern Mortality Decline', pp. 15–48; Haines and Shlomowitz, 'Maritime Mortality Revisited'; pp. 133–72; Haines, *Life and Death in the Age of Sail*; Haines, *Doctors at Sea*.

[18] Haines, *Emigration and the Labouring Poor*.

Table 8.1 Proportion of emigrants who embarked in the United Kingdom who died (loss rate) on voyages to New South Wales, Victoria, South Australia and Queensland, 1848–60 and 1861–9, in percentages

	NSW			VIC			SA			QLD		
	Adults	Children	All	Adults	Children	All	Adults	Children	All	Adults	Children	All
1848–60	0.6	5.2	1.7	0.7	6.2	2.1	0.5	5.5	1.9			
1861–9	0.4	2.0	0.6	0.2	2.7	0.5	0.2	4.3	1.0	0.6	5.4	1.4

Notes: Children include ages 0–13 before 1856, 0–11 thereafter. Higher child mortality on South Australia ships (1861–9) may be related to the higher proportion of children (20 per cent), than on New South Wales (15 per cent) and Victoria (13 per cent) ships, leading to a greater number of susceptibles for the transmission of infection. No tables were included for South Australia in CLEC appendices for 1848, therefore South Australian data are inclusive of 1849–60 and 1862–7. No ships were dispatched to South Australia by the CLEC in 1861, 1868 or 1869, hence gains made in New South Wales and Victoria in 1868–9 are not reflected in South Australian figures. Queensland-bound ships were included in New South Wales data before 1861, and only twenty-seven ships were dispatched to Moreton Bay by the CLEC between 1861 and 1867. Thereafter Queensland's Agent General was responsible for mobilisation and record-keeping. For a complete analysis of his data, 1860–1900, see Woolcock, *Rights of Passage*. So few ships were dispatched to Tasmania and Western Australia that they have not been included here. New South Wales data are inclusive of 1861–8; no ships were dispatched in 1869.

Source: Appendices to annual reports of the Colonial Land and Emigration Commission (CLEC); Robin Haines, *Life and Death in the Age of Sail* (London, 2006).

proved so efficacious on assisted voyages, in response to the high reputation of the Emigration Commission's regulated ships.[19]

The Provision of Surgeons and the Imposition of a Sanitary Regime

Another of the Emigration Commission's duties was to recruit and employ qualified, energetic and experienced medical practitioners capable of supervising a large body of people on a long ocean voyage. The origins of medical and sanitary regulation of emigrant vessels date back to the reforms introduced by Assistant Colonial Surgeon William Redfern's report to Governor Lachlan Macquarie on 30 September 1814, in response to the calamitous mortality on three convict ships recently arrived in New South Wales. Redfern had joined the Royal Navy in 1797 as a surgeon's mate, but was transported to New South Wales in 1801 for his part in the mutiny at the Nore. He worked as an assistant surgeon at the Norfolk Island penal settlement, for which he was given a free pardon in 1803. He was therefore well placed to make recommendations for the improvement of medical treatment of convicts. Death rates on convict ships plummeted following implementation of Redfern's recommendation that adequately trained, competent surgeons be endowed with the authority to challenge brutal, incompetent, or drunken captains. Dubiously qualified medical men were to be shunned. Surgeon superintendents who abrogated their responsibilities were to be punished severely. Equally important, he insisted that surgeons be given enough power to oversee

---

[19] On surgeons and the Passenger Acts, see Haines, *Doctors at Sea*, pp. 54–6.

Table 8.2 Emigrants who embarked in the United Kingdom who died on voyages to New South Wales, Victoria and South Australia, 1855–69, and to Queensland, 1860–6, by age

	Number embarked	Total deaths	Ages							
			Under 1	1–3	4–6	7–9	10–19	20–29	30–39	40–60
NSW	60,239	643	177	222	32	11	42	94	30	35
VIC	51,264	373	94	128	12	13	27	66	15	18
SA	37,056	421	149	154	14	8	20	45	14	17
QLD*	9,112	124	21	48	4	4	7	27	5	8
Total	157,671	1,561	441	552	62	36	96	232	64	78

	Voyage loss rate %	% of all deaths								
		Under 1	1–3	4–6	7–9	10–19	20–29	30–39	40–60	Total
NSW	1.1	25	34	3	3	7	18	4	5	100
VIC	0.7	28	35	5	2	7	15	5	5	100
SA	1.1	35	37	3	2	5	11	3	4	100
QLD*	1.4	17	39	3	3	6	22	4	6	100
All	1.0	28	35	4	2	6	15	4	5	100%

Notes: Victoria's lower percentage loss rate is probably related to the composition of ages on board: fewer children and higher proportions of adolescent and adult women.
* Queensland includes 1860–6 only (twenty-seven vessels dispatched by the CLEC).

Source: Appendices to annual reports of the CLEC; Robin Haines, *Life and Death in the Age of Sail* (London, 2006).

strict sanitation and hygiene procedures. At the forefront of ways of thinking about naval health and hygiene, Redfern pointed towards firm but kind discipline, daily exercise, personal and group hygiene, and co-operation over daily chores.[20]

Redfern, in effect, introduced the routines that were later to dominate the emigration service from its inception in 1831. The Colonial Office, learning from the experience of the Admiralty and Home Office, was in a good position to use the health and dietary regimes on convict ships as a template for the movement of families from one hemisphere to another. As we have seen, the diseases of child-

---

[20] After the introduction of such measures, deaths declined almost immediately, from eleven to two deaths per thousand per month. The rate was further reduced to one death per thousand after the mid 1850s on convict voyages to Western Australia. For Redfern's report, see *Historical Records of Australia*, Series I, vol. viii (n.d.), pp. 274–327. For death rates, see John McDonald and Ralph Shlomowitz, 'Mortality on Convict Voyages to Australia, 1788–1868', *Social Science History*, 13 (1989), pp. 285–313; John McDonald and Ralph Shlomowitz, 'Mortality on Immigrant Voyages to Australia in the Nineteenth Century', *Explorations in Economic History*, 27 (1990), table 6, p. 96. These and other articles on maritime mortality can be found in Ralph Shlomowitz, *Mortality and Migration in the Modern World* (London, 1996).

hood were of far greater consequence on emigrant ships, and mortality was bound to be far higher. Hence, as the emigration service progressed, surgeons and their policy makers were forced – by experimentation – to adapt their routines to take into account the health of the more vulnerable of their charges.

The maxim of 'cleanliness being next to godliness' governed attitudes to health and hygiene at sea, and meant that the steady reduction of adult mortality by 1850 on Australia-bound ships was in advance of that on land: a triumph by any standards.[21] This could not have been achieved without the supervision (and co-operation) of emigrants and the imposition of mandated procedures at sea by surgeons who wielded the sort of power that could only be envied by official medical officers of health on land.

During the first decade or so of assisted migration – the 1830s – naval surgeons were often employed on emigrant ships. They came with expertise gleaned from their supervision of Royal Navy vessels and sometimes also of convict transports. However, whereas the latter carried mainly adults, as we have seen, a large proportion of the human cargo on assisted migrant ships were children, often very young children and babies, who were most at risk of death at sea. Surgeons from the Royal Navy had little experience of caring for children, or of dealing with pregnant mothers and childbirth (whereas those employed on female convict vessels may have been more familiar with such matters). Hence a few voyages in the late 1830s, where childhood infectious disease prevailed, suffered horrifyingly high mortality, as we shall see. Thereafter, the newly formed Emigration Commission turned to private practitioners with appropriate qualifications to supervise families at sea.

For over a century maritime surgeons had learned both from each other, and from the extensive literature published by experimenting surgeons in the military, in the prison service, and on slave and merchant vessels. In the spirit of enquiry and humanitarianism adopted by surgeons in all these fields – including Thomas Trotter, Jeremiah Fitzpatrick, James Lind, John Pringle, and Gilbert Blane – a growing body of knowledge on disease prevention emerged. Innovations in medical science were sometimes based on novel experimentation and implementation, under their own auspices, by officers and surgeons who used their ships, quite consciously, as laboratories.[22] Not only did these pioneering practitioners experiment with the efficacy, for example, of various citrus fruits and other antiscorbutics, and cinchona, also known as Jesuit's bark (raw, unrefined quinine), for the treatment of malarial fevers, but also with ventilation, water purification, and dietary improvements. Most significantly, they argued – in numerous parliamentary inquiries and in their publications – that cleanliness was essential not only for good housekeeping practice, but for the prevention of disease. So numerous were their publications on various aspects of the health of seamen that,

---

[21] Haines and Shlomowitz, 'Explaining the Modern Mortality Decline', p. 15.

[22] For an extensive analysis of the influence of these famous reforming maritime and military surgeons, and their publications, and those of their less famous, but equally enthusiastic peers, see Haines and Shlomowitz, 'Explaining the Mortality Decline in the Eighteenth-century British Slave Trade', *Economic History Review*, 53 (2000), pp. 262–83.

in 1793, one publisher (John Murray) was moved to print a catalogue, available for maritime surgeons, of books and pamphlets on disease prevention at sea.[23]

It appears that the views of maritime and military reformers were not read just by maritime and military practitioners, but by their colleagues in the burgeoning public health fields, and by lay readers as well.[24] And it is precisely because the surgeons treated their ships as laboratories that they were later so influential. Theirs were empirical successes, not just models for potential action. Of course, not every maritime or military surgeon was motivated to observe and experiment. But published texts often gained official sanction, and were distributed to the Navy and merchant services, where surgeons were expected to follow the advice and superintend the regulations that were gradually mandated. A diligent surgeon might be in possession of an extensive library of books emphasising connections between the health of prisoners, slaves, convicts, soldiers, crews, emigrants, and civilians. Consequently, superintending surgeons on voyages to Australia in the nineteenth century were the inheritors of a well-established tradition of experimentation and dissemination of ideas and practice.[25] By the 1840s, medical practitioners employed on Australia-bound assisted emigrant ships were thus at the forefront of their rising profession. Most of the surgeon superintendents on migrant ships (from the mid 1840s when, after a hiatus of a few years, assisted emigration recommenced in earnest) were more correctly physicians rather than surgeons. They were often graduates of the University of Edinburgh – then at the forefront of medical training – or had studied abroad in highly regarded German or Dutch universities. The term 'surgeon' for maritime practitioners was adopted from the Royal Navy, where it was used to describe all medical staff whatever their training – whether as surgeons, apothecaries or physicians.

Most important was the focus on preventative medicine. The emphasis on prevention was stimulated by a new wave of interest in public health promoted by many medical practitioners and other reformers determined to improve the lot of the urban poor, particularly following the devastating outbreaks of Asiatic cholera in Britain in 1831–2, 1848–9 and 1853–4. This reforming zeal was transferred to convict and emigrant ships bound for Australia in response to the expectation, in London and the colonies, that immigrants required for the economic advancement of these remote outposts of empire would arrive in a healthy condition.

The degree of importance attached to the role of surgeon superintendents is demonstrated by the fact that they were paid extraordinarily well. Their gratuity rose in incremental steps (of two shillings) with each voyage successfully supervised, from ten shillings for the first, to a maximum of one pound per immigrant landed alive. This sum, guaranteed to be an incentive to deliver emigrants alive and well to their destination, netted experienced surgeons hundreds of pounds per

[23] John Murray, *A Catalogue of Medical Books, Chiefly those upon Diseases of Seamen: As well as those Incident to Hot Climates and in Long Voyages* (London, 1793).
[24] See for example Hector Gavin's *Sanitary Ramblings: Being Sketches and Ramblings, of Bethnal Green* (London, 1848).
[25] Haines, *Doctors at Sea*, ch. 4.

voyage, a fortune for doctors in the over-endowed medical profession in Britain where it was relatively difficult to make a living. (By comparison, surgeons on the unregulated Atlantic run earned just a few pounds per voyage.) Surgeons were also permitted to charge fees on the return voyage for attending well-off passengers returning to Britain, supplementing their earnings substantially.[26]

Pre-emigration Screening and Training of Passengers

The authorities regulated migration from the point of application. Since the 1830s, experience had shown that limiting the number of very young children per family on individual ships paid dividends in terms of health and welfare, given the prevalence of childhood disease at the ports of departure which could subsequently endanger the lives of everyone on board. Consequently, by the late 1840s, families with no more than three children under the age of 10, or two children under 7, were sought as applicants, though from time to time these regulations were relaxed, at a tragic cost when epidemics of measles, diarrhoea, whooping cough or croup broke out.[27]

At the emigrant depot prior to departure, the surgeon inspected his charges for health and signs of illness, rejecting those he believed could not survive the arduous voyage, or families with a child visibly suffering from an infection such as measles, or who could not provide evidence of having been vaccinated against – or show signs of having recovered from – smallpox. Those who had not been vaccinated, but who were willing, were vaccinated on the spot by the surgeon, who carried vaccine with him for further vaccinations at sea if necessary. Emigrants were domiciled in the depot for days, or occasionally weeks, before the departure of their vessel (mainly from Plymouth, but also from Southampton, from Nine Elms on the Thames, and, less often for Australia-bound emigrants, from Liverpool). There, they were introduced to mess dining, bathing, and the use of water closets, which were a novelty to the vast majority of emigrants. Most emigrants were convinced by the lectures of officials and chaplains stationed at the ports of departure that it was to their advantage to defer willingly to the authority of the surgeon.[28] Often, one or more of the Emigration Commissioners travelled to the quayside to lecture and give a farewell to emigrants. Homilies and other improving literature on Christian duty, and pamphlets on basket-weaving, rope-making, physical exercise and other ways of keeping busy on board in preparation for a life in the colonies, were distributed by various Church of England organisations.[29]

---

[26] Ibid., pp. 76–9.

[27] See regulations governing passengers in Haines, *Emigration and the Labouring Poor*, appendix 4, pp. 272–81; and also Haines, *Doctors at Sea*, p. 19.

[28] Many emigrants refer to the significance of the surgeon and his regulations, and the formal technique of their letter writing suggests that the emigrant pamphlets published in bulk by various Church of England charitable organisations were well read, and their letter- and journal-writing templates well used. See the emigrant testimonies in Haines, *Doctors at Sea* and *Life and Death in the Age of Sail*.

[29] On the work of the port-side chaplains and religious charities, including the Societies for the Propagation of Christian Knowledge and Propagation of the Gospel, and their associations,

Adults were expected to take advantage of the presence of a schoolmaster on board, and to improve their reading and writing and, especially, their letter-writing skills. That many followed the urging of the lectures and pamphlets is manifest in their diaries and letters. The depots were an important introduction to the voyage, instilling the expectations of the colonial authorities who, in return for offering a free passage, counted upon co-operation between the emigrants themselves, and with the surgeon and his volunteer assistants.

These assistants – usually respectable married men – were chosen from among the passengers by the surgeon at the depot. They earned the considerable sum of two to five pounds for satisfactory work as sanitary constables on board, and at the end of the voyage they were also issued with a character reference, enhancing their chances of the best employment opportunities on shore. Married men eagerly sought a position as a voluntary constable, both because of the status endowed and because of the prospect of earning money on the voyage out.[30] At the depot the surgeon also chose a matron from volunteers amongst the married women. The matron helped in the hospital ward and supervised the single women, for a similar gratuity distributed upon arrival if her performance was deemed satisfactory.

Regulation of Shipping Routes, Passenger Numbers and Size of Vessels

Another way in which the authorities regulated voyages was in the routing of voyages and in the size of vessels and passenger numbers. Some ships' masters – in pursuit of records and fame perhaps – defied the regulations and sailed the extreme Great Circle route, causing great discomfort to the emigrants in the gigantic, freezing, seas of the Southern Ocean around the 50th parallel. To ensure successful voyages, and with the comfort of emigrants in mind, the Emigration Commissioners therefore enforced new regulations upon masters who were instructed to follow a modified Great Circle route.[31]

The correlation of passenger numbers to size of vessels was also critical to health and mortality on board. As noted above, ordinarily, under the Emigration Commission's regulations, families with more than two or three young children were not permitted to embark. However, at a time when Australian demands for agricultural labour were unremitting, in 1852 the Commissioners reluctantly bowed to pressure from deputations of land-owning colonists in London for a relaxation of these rules to allow for an increase in recruitment. The Commis-

---

see Haines, *Emigration and the Labouring Poor*, ch. 6, where the work of the much revered Revd Thomas Cave Childs is also discussed. For the work and proselytising on board before departure of the British Ladies Female Emigration Society, see Haines, *Doctors at Sea*, ch. 8.

[30] For just two examples of eager voluntary constables, see the diary of Edward Allchurch, in Haines, *Life and Death in the Age of Sail*, p. 242, and that of Hugh Wilson, in Haines, *Doctors at Sea*, pp. 127–8. The chance of earning money on the voyage out was a great incentive to volunteer, although a strict code of conduct was expected and demanded by the surgeons, the Commissioners, and the immigration agents in Australia.

[31] On the record passage of the *Constance* in 1849, see Haines, *Doctors at Sea*, pp. 163, 336–7, notes 96 and 97; Haines, *Doctors at Sea*, pp. 36, 105; and for Great Circle sailing, see ch. 7.

sioners made two critical errors of judgement which were to shatter them (and ultimately bring about a tightening of their regulations thereafter): first, with great apprehension, they allowed the recruitment of large families with several very young children; and secondly, they reluctantly chartered some American-built double-decker vessels. The risks, they knew, were compounded by the fact that the ships would be leaving from Liverpool, a city then raging with disease and which was rarely the port of embarkation for Australia-bound assisted emigrant vessels. Moreover, the ships would be carrying large numbers of children from the peripheries of the British Isles, mainly from the poverty-stricken Scottish Highlands, and the famine-weary west of Ireland – people already under stress.

Thus in 1852, amongst ten ships bound for Australia (each of at least a thousand tons), were eight American-built double-deckers.[32] Once the first four vessels had sailed, the Commissioners waited anxiously for news of the ships' arrival. They were appalled when they heard of the catastrophic, though not altogether unexpected, voyage of the *Bourneuf*, the first to arrive, a 1,495-ton double-decked ship carrying 754 emigrants. Eighty-four had died at sea, and a further four in quarantine. All but five of the dead were children. The *Marco Polo*, a 1,625-ton vessel, arrived with 887 passengers, having buried fifty-two emigrants at sea on its seventy-eight-day voyage. On just four of the double-decked ships, the *Bourneuf*, *Marco Polo*, *Wanata* and *Ticonderoga*, the combined deaths at sea and in quarantine amounted to 356.[33]

Significantly, however, the *Europa*, at 1,088 tons and carrying 492 migrants, lost just eight passengers on its ninety-day voyage, confirming the benefits of the greater space available on high tonnage ships when far fewer emigrants were carried. The Emigration Commissioners, chastened by their lack of judgement in allowing the colonial governments to bully them into chartering the double-deckers, in a year when colonial demands for rural labour were particularly strident and ships available for charter scarce, were never again to contemplate such a rash decision. They resolved to charter no more double-deckers, and death rates immediately plummeted. They recognised the benefit of large ships, however, which were faster and more spacious, offered greater comfort, and reduced the risk of mortality at sea. They were much favoured by both the Emigration Commissioners and the colonial immigration agents, but only so long as they kept to a reasonable passenger/tonnage ratio, similar to that on the *Europa*, and restrictions on the number of children in each family under the age of 7 were observed. Nevertheless, epidemics were to continue, and one of the more notable findings of my time-patterning of deaths over the length of voyages to South Australia between 1848 and 1885 demonstrated that, contrary to expectations, childhood infections such as measles, scarlatina/scarlet fever, and whooping cough appear not to have died down before

[32] The ships were the *Marco Polo*, *Wanata*, *Bourneuf*, *Ticonderoga*, *Hercules*, *Dirigo*, *Shackamaxon* and *Europa*.
[33] Annual report of Victorian Immigration Agent Edward Grimes, 9 June 1853, Appendix No. 4, in 'Correspondence Relating to Emigration to the Australian Colonies', BPP, 1854 (436), vol. XLVI, p. 164. See also Haines, *Doctors at Sea*, pp. 20–4.

the end of the passage on voyages where epidemics occurred; there were enough susceptible passengers on board to keep the infections active. Hence it is likely that children with incipient measles, for example, walked, or were carried, up the gangway and onto Australian soil as voyage times shortened in the early 1840s. By the end of the decade, numerous vessels were quarantined, having arrived with passengers still presenting with measles and other infections.[34]

Supervising Health on Board: The Role and Responsibilities of the Surgeon

The day-to-day regulation of state-assisted emigrant voyages can be examined through the prism of the responsibilities of the medical officers on board. As superintendents with special authoritarian powers, they were responsible for the safe carriage of between 150 and 1,000 men, women and children travelling in steerage on individual ships. Like those on convict ships, which mainly carried adults, the housekeeping and sanitary regulations embodied in the official 'Instructions to Surgeons' governing assisted emigrant vessels were designed to lower mortality and to promote the comfort and well-being of families travelling in steerage. In many ways, it was the success of their pastoral care and supervision of the daily regimes on board, and their disciplinary role as the agent of the state at sea (submission to the strict supervision of authority – the surgeon superintendent – was mandatory), rather than their medical training and skill as surgeons, which made all the difference in the sphere of maritime health.

Medical Work
Surgeons' medical skills were, of course, important: they dispensed medicine for a range of complaints, especially chronic indigestion and constipation, and acted as resident obstetricians and paediatricians, often successfully delivering a number of infants at sea while caring for ante- and post-natal mothers and their newborn infants, usually with the help of a matron. At their daily clinics, doctors attended to every kind of illness, mainly digestive problems for adults, and infections, worms, and irritability in children. They put into practice isolation procedures when an infection erupted on board, and they were sometimes called upon to set limbs sprained or broken in falls, suture wounds, and occasionally perform operations for hernias, or internal obstructions, or a tracheotomy on a child with diphtheria. Post-mortems were sometimes called for.

The extent to which emigrants relied on doctors for comfort and relief at sea, as their letters and diaries attest, meant that at their daily clinics on board,

---

[34] Robin Haines and Ralph Shlomowitz, 'Causes of Death of British Emigrants on Voyages to South Australia 1848–1885', *Journal of the Society for the Social History of Medicine*, 16 (2003), pp. 193–208; *Doctors at Sea*, especially pp. 5, 140. Measles was endemic in Melbourne by mid-century, and measles and scarlatina, for example, reached Sydney on quarantined ships in the late 1840s. See Jean Duncan Foley, *In Quarantine: A History of Sydney's Quarantine Station, 1828–1984* (Sydney, 1995).

many surgeons were faced with a long line of patients who were unaccustomed to medical care at home but determined to take advantage of his obligations to them. Ellen Moger, laid low by seasickness and her children's deaths, called on her doctor for a good deal of bleeding, blistering, and plastering during the voyage, and the doctor paid her much attention.[35] The emigrants, far more literate than generally understood, knew their rights regarding medical care on board, and took full advantage of them.

Many newborn infants and their mothers thrived under the surgeon's care; some infants wasted away in spite of their attention, owing largely to the dreadful seasickness suffered by pregnant and nursing mothers. While many women, and men, found their sea legs quite quickly and thrived during the passage, their less robust fellow travellers found that the seasickness at the beginning of the voyage left them feeling weak and debilitated on and off for some time. Women seem to have suffered from motion sickness to a greater degree than men, suffering misery and weakness with constant nausea, often prostrate for days or weeks at the beginning of the voyage and at other times during heavy weather, especially upon entry into the boisterous Southern Ocean after the calm of the tropics.[36] The surgeon could do little for seasickness apart from prescribe aperients and encourage his patients to go on deck as soon as they were able. Most, though, were comforted by the surgeon's attention. It is, perhaps, surprising that on South Australia-bound ships between 1848 and 1885 – voyages for which we have individual causes of death – just two were attributed to seasickness. However, it is likely that maternal seasickness was responsible, indirectly, for the death of infants who were prematurely delivered or whose mothers were too ill to nurse or care for them, as in the case of Ellen Moger. She recorded that, 'for the first five weeks I was scarcely able to move my head from my pillow with sea-sickness, which brought me so low that I could render but very little assistance to the dear children' – who, as we know, subsequently died.[37]

Supervision of Ventilation and Cleaning

One of the greatest boosts given to maritime health, as we have seen, was the report submitted by Assistant Colonial Surgeon Redfern in 1814. Redfern's recommendations included strict supervision of daily scrubbing of decks, cooking gear and mess tables, and daily fumigation between decks. By the 1840s, a decade of experience had both endorsed Redfern's recommendations and shown that the health of children, especially infants, would be the major concern of surgeons at

[35] Letter from Ellen Moger to her parents.
[36] See the diary of Ellen Moger on the subject of seasickness, cited below, and see also Edward Allchurch's descriptions of his wife's seasickness, and the misery of the women under his care as voluntary constable: 'Our dinner table is a melancholy sight, the women sitting with their heads hanging down, Babys crying etc., such a scene, very rough night had to turn out, the children very sick, the ship rolling very heavily …', cited in Haines, *Life and Death in the Age of Sail*, p. 245. On the subject of the greater susceptibility of women to seasickness, see Haines, *Doctors at Sea*, pp. 9–10.
[37] Letter from Ellen Moger to her parents.

sea. Hence, in an attempt to prevent illness – or the spread of disease – surgeons were enjoined by the Emigration Commissioners to keep their vessels clean, scrubbed, well deodorized and ventilated; to supervise the emigrants' hygienic practices such as regular bathing and clothes washing; and to ensure that sanitation was of the highest standard.

As it had been on Royal Navy vessels since the eighteenth century, ventilation was deemed very important. During calm seas the hatches could safely be left open with wind sails directing air through them. Nevertheless the atmosphere between decks would have been fairly abhorrent, particularly after a night in which three to four hundred people had slept in cramped accommodation, serviced by only three or four water closets, and without the benefits of Navy discipline. Worse, on stormy nights, when the hatches were closed, only the air shafts were left for ventilation. Despite the attentions of the constables, the water closets often malfunctioned or overflowed, adding to the stench.[38] Competing with these, and the fetid air produced by numerous adults and children living in close proximity, were the daily fumigants smoking in charcoal and tar- or creosote-burning swinging stoves. Other malodorous disinfectants were sprinkled liberally on the decks and bottom boards of the berths, including chloride of lime or zinc mixed with vinegar and other solutions. Hugh Wilson, a voluntary constable on board the *Sarah* bound for Sydney in 1849, usually rose between 4 and 5 a.m. because the air was not very good by that time. As he explained,

> ... soon afterwards the deck is filled with washing parties the sailers busy washing and scrubbing the deck and the emigrants washing either their clothes or persons and by the time they have got themselves dressed and provisions for the day tis 8 o'clock and the Captains of the mess are busy getting down their tea or coffee [from the galley]. Imeddeately after breakfast two of each mess wash the things and scrub with dry sand and stones the whole of the floor & forms, the stones used are ... called holley stones [holy stones]. On the other days the deck is scraped with scrapers and swept clean after every meal, and as infection is feard they fumigate the t'ween decks every two days, the effect there of, is both apparent and pleasant and we feel much more comfortable thereafter. I hope they manage to prevent or stay the prospect of disease but if it is God's will that I am not to reach Sydney I say his Will be done.[39]

With the daily scrubbing and fumigating routines, ventilation, and strict housekeeping, most emigrants found that the deodorants freshened the air considerably. Many well-disciplined ships appear to have avoided the stenches reported on those high-profile pestilent vessels where order had disintegrated, seriously

---

[38] For problems related to water closets reported by surgeons, see Haines, *Life and Death in the Age of Sail*, pp. 115, 77, 263. References to overflowing cisterns and the wrongful use of WCs (such as throwing food or clothing into them, thus blocking them up) permeate the immigration agents' and surgeons' reports. See Haines, *Doctors at Sea*, p. 37.

[39] Diary of Hugh Wilson on the *Sarah*, 1849, Mitchell Library, Sydney, B1535 (CY 1024). For a comprehensive account of his commentary on the voyage, see Haines, *Life and Death in the Age of Sail*, pp. 146–65, and *Doctors at Sea*, p. 128.

testing the patience and temper of their human cargo (and of the authorities who examined the ships on arrival).

It was the voluntary constables' job to ensure that rostered emigrants took it in turn to fetch water and meals from the galley at appointed times, sweep and clean the decks, berths and tables, and check that the water closets were working, beds made and so forth. They also took it in turns to guard the single women's quarters against the predations of male emigrants and sailors. Their supervision, under the governance of the surgeon, was crucial to the outcome of the voyage. Constables whom the surgeon deemed to lack the energy or initiative for the task were dismissed and replaced by a more worthy volunteer. Hugh Wilson noted, however, that on board the *Sarah* 'the Drs orders are not complied with'. Unfortunately, the doctor was 'inexperienced' and making 'his first trip to sea', and could have done little to combat the outbreak of Asiatic cholera that engulfed the ship.[40]

Supervision of Washing and Diet

Supervised clothes washing was allowed on deck only twice weekly, including the washing of soiled nappies. Passenger baggage allowances, including regulations on clothing, had an indirect influence on hygiene. Adults were allowed to take the tools of their trade, but total baggage was not to weigh more than half of one ton, or exceed twenty cubic or solid feet in measurement. Boxes were not to exceed ten cubic feet. The compulsory outfit of clothes need not be new, but was to be sufficiently robust to endure a long passage. Inspected for quantity and quality before departure, it was to contain not less than the following items. For males: six shirts, six pairs each of stockings and shoes, and two complete suits of exterior clothing. Two or three serge shirts for men and extra flannel for women and children were also recommended. For females: six shifts, two flannel petticoats, six pairs of stockings, two pairs of shoes, and two gowns: 'the larger the stock of Clothing the better for health and comfort during the voyage'.[41] Sheets, towels and soap were also to be included, suitable for very hot and very cold climates. Emigrants with insufficient or poor quality clothing were obliged to purchase new items, or they would be refused permission to embark. Yet, either for the sake of delicacy, or because officials assumed that women would automatically take care of such personal items, no provision was made in the regulations for nappies (diapers) or sanitary napkins.[42] Emigrant manuals encouraged mothers to bring dozens of disposable nappies made from old linen but, for those travelling in steerage, space was severely limited, probably leading to infrequent nappy changes and hence increasing the potential for serious illness. One manual advised its better-off readers as follows:

[40] Ibid.
[41] See table 2.3 in Haines, *Emigration and the Labouring Poor*, p. 26.
[42] For a full review of the kit and clothing regulations, see Haines, *Emigration and the Labouring Poor*, p. 26.

The mother who has to take an infant on board, or she who expects to be confined on the voyage, should, for some time before her embarkation, obtain from her friends all the old cotton or linen she can procure, and manufacture them into napkins, of which she must have very many dozens; for, as these cannot be used again on board ship, and must, the moment they are removed, go through the port-hole, unless she be *well* supplied, the mother will be very unpleasantly situated.[43]

It was also the surgeon's duty to ensure that the emigrants (especially children and infants) received their mandatory rations, including special infant foods, and that their food was well cooked. Like most emigrants, Sarah Brunskill found the diet palatable and abundant:

Our provisions are of the best kind and more than we ever can consume. Twice a week we have 3 lb ½ of preserved meat to which we put a quart of water and it makes a most excellent soup ... we bake fresh bread every day, a great luxury I can assure you. Twice a week we have salt beef which is not good – the other days pork and as fine meat as I ever wished to eat; potatoes one day, and rice the next; a plentiful supply of raisins, so we often have good puddings. The flour and suet are as good as I ever had at home. In short our provisions are of the best kind.[44]

Conversely, Ellen Moger's voyage was not so well provisioned. She says of her children when they sickened:

They could eat none of the ship's provisions and our vessel was not like many that are sent out, provided with one or more cows for the accommodation of the sick; and had I the voyage to take again, I would make that a first consideration as I firmly believe that the dear children would have lived, and much sickness been spared, had we experienced proper attention from our Doctor and been provided with a little natural nourishment.[45]

The testimony of many emigrants confirms that, overall, the cleanliness and hygiene routines generally worked well. It can also be inferred – from the conditions under which they lived on shore – that life below decks was tolerable for most emigrants and their surgeon superintendents. Australia-bound emigrants were self-selecting individuals who were screened for their health and respectability before departure, but life at home was generally crowded, odiferous and

---

[43] *The Dictionary of Medical and Surgical Knowledge and Complete Practical Guide in Health and Disease for Families, Emigrants, and Colonists* (London, 1864), p. 277. The manual also advised families to bring some quires of common brown paper to be made ready for use and kept handy, but did not mention what 'this most requisite article' was to be used for. Undoubtedly, its readers understood. The author's insistence that soiled nappies (and menstrual napkins) go through the port-hole suggests that cabin passengers, rather than emigrants for whom there was no accessible port-hole in steerage, were expected to take note of this advice.

[44] George and Sarah Brunskill, 'Letter written on the Voyage'.

[45] Letter from Ellen Moger to her parents.

domestic arrangements uncomfortable, even wretched, for the poorer rural classes from whom the majority of migrants were drawn. They were accustomed to living in close quarters with large families; their incomes were low and they had little to spare for even the humblest luxury. Indeed, many people, as their letters and diaries confirm, enjoyed the voyage, treating it as a temporary retreat from the grind of daily work. Despite losing her children, Ellen Moger declared that she had had 'a safe, and many would say, a delightful voyage', and even found time in her letters to describe the magnificence of the marine scenery.[46]

Redress against Incompetent Surgeons

Surgeons on ships bound for Australia in the nineteenth century have generally received a bad press. Some surgeons were indeed incompetent, drunken, and idle. Their filthy, smelly ships – when inspected upon landing – infuriated and disgusted local officials and elicited outrage in official correspondence to London, and in the Australian and British press. But these surgeons did not, as a rule, go unpunished. Even vessels that arrived in a clean and tidy state, whose surgeons were reported by emigrants or immigration department officials as incompetent or unworthy of the confidence placed in them, could be fined extraordinarily large sums of money, as we shall see.[47] The public shaming of such surgeons, via the press, the various Government Gazettes, and in official reports, served as a warning to others to take their position, and the authority vested in them, seriously.

In the interests of tightening procedures to reduce illness and death on their chartered vessels, the Emigration Commissioners continuously evaluated the performance and efficiency of surgeons. They compiled and published reports in parliamentary blue books based on comments and enquiries made at the ports of departure by the immigration agents. Most often surgeons were considered to be 'most efficient', 'very efficient', 'humane', 'well spoken of by the emigrants'. Negative comments included, 'inefficient and intemperate habits', 'highly unsatisfactory', 'not equal to his duties', 'surgeon not sufficiently energetic in enforcing cleanliness'. The Commissioners made it clear when a surgeon was ineligible for further employment in the service, with comments such as 'unfitted by temper and health for re-employment'.[48]

Upon arrival, surgeons who had breached the trust placed in them, or shirked their responsibilities, were not only recorded as unemployable in the future, but could be fined large sums as high as £20 for allowing communication between sailors and single women. Punishment was sometimes even more drastic. The Queensland Supreme Court, in 1864, jailed one surgeon for six months for having lied to the Health Officer at Moreton Bay about the presence of infection among

---

[46] Ibid.

[47] Haines, *Doctors at Sea*, pp. 85–91.

[48] Sub-enclosure 2, to enclosure 1, in no. 3, Earl Grey to Governor Fitzroy, 11 March 1850, in 'Papers Relative to Emigration, NSW', *BPP*, 1851 (347), vol. XL, pp. 84–8.

immigrants on the *Flying Cloud*. His false declaration had led, or so it was believed at the time, to the spread of typhoid fever in Brisbane, after pratique (permission to enter port) was granted prematurely to his ship. Some surgeons were fined in consequence of emigrants' complaints against them. South Australia's Immigration Agent, upon receiving any complaints from emigrants, summoned the Immigration Board to examine the complainants. In the case of the *Mallard* in 1855, the surgeon was fined one-quarter of his gratuity (his pro rata fee for each immigrant landed alive, hence a considerable sum) for multiple misdemeanours. His transgressions included neglecting his duty regarding the sick, failing to enforce a proper issue of rations, especially to young children, failure to keep a medical journal as instructed, and want of discipline.[49]

Others who fell foul of the Immigration Agent were deprived of their return passage money, and the surgeon of the *Lord of the Isles* in the same year had proven so incompetent that the Immigration Board insisted that 'he should not again be entrusted with the charge of an emigrant ship'. He had 'greatly neglected his duty in not attending to the cleanliness of the ship ... consequently filth and vermin prevailed among the people'. Not only was he sacked, but his gratuity was reduced from ten to seven shillings and sixpence per immigrant landed alive.[50] Punishments such as this reflected the standards demanded by officials in Britain and Australia. Ineffectual surgeons were occasionally docked their entire gratuity, and ship owners were fined from £50 to £2,000 for failing to honour the charter party. That these fines were imposed ought not suggest that incompetence was widespread but, rather, that management of government-chartered vessels remained under scrutiny by both officialdom and the press, who demanded accountability. The transgressions of a minority of surgeons thus indicate that mortality might have been far higher had it not been for tight scrutiny in both hemispheres. The failures of a few, sensationalized in the press, served as a warning to others, but ought not to overshadow the performance of the majority.[51]

Though cases of gross ineptitude are often chosen to illustrate emigrant voyages, they are, fortunately for Australia's pioneer immigrants, relatively rare. Even without the huge amount of individual information that exists, on the ships, the surgeons and the immigrants, this could be deduced from the fact that all but 2 per cent of assisted migrants who boarded vessels in the United Kingdom arrived at a colonial port alive and in reasonable health. Many diarists delighted in boasting about their weight gain during the voyage. Some of the disastrous voyages – those with the highest death rates – were supervised by competent medical practitioners who could do little in the face of an unforeseen epidemic against which no doctor, with all the medicines at his disposal, could fight, especially on a double-decked vessel with up to one thousand or more people on board, and with just one or two assistant surgeons.

---

[49] Immigration Agent's quarterly Report, *South Australian Government Gazette*, 12 July 1855.
[50] Ibid., 1 February 1855.
[51] See Haines, *Doctors at Sea*, chs 5 and 11.

Many emigrants often mention their surgeon in their diaries and letters. Some blamed doctors for lack of proper care during their children's illnesses. Ellen Moger described her surgeon as a 'young and austere man'. He was, she wrote, 'during the first half of the passage very careless and inattentive to the health of the passengers, till there were many alarming deaths, when he became more solicitous, respecting them'. In her letter she partly blamed the surgeon for the deaths of her own children, saying that he had not paid them 'proper attention'.[52] However, many eulogised the surgeon who supervised their voyage. Women – many of whom told correspondents that their confinement at sea had been their easiest, and expressed great confidence in their surgeon and his treatment before and after the birth – named children born at sea after him, celebrated his birthday at sea, and sewed counterpanes and shirts for him in gratitude for his services. Emigrants delivered petitions to colonial authorities upon arrival, praising the surgeon, and some women were loath to take their leave of him at the journey's end. Far more surgeons appear to have been truly revered than feared.

Surgeons' Careers and Medical Expertise in Australia

The extent to which expertise gained at sea found its way into medical practice in Australia is difficult to establish. But given that many colonial practitioners made their way to Australia as a superintendent on an emigrant vessel, it is probable that their sanitary supervision, and experience gained in their daily clinics attended by queues of patients, and their management of childhood diseases on board, did not go to waste in Australia.

Many surgeons stayed in the service for decades, undertaking twenty or more voyages. Some superintended one or two voyages, saving enough money to establish a private practice at home. Others made just one voyage, settling in Australia either to practise privately, or to take up positions in the colonial public service, or in departments of health. One much admired surgeon, Dr John Sprod, who arrived on the *Forfarshire* in 1874, went on to become a senior health officer in Adelaide, typifying the careers of numerous surgeons who worked their passage to Australia in the expectation of finding a position in the colonies.[53] Others took up posts in the immigration departments, where their knowledge of disease-containment and supervision of families undoubtedly enhanced public health measures in the rapidly growing cities of Australia. South Australia's Immigration Agent and Health Officer for the Port of Adelaide for nearly three decades from the late 1840s was a zealous Scots medical practitioner, Dr Handasyde Duncan, who encouraged surgeons on Adelaide-bound ships to bring him the latest information on every aspect of sanitation, public health, diet, and more. From about 1850 he chemically tested the new dietary foods and infant formulas carried by ships,

52 Letter from Ellen Moger to her parents.
53 Haines, *Doctors at Sea*, p. 91.

wrote lengthy reports on their efficacy or otherwise, promoted some brands over others, and made his views heard in London in his regular reports, which were forwarded to the Commissioners.[54]

Medical innovation could reach Australia with extraordinary speed, as shown by the importation of chloroform by an Adelaide doctor in May 1848, just six months after its success was first publicly confirmed in Edinburgh the previous November.[55] As news of the discovery cannot have reached Australia before February, Dr Kent's consignment must have been sent by a colleague aware of his interest in anaesthesia, or brought to him by a ship's surgeon for similar reasons. Shortly afterwards, Dr Kent and his colleague, Dr Mayo, demonstrated chloroform's efficacy in anaesthetising their patients.[56] This was not a one-way process. By the 1870s medical practitioners in Melbourne were at the forefront of surgical treatment for diphtheria and at least one surgeon superintendent performed a tracheotomy on a patient at sea, a procedure he had most likely learned in Melbourne.[57] In this way, pioneering medical practice in the colonies migrated, via surgeon superintendents who adopted ideas and practice learned during their sojourn in the colonial capitals, back to Britain and elsewhere.

Conclusion

To recapitulate: of the 2 per cent of assisted migrants who died at sea in the nineteenth century *en route* to Australia, three-quarters were under the age of 6. Ninety per cent of these victims were under the age of 3; half were under the age of 1. These young children embody the tragic costs to parents of migration from one hemisphere to another in the age of sail. Nevertheless, infant and childhood mortality on land was also exceptionally high. For the majority of children and their parents, the voyage represented an introduction to a new world, where their labour was in demand, and where opportunities for social and economic advancement abounded. If it had not been for dedicated, dutiful, and often sympathetic supervision by over two thousand surgeon superintendents, this extraordinarily successful delivery of nearly three-quarters of a million people to Australia could not be celebrated today.

Without doubt, government intrusion into the lives of travellers really mattered in drastically reducing mortality at sea. By systematically monitoring the ships, the

---

54 On Dr Duncan's close interest in improving the lot of migrants, see Haines, *Doctors at Sea*, especially pp. 99–102 on infant feeding and testing of new methods of bunks and bedding.
55 First discussed in the *Medico-Chirurgical Society of Edinburgh* on 10 November 1847, its efficacy was described by James Young and J.Y. Simpson, in 'On a New Anaesthetic Agent, more Efficient than Sulphuric Ether', *The Lancet*, 21 November 1847.
56 *The South Australian*, 30 May, 18 July 1848.
57 For diphtheria and its treatment in Australia, see F.B. Smith, 'Comprehending Diphtheria', *Health and History*, 1 (1999). For an account of Surgeon Superintendent Kynsdon's treatment of a 5-year-old child with diphtheria on the *Queen of Nations* in 1877, see Haines, *Doctors at Sea*, p. 49.

equipment, the health of emigrants and the performance of surgeons, the imperial and colonial governments were able to oversee the successful delivery of Australia's free settlers in the Victorian era. And, from the 1850s, the remarkable decline in mortality on ships carrying families over fourteen thousand miles was in advance of a similar decline on land. In the absence of sophisticated medical science, attention to the virtues of clean water, an adequate diet, and strict attention to sanitation and hygiene, were shown to be the quickest route to low mortality. The surgeons' superintendence of the health, hygiene, and sanitary routines on board meant that convict and emigrant voyages to Australasia, in spite of the far longer duration of the voyage, were the most successful of all transoceanic crossings in the nineteenth century.[58]

---

[58] Haines and Shlomowitz, 'Explaining the Modern Mortality Decline'.

9

Medical Encounters on the Kala Pani: Regulation and Resistance in the Passages of Indentured Indian Migrants, 1834–1900

Laurence Brown and Radica Mahase

During the nineteenth century, over one million migrants left the Indian sub-continent to cross the *Kala Pani* ('dark waters') as indentured workers for the tropical colonies of the Atlantic, Pacific and Indian Oceans. For many of these migrants, the voyage marked a profound rupture with the social and cultural worlds which defined their lives in India. Emigration across the *Kala Pani* was seen as breaking Hindu prohibitions, resulting in the migrant's loss of caste.[1] In early 1898, as he was just about to board the ship *Avon* heading to Dutch Surinam, Munshi Rahman Khan observed how caste, class and religious divisions had already begun to break down in the depot in which migrants were gathered before embarkation from Calcutta. Rahman Khan described how an earthen pot,

> was used to keep water for multifarious activities like drinking, washing hands and face, and washing after defecation, etc. This was highly unhygienic and especially against the habits of the *Sanatans* [orthodox Hindus] who had earlier followed their beliefs rigidly.[2]

As Rahman Khan's fellow passengers removed the ceremonial threads and jewellery that marked their social status in India, they faced the uncertainties of a maritime passage that was often an exceedingly harsh physical experience dominated by the dangers of the ocean, disease and violence at the hands of the ships' crews.

It was these threats of coercion and death that led many British and colonial abolitionists to label Asian indentureship as a 'new system of slavery' in the 1830s and 1840s. The fluctuating mortality of Indians on the *Kala Pani*, and upon arrival, stirred repeated debates over the legitimacy of indentureship and resulted in its

---

[1]   David Dabydeen and Brinsley Samaroo, 'Introduction', in David Dabydeen and Brinsley Samaroo (eds), *Across the Dark Waters: Ethnicity and Indian Identity in the Caribbean* (London, 1996), pp. 3–10.
[2]   Munshi Rahman Khan, *Autobiography of an Indian Indentured Labourer*, trans. Kathinka Sinha-Kerkhoff, Ellen Bal and Alok Deo Singh (Delhi, 2005), p. 78.

temporary suspension in 1839 and 1856. Facing the spectre of the horrific maritime mortality that had afflicted the Middle Passage of the trans-Atlantic slave trade, British imperial authorities defended Asian indenture by emphasizing their close medical management of the oceanic passage from India. The debates over maritime mortality during the nineteenth century have remained a central focus for historians exploring indentured migration from South Asia, as they raise fundamental issues over the nature of indentureship, including the extent to which it was a coercive or voluntary form of migration, and the role of the colonial state in its regulation and expansion. This chapter explores how the medical and sanitary regulation of indentured migrants was transformed during the nineteenth century, and how such changes were affected by the encounters between European and Indian visions of medical practice.

Debating Maritime Mortality and Colonial Medicine

The voyages of indentured migrants during the nineteenth century are almost unique in the intrusive range of state record-keeping they produced on the medical regulation and material conditions experienced at sea. Only the transport of nineteenth-century migrants to Australia produced similar – if not quite as extensive – levels of bureaucratic state involvement. The standardized forms completed and paperwork generated for each crossing by the surgeons appointed to migrant ships have been heavily relied on by historians such as Hugh Tinker, who argued that the violence and constant abuses of indenture represented systemic coercion.[3] Rejecting this interpretation, Ralph Shlomowitz, Pieter Emmer and David Northrup have used the statistical tabulations from the same medical records to contend that such abuses were effectively countered by state regulation, and that indentureship offered real material advancement for the migrants themselves.[4]

Comparing different forms of trans-oceanic migration during the nineteenth century, Shlomowitz has emphasized how the crude death rates (that is, the overall death rate presented over a constant period of time) of indentured Indians at sea were much closer to other forms of non-enslaved migration (such as the voyages of British convicts or European emigrants to Australia) than to the trans-Atlantic slave trade. Maritime mortality on indentured vessels declined during the last quarter of the nineteenth century (Figure 9.1), which Shlomowitz has argued was due to sanitary reforms caused by state intervention.[5] Drawing

3   Hugh Tinker, *A New System of Slavery: The Export of Indian Labour Overseas, 1830–1920* (London, 1974).
4   Ralph Shlomowitz, *Mortality and Migration in the Modern World* (Vermont, 1996); David Northrup, *Indentured Labor in the Age of Imperialism, 1834–1922* (Cambridge, 1995), P.C. Emmer, 'Caribbean Plantations and Indentured Labour, 1640–1917: A Constructive or Destructive Deviation from the Free Labour Market', *Itinerario* (1997), pp. 73–89.
5   Ralph Shlomowitz and John McDonald, 'Mortality of Indian Labour on Ocean Voyages, 1843–1917'. *Studies in History*, 6:1 (1990), pp. 35–59.

Figure 9.1 Death rate (per 1,000 people per month) on voyages
from Calcutta by destination

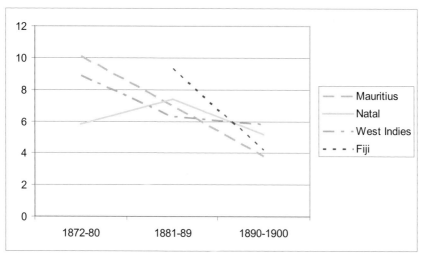

Source: Ralph Shlomowitz and John McDonald, 'Mortality of Indian Labour on Ocean Voyages,
1843–1917', *Studies in History*, 6:1 (1990), p. 63.

on this research, David Northrup presented a progressive chronology of indentured migration, marked by 'larger and better equipped and regulated ships,
faster voyages, improved experience in handling large seaborne populations and
increased medical knowledge'.[6] However, social historians such as Marina Carter
have contested the effectiveness of these measures, arguing that it was the changing
demographic composition of the migrant groups from India which, perhaps, had
the greatest impact on variations in mortality rates at sea.[7]

In contrast to the quantitative histories of maritime mortality which endorse
the effectiveness of naval sanitary reform, historians of colonial India have adopted
a far more critical approach to the imperial archive, focusing on the contested
nature of medical intervention in the nineteenth century. David Arnold has shown
how European medical practice in India was constantly reshaped by its inter-
actions with the changing imperatives of colonial rule, its relations with Indian
medical knowledge and subaltern resistance.[8] Mark Harrison has explored the
limitations and internal conflicts of British public health projects in India, highlighting the gap between imperial rhetoric and regulation on the ground.[9] Inspired

6 Northrup, *Indentured Labor in the Age of Imperialism*, p. 103.
7 Marina Carter, *Servants, Sidars and Settlers: Indians in Mauritius 1834–1874* (Oxford, 1995),
pp. 137–8.
8 David Arnold, *Colonizing the Body: State Medicine and Epidemic Disease in Nineteenth-
century India* (Berkeley, 1993).
9 Mark Harrison, *Public Health in British India: Anglo-Indian Preventive Medicine, 1859–1914*
(Cambridge, 1994).

by these works, this chapter seeks to develop a new perspective on indentured voyages by moving beyond the statistical registers of maritime mortality to explore the changing medical practices that shaped the Indian experience of migration.

The emigrant ships that traversed the *Kala Pani* were not dominated by one monolithic, static form of Western-inspired colonial medicine. Rather they were the site of shifting encounters between British and Indian understandings of medicine. Naval surgeons faced pressures from above for the constant recording and regulation of migrant conditions, and for a decisive response to the threat of epidemic disease. This resulted in many focusing their energies on sanitary management and mortality rates rather than on other aspects of migrant health. As doctors, assistants, translators, and patients, Indians often followed their own medical practices and networks rather than merely becoming the passive and fatalistic victims depicted in the imperial archives. Re-reading these sources from a patient-oriented perspective reveals the tensions of power that shaped migrant responses to the new regimes of therapeutic treatment and sanitary regulation they encountered at sea.[10]

Regulating the Indentured System

In September 1838 the Calcutta authorities launched a public inquiry into the emerging mass migration of indentured workers which had developed through the port. The testimony of Abdoolah Khan was vital in allowing the investigation to access the experiences of the subaltern migrants. He had studied medicine a decade earlier in the 67th Regiment Hospital and had then begun practising in Calcutta.[11] In late 1837 and early 1838 he had served on two immigrant vessels carrying indentured labourers to Mauritius. Khan described these as traumatic journeys, with the passengers confined below decks and disturbed by lack of bedding, space, and clean water. On one of his voyages to Mauritius, the indentured migrants were fed with tamarind and rice, and limited to a daily ration of only a quart of water (two pints) to drink.[12] There was also the mental anguish for many of the emigrants in finding themselves contracted to labour for five years, rather than the two-month period to which they had initially agreed in India. Khan witnessed how captains – habituated to the use of corporal punishment on their lascar crews – would order that migrants be flogged or beaten for breaches of the ship's discipline, such as urinating below decks.

In his testimony, Khan talked little about the therapeutic treatments he used at sea. On his first voyage, two emigrants died of an overdose of opium which

---

[10] Roy Porter, 'The Patient's View: Doing Medical History from Below', *Theory and Society*, 14 (1985), pp. 175–98.

[11] British Parliamentary Papers, 1841, Session 1 (45), 'Letter from Secretary to Government of India to Committee on Exportation of Hill Coolies; Report of Committee and Evidence', p. 321.

[12] Ibid., p. 324; The consumption of dhal was also limited to every fourth day as its preparation was seen as consuming too much water.

they had purchased before boarding, although Khan was silent over whether this was suicide, self-medication or addiction. Later, serving on the 457-ton vessel, the *Christopher Rawson*, he clashed with the captain, Charles Edwards, over the medical care of its 290 indentured passengers, resulting in him being assaulted by Edwards.[13] Edwards claimed that Khan was incompetent after watching him administer mercury pills to members of his crew. The captain therefore decided to determine the drug and dosage himself, which he then forced Khan to administer, arguing that 'this doctor could not bleed and was wholly unaware of the properties of English medicine'.[14] Such claims were contradicted by Khan's Western medical training, although they also reveal the tensions that were caused within colonial racial hierarchies when Indian doctors, interpreters or nurses were responsible for the medical management of vessels at sea. In Khan's opinion, it was the interference of Edwards which ultimately cost the lives of the five passengers who died *en route* to Mauritius.

Another medical witness appearing before the Calcutta commission was former Royal Navy surgeon A.S. Wiseman. In July 1839 he had travelled on the 437-ton *Whitby*, a vessel owned by the merchants Gilders, Arbuthot and Co., who had intensively lobbied both for the establishment of indenture to Mauritius in 1834, and for its extension to the Caribbean in 1838.[15] The *Whitby* carried 250 immigrants, although Wiseman believed that it provided enough space and ventilation for its passengers. Before the vessel left Calcutta for British Guiana, the immigrants suffered a wave of bowel complaints, which Wiseman argued was due to the generosity of food provision on the vessel. A year earlier, a similar diagnosis was made by J.P. Richmond, doctor on board the *Hespersus*, which had travelled the same route from Calcutta to British Guiana. Richmond noted that for his Indian passengers the first week of the voyage was dominated by diarrhoea and dysentery due to the change of diet, with vomiting, cramps and what he saw as other cholera-like symptoms.[16] Yet the reality of these early voyages was that rations were often extremely limited, restricted to rice and vegetables, as captains sought to maximize profit from these privately chartered voyages. By presenting mortality as due to the fragility of Indian bodies and the generosity of the rations provided at sea, the responsibility of those managing the transportation of migrants for Indian ill health was minimized.

Significantly, Khan's account of the abuse and privations that existed on indentured vessels carried considerably more weight for the Calcutta commission than the more positive view of Wiseman, as they recommended that indentured recruitment for Mauritius and the British West Indies should be suspended. Dissenting from these findings, J.P. Grant argued that indentured immigration was a form

---

[13] Ibid., p. 326.
[14] Ibid.
[15] Ibid., p. 313.
[16] British Parliamentary Papers, 1839 (463), 'Hill coolies, British Guiana. Correspondence relative to the condition of the hill coolies and other labourers introduced into British Guiana', pp. 156–60.

of free labour, and he focused his critique of the commission's proceedings on a rejection of Khan's evidence.[17] He argued that as the 'country ships' that sailed the Indian Ocean did not need an Indian doctor for their native crews, so there was no need for an equivalent on the emigrant vessels. In Grant's view, Indians had lived for generations without medical attendance and therefore they did not need to be subject to 'European medical discipline'.[18] However, it was precisely the intensive management of migrant health which was central to the re-emergence of indentured immigration to Mauritius from 1842 and to the Caribbean from 1844. Facing the prospect of migrant mortality, the involvement of the imperial state shifted from the detached regulation of private recruitment before 1838 to direct responsibility for the recruitment, transportation and employment of labourers. This was symbolized by the expanding role of naval doctors in not only super-vising the health of migrants, but recording their conditions, directing their diet and daily routines, and determining whether the ship's charter had been carried out in full.

The importance of 'European medical discipline' in legitimizing the expansion of Indian migrant labour was reflected in the increasing regulations for carriage of indentured workers. In 1837 local legislation passed in Mauritius required private vessels carrying more than twenty labourers to have sufficient accommodation, food and 'medical attendance', which was interpreted as the need for either a Euro-pean or Indian doctor.[19] The obligation for either a naval surgeon or a native doctor was maintained by the Mauritius Act XV of 1842, which marked the state's resumption of indentured immigration with more detailed requirements for diet, accommodation and medical inspection.[20] This legislation was then taken as the model for the carriage of indentured immigrants to the Caribbean, although the voyage of twenty weeks from Calcutta was twice as long as that to Mauritius.[21]

Facing the Spectre of Maritime Mortality

During the second half of the 1850s, emigration from India reached a new peak, fuelled by demand from the colonies and by famine, social dislocation and repres-sion of the Great Revolt. At the same time there was a dramatic increase in mari-time mortality, especially on voyages to the West Indies during the 1856–7 season. Twelve vessels left Calcutta carrying a total of 4,094 indentured immigrants to

---

[17] British Parliamentary Papers, 1841 (427), 'Hill coolies. Copies of papers respecting the exportation of hill coolies, received from the government of India; in continuation of those presented to the House of Commons on the 11th day of February last', pp. 7 and 36.
[18] Ibid., p. 30.
[19] British Parliamentary Papers, 174 (314) 'Copy of Mr Geoghegan's Report on Coolie Emigra-tion from India', pp. 3–4.
[20] Ibid., pp. 10–11.
[21] Such regulations differed from the Passengers' Act in requiring only twelve feet of space per indentured Indian compared to fifteen feet for European passengers, and in identifying the age of adulthood as 10 years for Indians compared to 14 years under the Passengers' Act. Ibid., p. 15.

the West Indies, of whom 17.3 per cent died at sea. The government of Bengal appointed Dr Frederic Mouat, Inspector-General of Jails, to investigate the escalating death rate. Having studied medicine in London, Edinburgh and Paris, Mouat had spent seventeen years in India teaching clinical medicine, chemistry and materia medica, as well as translating key texts in anatomy and pharmacy into Hindi.[22] His report absolved the authorities in Calcutta from responsibility for the deaths by rebutting the accusations of ship captains and surgeons that emigrants had been unfit for passage due to the conditions in the depots in which they were housed before embarkation, and the failure to properly identify those who were already ill.

At the heart of the debates that generated Mouat's report was the environmental understanding of disease causation which located the origins of indentured immigrant ill health in their immediate physical environment or surrounding atmospheric conditions. As a result, surgeons' journals tended to argue that oceanic mortality had been caused by conditions before embarkation (such as contaminated water supply in Calcutta's immigrant depot), or to locate the causes of ill health as lying with migrants themselves due to their perceived inherent fragility, unsanitary customs or resistance to Western medicine. Defending medical services in India, Mouat provided a much more critical analysis of shipboard medical practices, arguing,

> That the lamentable sickness and mortality under investigation were caused by the increased proportion of women and children [carried by these vessels], by the neglect of proper sanitary precautions on board most of the vessels, by the shipment of water of the River Hooghly when it was unwholesome, by the absence of the means of separating the healthy and the sick, by the change in the diet of the emigrants, by the absolute want of suitable food for young children and infants, by the presence of grain cargoes, by the probable foul state of the bilge, and in some instances by the inexperience of the medical officers, in others by their being unable to communicate with the emigrants, and being unaccustomed to the treatment of the diseases of natives of India.[23]

Rather than providing remedies for the limitations of medical personnel, Mouat's report was particularly concerned with limiting the numbers of women and children carried at sea, because he believed that these contributed disproportionately to mortality rates.[24]

The voyage of the *Salsette* from Calcutta to Trinidad in early 1858 exemplified the dangers faced by young and elderly passengers on the long passage to the Caribbean. Over 111 days at sea, 42 per cent of the indentured passengers died

[22] 'Dr Frederic John Mouat, M.D., LL.D.', *Journal of the Royal Statistical Society*, 60:2 (1897), pp. 434–7.
[23] 'Copy of Mr Geoghegan's Report on Coolie Emigration from India', p. 24.
[24] For example, in a survey of 280 voyages to Mauritius between 1860 and 1872, Shlomowitz and McDonald found that the death rate of adults was 12.6 per 1,000 while for children it was 40.4 and for infants 90.4. See Shlomowitz and McDonald, 'Mortality of Indian Labour on Ocean Voyages, 1843–1917', p. 139.

(142 out of a total of 342). For British abolitionists, the extreme mortality on the voyage of the *Salsette* symbolized the systemic failings of indentureship, as they argued that it could not be blamed on any exceptional epidemic, nor on the deliberate mismanagement of the vessel.[25] The early entries in the diary of the *Salsette*'s captain, Edolphus Swinton, are dominated by descriptions of the elderly and young dying from cholera, dysentery and diarrhoea. Swinton blamed this mortality on poor selection at the depot in Calcutta, claiming that many of his passengers were already ill and emaciated before boarding his ship. Describing Indian habits as beastly and unclean, he implied that it was the immigrants themselves who were responsible for their own ill health.[26]

During the first fortnight at sea, Swinton noted, 'it appears they are sinking for want of food suited to them', as although many of the children on board were thin, they refused to eat.[27] However, elsewhere in his diary he noted complaints by the indentured immigrants that their daily rations of twelve ounces of rice were insufficient.[28] Infant mortality was blamed by the captain and his wife on lack of preserved milk. The river water from Calcutta that was filtered for passengers was described as unfit to drink. Also, there was an insufficient supply of clothing for the voyage.[29] After a month at sea, during which twenty-eight adults had died, Swinton recorded:

> Got the launch boat cleared to convert it into an hospital for the sick; the smell below being so dreadful, though everything done to prevent it. I regret it was not done on leaving Calcutta, as I believe many would have been saved, the sickness arising entirely from bad smells. Each time I go below the smell makes me sick.[30]

By 28 May, the ship's doctor had run out of the chalk-mixture and laudanum which he was using to treat the many cases of diarrhoea and cholera. Despite his protests, Swinton was forced to divert to Saint Helena to pick up more medicine.[31]

Throughout the passage, the captain's diary contains frequent references to the resistance of Indians to inspection and treatment by the ship's doctor:

13 May: 'Doctor found several sick not reported.'[32]
16 May: 'Boy of fifteen died to-day, who would not come for prescription before yesterday morning. Doctor suggests the propriety of not giving any more of these people medicine, they having such an objection and aversion to it that they will

[25] Jane Swinton, *Journal of a Voyage with Coolie Emigrants, from Calcutta to Trinidad* (London, 1859), pp. 3–4.
[26] Ibid., p. 8.
[27] Ibid., pp. 5–6.
[28] Ibid., p. 8.
[29] Ibid., p. 13.
[30] Ibid., p. 8.
[31] Ibid., p. 9.
[32] Ibid., p. 8.

rather pine and die than apply for it in time; but as we had no country medicine (i.e. herbs), which their faith lies in, I think it is well to continue now.'
26 May: 'This mortality is dreadful, and without any means of being checked ... An old woman died, who would not confess that she was ill, and only came before the doctor a few hours before her death.'[33]

Hiding symptoms such as extreme diarrhoea, or explicitly denying they were sick, were common forms of resistance on board.[34] Swinton repeatedly complained that female indentured immigrants actively sought to evade medical observation, revealing the extent to which physical inspection or treatment by white male doctors could be seen as 'either polluting or tantamount to sexual molestation.'[35] The opposition of Indian women on the *Salsette* to Western medical treatment resulted in Jane Swinton, the captain's wife, calling for female nurses on indentured immigrant ships, although such a measure was never implemented.[36]

In reflecting on the traumatic passage of the *Salsette*, Jane Swinton noted that the ship's doctor was wholly reliant on his Indian interpreter.[37] Such concerns were also articulated three decades later by James Laing, who stated that his *Handbook for Surgeons Superintendent of the Coolie Emigration Service* was intended to make surgeons less dependent on their Indian medical assistants. Laing advised other surgeons on the importance of maintaining colonial racial hierarchies at sea, recommending that Indian compounders, hospital attendants, nurses and interpreters should be treated well, but also kept in their place.[38] However, the balance of power between white surgeons and their Indian staff was often weighted towards the latter due to their previous experience on indentured immigrant ships and the sheer numbers of passengers needing surveillance.[39]

Medical Practice on the *Kala Pani*

The intensification in state regulation of the oceanic passage of indentured migrants after 1842 resulted in the increasing standardization of drugs available on the voyages. In 1846, vessels sailing to the West Indies were issued with a list of required medicines which included thirty-six specific articles and the acknowledgement that doctors may also choose to carry 'country medicines' from

---

[33] Ibid., p. 9.
[34] Ibid., p. 10. The fear of purgative treatments resulted in Indian convicts hiding their symptoms from European doctors. See Clare Anderson, '"The Ferringees are Flying – the Ship is Ours!" The Convict Middle Passage in Colonial South and Southeast Asia, 1790–1860', *Indian Economic and Social History Review*, 41 (2005), p. 157.
[35] Arnold, *Colonizing the Body*, p. 10.
[36] Swinton, *Journal of a Voyage*, p. 13.
[37] Ibid., p. 12.
[38] James M. Laing, 'Handbook for Surgeons Superintendent of the Coolie Emigration Service' (1889), TNA, CO 885/5/32, p. 11.
[39] Ibid., p. 34. Laing specified a staff of four Indians for 500 passengers.

Table 9.1 Quantities of selected medicines required for indentured immigrant ships, per 100 passengers, 1846 and 1863 (in grams)

Medicine	1846	1863	Difference
Blistering ointment	740	120	-620
Senna leaves	500	240	-260
Calomel	240	120	-120
Camphor	180	120	-60
Copper sulphate	90	30	-60
Zinc sulphate	90	30	-60
Blue pill	120	90	-30
Cubeb powder	0	30	+30
Grey powder	0	60	+60
Magnesia	0	60	+60
Ginger powder	0	60	+60
Alumen	180	240	+60
Opium	90	180	+90
Quinine	22.5	120	+97.5
Potass nitrate	0	120	+120
Catechu	0	180	+180
Jalap powder	120	360	+240
Copaida	0	240	+240
Mercurial ointment	0	240	+240
Camphor liniment	0	500	+500
Lime chloride	2,240	15,000	+12,760

Source: British Parliamentary Papers, 1846 (706), 'Colonial Land and Emigration Commission Sixth General Report', p. 57; and British Parliamentary Papers, 1863 (3199), 'Colonial Land and Emigration Commission Twenty-Third General Report', pp. 195–6.

India.[40] Within two decades, this generic category for Indian drugs or herbal remedies, which had been left to the discretion of individual practitioners, had been removed from the list. Instead, the formal inventory of required medicines had been extended to eighty-one articles (some of which were of Indian origin).[41] Comparing the two lists of required medicines suggests that therapeutic regimes at sea did change significantly during this period (see Table 9.1).

The largest reduction between the 1846 list of medicines and that of 1863 is in the amount of blistering ointment carried per vessel. This would suggest that its

[40] British Parliamentary Papers, 1846 (706), 'Colonial Land and Emigration Commission Sixth General Report', p. 57.
[41] British Parliamentary Papers, 1863 (3199), 'Colonial Land and Emigration Commission Twenty-Third General Report', pp. 195–6.

use as a therapeutic practice at sea had become relatively minor. During the same period, calomel and camphor appear to have been increasingly administered via the skin as ointments rather than orally. Calomel was seen at the time as a 'mild but sure mercurial' which could be used as either a purgative or a sedative in cases of cholera and dysentery.[42] Calomel was also seen as promoting the effectiveness of other drug therapies. Mercury was also a core ingredient of 'Blue pills', which vessels carried as a purgative treatment for cholera. While the 1863 regulations decreased the quantities of these mercury-based medicines, they increased the total of 'Grey powder' carried, which was seen as the weakest form of mercury to be used on the young or for those with feeble constitutions.[43] The turning away from the more violent mercury-based purgatives suggests that the perceived frailty of Indian bodies did impact on therapeutic practices at sea.

Camphor (derived from the Camphora tree) was another drug which was increasingly used as an ointment rather than administered orally. Identified as a stimulant when taken orally, it was used as a remedy for typhoid to increase the patient's temperature or pulse, and employed as a sedative it was applied to the skin to cool patients suffering from fever.[44] It was also commonly used in cases of venereal disease. Other medicines whose supply was decreased by the regulations of 1863 were blue vitriol (copper sulphate) and white vitriol (zinc sulphate), both of which were used as emetics to induce vomiting in cases of dysentery. The reduced quantities of inorganic purgatives and emetics in the 1863 regulations were more likely to have been due to concerns about their effectiveness on Indian bodies, rather than considerations of cost or subaltern resistance (which would have been reflected in the increased adoption of Indian herbal medicines).[45]

The expanded list of required medicines in 1863 gave more prominence to organic drugs. Amongst these newly listed remedies in 1863 were chirata, from Northern India, and jalap powder, from Mexico. The former was described as a tonic that was effective in treating anaemia and diarrhoea. Jalap powder was a powerful purgative, though it was also seen as safe to be used on children and weak patients.[46] Ginger powder was often combined with other purgative drugs to mask their taste. Other new organic drugs included cubeb powder for gonorrhoea, and copaida from Brazil, which was seen as providing a mild treatment for stomach illnesses. The amount of opium carried by immigrant vessels was doubled in 1863 to 180 grams; this was supplemented with 240 grams of opium tincture. It is possible that some of these drugs were carried to sea in the 1830s and 1840s as 'country medicines' by doctors acting on their own discretion; however, their

[42] Robert Scoresby-Jackson, *Note-Book of Materia Medica, Pharmacology and Therapeutics*, 4th edn (Edinburgh, 1880), p. 151.
[43] Ibid., p. 145.
[44] Ibid., p. 322.
[45] During the 1850s and 1860s in Bengal, indigenous drugs were promoted by colonial administrators on the grounds of economic cost, despite objections from practitioners who preferred standardized Western medicines. See Poonam Bala, *Imperialism and Medicine in Bengal: A Socio-historical Perspective* (New Delhi, 1991), pp. 49–51.
[46] Scoresby-Jackson, *Note-Book of Materia Medica*, p. 300.

formalized inclusion in the list also reveals the extent to which other Indian herbal remedies were not recognized by colonial authorities.

Comparing the pharmaceutical inventories of 1846 and 1863 reveals how the expansion of formalized regulation excluded Indian drugs which would have been more prevalent in the 1830s when vessels relied on private suppliers in India. By the late 1880s, James Laing noted that a complete chest of medicines was supplied to surgeons on indentured immigrant ships direct from Apothecaries' Hall in London, which could simply be set up next to the dispensing table on board.[47] Amongst those Indian drugs in decreasing use were senna leaves, a laxative from southern India, which would have been familiar to some of the indentured, so it is unlikely that their reduced supply would have been due to migrant resistance. European doctors tended to see senna leaves as weak purgatives which needed to be used with other drugs to be effective. The construction of Indian bodies and herbal medicines as fragile and feeble, therefore, powerfully shaped not only the understandings of causation of migrant mortality and morbidity but also the nature of pharmaceutical treatments experienced by migrants.

Laing's 1889 *Handbook for Surgeons* provided just a few pages describing the possible medical treatment of immigrants, but these strongly emphasized how the administration of drugs was shaped by the racial construction of the Indian body. Laing advised other surgeons that, in Indians, 'the pulse (radial artery) is sometimes very small and hardly to be felt in these people even when in perfect health, which used to startle me considerably till I found it was natural'.[48] The Indian diet was also criticized by Laing:

> Like all vegetarians, they are very liable to have intestinal parasites, especially the children, and if you find any coolie suffering from irregularity of the bowels, foul tongue, and general malaise which you cannot account for, a dose of calomel and santonine followed by a purgative will often relieve your mind and his 'tumjack'.[49]

According to Laing, this fragile physiognomy was matched by native fatalism, and, as a result, 'the people will not bear the use of depressing medicine for any length of time, and, if you miss the proper time for tonics and stimulants you lose your patient'.[50] The importance of 'judicious stimulation' through chloral or calomel revealed how some European surgeons tended to rely on stimulants due to their perceptions of the frailties of Indian constitutions.

[47] Laing, 'Handbook for Surgeons Superintendent', pp. 10 and 20.
[48] Ibid., p. 41. Revealingly, Laing's description of his medical inspection of immigrants before they boarded the ships focused on their value as labourers, and the potential threat of epidemic disease, rather than a concern for their overall health. He particularly emphasized examining the face and arms as indicators of health, especially the palm of the hands to see whether the migrant's skin had been toughened by rural labour. See ibid., pp. 16–17, for this description.
[49] Ibid., p. 40.
[50] Ibid.

The voyage of the *Jeune Albert* in 1859 from Pondicherry to the French Caribbean provides a contrasting account of the use of mercurial medicines. The ship's surgeon, Hippolyte Bernavon, had served in military hospitals in the French naval bases at Marseille and Toulon where he had been decorated for his work during Asiatic cholera epidemics in France. In late June 1859, Bernavon boarded the 518-ton *Jeune Albert* with 502 indentured Indian passengers. At Karikal, the ship had taken on large numbers of emaciated women who were visibly suffering from famine, although the depot authorities had assured Bernavon that his passengers would recover once on board.[51] Instead, within a week at sea his sick bay was full, and within three weeks there were over ninety sick passengers, of whom a third were suffering from dysentery. The same illness immobilized half the ship's crew and its captain, while many of the passengers were so completely prostrate with seasickness and dysentery that they were unable to eat, take medicine or even venture out of the ship's hold.[52]

As the *Jeune Albert* traversed the Indian Ocean, Bernavon feared that no medication would stop the march of dysentery.[53] Mercurial medicines seemed to have no effect, although calomel mixed with opium seemed to slow its progress. On the most serious cases he used high doses of silver nitrate (up to eight milligrams) as an extreme purgative.[54] Of the forty-one patients suffering from dysentery, only four died. Facing six times the number of patients that could be held in the ship's hospital, Bernavon's account of the desperate resort to heroic purgatives in the face of uncertainties and crises at sea contrasts with the confident interventionism of Laing.

Even where voyages experienced relatively low rates of mortality, the pharmaceutical resources provided for surgeons could be stretched to breaking point. After 1860, British authorities allowed the recruitment of indentured migrants from British India for France's colonies as long as they were transported and managed at sea under the same regimes that existed within the British Empire. The surgeons of the French Navy who served on these indentured immigrant vessels were often critical of British regulations. The British consul in Martinique reported that the doctor on board the *Oncle Félix*, which had carried 450 immigrants from Pondicherry, had complained of

> the medicines provided by the present scale as being wholly inappropriate to many of the maladies most prevalent during such voyages. It is a complaint that is usually preferred by the Surgeons arriving here in charge of Indian Immigrants.[55]

---

[51] Hippolyte Bernavon, *Rapport Médical adressé a Monsieur Le Docteur Petit sur l'état sanitaire des passagers indiens du navire le Jeune Albert, depuis leur emparqument à Pondichéry jusqu'à ce jour* (Paris, 1859), p. 2.

[52] Ibid., p. 6.

[53] Ibid., p. 7.

[54] Ibid., p. 8

[55] Lawless to Sailsbury, 3 December 1879, BL, India Office, L/PJ/6/1.

On the 107-day passage to Martinique, outbreaks of measles, fever and severe 'stomach affections' had been succeeded by colds and pneumonia in traversing the Atlantic. These resulted in seven deaths.

Sanitary Regimes at Sea

Claims that the pharmaceutical inventories required at sea were inadequate re-emerged in 1870 with the debates over an upsurge in mortality on vessels carrying indentured immigrants to British Guiana. During late 1869 and early 1870 approximately 2,330 indentured Indian migrants were transported to British Guiana on board six vessels; however, 197 of these immigrants died at sea. The surgeon superintendent on the *Arima* was Indian-born Dr Raheen, who had received his MD in America. Although the *Arima's* voyage was only eighty-two days, Raheen claimed that 'the medical comforts (stimulants) were not supplied for the latter part of the voyage', while there were also shortages of firewood, vegetables and fresh water. He also claimed that the space reserved for immigrants had been used to store cargo.[56] In response, the Agent General of Immigration in British Guiana sought (unsuccessfully) to blame the high mortality on the incompetence of racially inferior 'native surgeons'. Elsewhere, emigration authorities in London noted that 'The Jamaican Emigration Agent is in favour of the employment of <u>Indian</u> doctors on board ship [underlining in original]'.[57]

The debates over the mortality of immigrants to British Guiana in 1870 reveal the extent to which the effectiveness of surgeons was judged by the sanitary state of their vessel. The *India*, which suffered twenty-two deaths on its 112-day voyage, was described as being dirty and in bad order, resulting in its landing more 'non-effective' or sick immigrants. Indian-born surgeon Robert Sinclair was blamed for failing to maintain a proper sanitary regime. Yet the relationship between sanitary order and mortality was not always direct. The next immigrant vessel to reach British Guiana, the *Arima*, was described as having a dirty deck and being disorderly; however, it had only experienced nine deaths on its voyage. Its passengers were described as 'dirty in their persons but in good health and in very fair condition'.[58] Although accusations of incompetence against Indian doctors were rebutted by the Colonial Office, there had been a steady Europeanization of medical personnel on board the indentured immigrant ships. Reflecting the mid-century professionalization of medicine in England and India, naval surgeons often had considerable training which compared favourably to that of their peers in the India medical service.[59]

[56] Walcott to Rodgers, 29 April 1870, TNA, CO 318/257.
[57] Ibid.
[58] Ibid.
[59] British Parliamentary Papers, 1874 (293), 'Return of Number of Ships employed in conveying Coolies from India and China to W. Indies, 1872–74'; Mark Harrison, *Public Health in British India*, p. 235.

While the causes of high migrant mortality were at times blamed on the distinctive environmental conditions of India (particularly the port facilities of Calcutta), native medicine and the physical constitutions of Indians, the indentured immigrant ship itself was also seen by some as the source of ill health. Focusing on the miasmas that circulated below decks, surgeons and colonial officials complained that immigrants were exposed to a 'nasty steam' which originated in the hold of vessels that carried cargoes of rice. Another interpretation held that as some ships had carried a cargo of salt from England, their decks had become impregnated with salt which held in the damp.[60] The *Shand*, which lost ninety-eight out of 462 passengers in 1870, was seen as a particularly problematic 'salted' vessel. The Agent General of Immigration in British Guiana argued that such 'salted ships' were

> Not uncommon in the Australian immigration. They were for the most part of American build and usually the most commodious, and in other respects the most eligible class of vessels for the carriage of passengers.[61]

Receiving these reports, emigration officials in London stated, 'they do not attach much importance to the vessel being "salted"', and blamed the high mortality on the *Shand* on the physical condition of the immigrants, the quality of provisions carried and the 'incapacity' of medical personnel on the vessel.[62]

The miasmic tradition, however, led naval surgeons to concentrate their sanitary intervention on the hold, where migrants lived for most of the voyage. Dr Adolphe Allanic, who twice completed the voyage from Pondicherry to Guadeloupe as ship's medical officer between 1867 and 1871, believed that sickness was caused by emanations from migrants' clothing, describing them as naturally dirty. Both Allanic's voyages were on English ships, which he argued had generally better dimensions and internal structure than the smaller French merchant ships. In 1867, he sailed upon the 800-ton *Dunphaile-Castle* and at the end of 1870 he completed another three-month voyage, this time on board the 1,120-ton *The Contest*. This was a three-masted clipper from Liverpool built in 1855, which had been recast in 1869. Allanic was full of praise for the space and ventilation on *The Contest*, with its two mechanical ventilators.[63]

The use of mechanical ventilators (which had been used on board some Royal Navy ships in various forms since the eighteenth century) was thought to reduce the threat of miasmic disease. But this was strongly contested in the late 1870s – not on medical grounds but due to economic pressures. The government of India advocated the adoption of the Thiers automatic ship ventilator as used on imperial troop ships. The Nourse shipping line, which ran some of the largest immigrant vessels under state contract, adopted the ventilator, but this was done as a measure

---

[60] Laing, 'Handbook for Surgeons Superintendent', pp. 4–6.

[61] Walcott to Rodgers, 5 May 1870, TNA, CO 318/257.

[62] Ibid; 'Copy of Mr Geoghegan's Report on Coolie Emigration from India', pp. 50–1.

[63] Adolphe Gustave Marie Allanic, 'Considérations Hygiéniques et Médicales sur les Transports des Immigrants Indiens', Thèse Médicine (Montpellier, 1871), pp. 9–13.

against other competing shipping lines. However, many of the colonies importing immigrants resisted these ventilators due to cost, arguing that the ventilator was disproportionately expensive and mechanically flawed as it was dependent on the motion of the sea.[64] Such concerns for economy could have tragic consequences, such as in the failure to properly service and man onboard water distillation apparatus which lay behind the horrific voyage of the *Shand* in 1870.

Financial constraints also shaped discussions over the recruitment of surgeons from the emigration service to Australia, with colonial governments such as that of Jamaica unwilling to agree to paying higher salaries for more experienced naval surgeons.[65] The repeated demands for cost efficiencies meant that new technologies were far slower to be adopted on indentured routes than on other forms of shipping, and this was reflected in the partial adoption of steam ships at the end of the nineteenth century. By 1891, of the twenty-seven vessels employed to convey 15,668 indentured Indians to the colonies, only a quarter were steamers; the remainder relied on sail as a cheaper means of travel.

Conclusion

At the end of the 1880s, James Laing, a surgeon superintendent with over a decade of service on vessels transporting indentured labourers from India to the Caribbean and Pacific, warned those taking up similar appointments that they should ensure that there was a good light and a sturdy table in their cabin. Not only were they responsible for the health of the human cargo of the 'coolie ship', but any prospective surgeon 'will find that he has a good deal of writing to do'.[66] Laing's inventory of the paperwork accompanying each surgeon to sea included:

1. Nominal List of coolies, No 1.
2. Surgeon's journal.
3. Admission and discharge book.
4. Case book.
5. Register of births and deaths.
6. Return of deaths for Emigration Agent (I keep a copy for myself)
7. Surgeon's report of arrival (three copies enclosed ...)
8. Summary of medical history of the voyage, or abstract report for the medical inspector at Calcutta. (I keep a copy of this for my own information).
9. Register of cholera cases, four copies ...
10. Return of coolies unsuccessfully vaccinated in the depôt (and who will have to be re-vaccinated during the voyage).
11. Book with counterfoils for requisitions for stores, medical comforts, and [et]c.

[64] TNA, CO 884/4.
[65] Walcott to Newcastle, 28 June 1861, TNA, CO 137/355.
[66] Laing, 'Handbook for Surgeons Superintendent', p. 15.

12. List, receipted by Surgeon superintendent, for extra clothing, and [et]c., to be issued.

13. Coolies' tickets, one for each man, woman, and child, signed by the Protector, the Emigration Agent, the Surgeon Superintendent, and the Depôt Surgeon …[67]

Such an array of documentation underlines the key role naval doctors played in regulating, recording and interpreting the maritime passage of indentured Indians in the nineteenth century. With the revival of indentureship after 1842, sponsored by the imperial state, medical practice at sea was transformed due to demands for standardization and the daily pressures of recording and managing such large human cargoes. The focus of Laing's handbook on sanitary regulation reveals the extent to which medical practice at sea followed the imperatives of limiting mortality and colonial bureaucracy rather than protecting the overall health of Indian migrants.

Almost two decades earlier, one such migrant, a man named Sébastien from the French entrepôt of Pondicherry, faced a similar regime of medical documentation, recording and inspection after signing an indenture to work in the Caribbean colony of Guadeloupe. With his wife and brother, they boarded the 1,120-ton three-masted British clipper, *The Contest*. Sébastien had suffered from severe dysentery before leaving India, and once the vessel sailed many of the other passengers were constantly seasick. On the water, they faced a new daily routine of feeding, cleaning, being ordered below deck and up again. As Sébastien became weaker, an Indian nurse noticed his frequent visits to the ship's latrines. Reported to the French doctor on board he was ordered into *The Contest*'s hospital on the twenty-fifth day of the voyage. The doctor became increasingly alarmed as Sébastien's pulse grew weaker, and gave him a warm punch containing laudanum to drink. At night, as Sébastien began to feel colder and colder, he was prescribed a mixture of mint and cinnamon spirits which seemed to improve his condition. The following night, 5 December 1870, he died.[68] For almost a month at sea, Sébastien had successfully avoided the intrusive medical intervention which Laing's paperwork implied, and it was only near death that his health was recorded and analysed.

As we have seen, naval doctors acted as key intermediaries in regulating migrant life on the *Kala Pani*, both in enforcing increasingly intensive sanitary regimes and through periodically intervening to protect indentured immigrants from abuse by captain and ship's crew. As scientific experts whose opinions were heard in Royal Commissions, Colonial Office reports and public debates, these doctors were prominent voices in legitimizing the state system of indentured migration through their recording of maritime mortality and migrant health. This regulatory role of naval doctors shaped their medical practice at sea as understandings of purgative medicine and sanitary intervention changed during the late nineteenth century. The threat of mortality caused by epidemic disease resulted in radical

[67] Ibid., p. 23.
[68] Allanic, 'Considérations Hygiéniques et Médicales', pp. 56–7.

purgative interventions or intrusive sanitary surveillance which were frequently resisted by indentured Indian migrants. Despite these regimes, the indentured were also able to carry their own medical practices with them, as James Laing still complained that the lascar crew of the immigrant ships would often supply ganga to the migrant labourers at sea.[69]

---

[69] Laing, 'Handbook for Surgeons Superintendent', p. 21.

Bibliography

Ackroyd, Marcus, Brockliss, Laurence, Moss, Michael, Retford, Kate and Stevenson, John, *Advancing with the Army: Medicine, the Professions, and Social Mobility in the British Isles, 1790–1850* (Oxford, 2006)

Allen, William and Thomson, T.R.H., *A Narrative of the Expedition sent by Her Majesty's Government to the River Niger in 1841 under the Command of Captain H.D. Trotter* (London, 1968, first published 1848)

Arnold, David, *Colonizing the Body: State Medicine and Epidemic Disease in Nineteenth-century India* (Berkeley, 1993)

Arnold, David (ed.), *Warm Climates and Western Medicine* (Amsterdam and Atlanta, 1996)

Atkins, John, *The Navy Surgeon; Or, Practical System of Surgery* (London, 1742)

Austen, M., *The Army in Australia, 1840–50* (Canberra, 1979)

Baldwin, Peter, *Contagion and the State in Europe, 1830–1930* (Cambridge, 1999)

Bateson, C., *The Convict Ships, 1787–1868* (Glasgow, 1985)

Baugh, Daniel A., *British Naval Administration in the Age of Walpole* (Princeton, 1965)

Bean, Richard N., *The British Trans-Atlantic Slave Trade, 1650–1750* (New York, 1975)

Behrendt, Stephen D., 'The Captains in the British Slave Trade from 1785 to 1807', *Transactions of the Historic Society of Lancashire and Cheshire*, 140 (1991), pp. 79–140

Behrendt, Stephen D., 'Crew Mortality in the Transatlantic Slave Trade in the Eighteenth Century', *Slavery and Abolition*, 18 (1997), pp. 49–71

Behrendt, Stephen D., 'Markets, Transaction Cycles, and Profits: Merchant Decision Making in the British Slave Trade', *William and Mary Quarterly*, 58 (2001), pp. 171–204

Behrendt, Stephen D., Eltis, David and Richardson, David, 'The Costs of Coercion: African Agency in the Pre-Modern Atlantic World', *Economic History Review*, 54 (2001), pp. 454–76

Bell, J., *Memoir on the Present State of Naval and Military Surgery Addressed to The Right Honourable Earl Spenser, First Lord of the Admiralty* (Yarmouth, 1798)

Bernavon, Hippolyte, *Rapport Médical adressé a Monsieur Le Docteur Petit sur l'état sanitaire des passagers indiens du navire le Jeune Albert, depuis leur emparqument à Pondichéry jusqu'à ce jour* (Paris, 1859)

Bewell, Alan, *Romanticism and Colonial Disease* (Baltimore and London, 1999)

Blane, Gilbert, 'On the Comparative Health of the Royal Navy, from the Year 1779 to the Year 1814, with Proposals for its Farther Improvement', in Gilbert Blane, *Select Dissertations on Several Subjects of Medical Science* (London, 1822), pp. 1–64

Booker, John, *Maritime Quarantine: The British Experience, c.1650–1900* (Aldershot, 2007)

Brockliss, Laurence and Jones, C., *The Medical World of Early Modern France* (Oxford, 1997)

Brockliss, Laurence, Cardwell, M. John and Moss, Michael, *Nelson's Surgeon: William Beatty, Naval Medicine and the Battle of Trafalgar* (Oxford, 2005)

Brumwell, S., *Redcoats: The British Soldier and War in the Americas, 1755–1763* (Cambridge, 2002)

Bryson, Alexander, *Report on the Climate and Principal Diseases of the African Station* (London, 1847)

Bynum, W.F. et al., *The Western Medical Tradition: 1800 to 2000* (Cambridge, 2006)

Carpenter, K., *The History of Scurvy and Vitamin C* (Cambridge, 1986)

Carter, Marina, *Servants, Sidars and Settlers: Indians in Mauritius, 1834–1874* (Oxford, 1995)

Christopher, Emma, *Slave Ship Sailors and their Captive Cargoes, 1730–1807* (Cambridge, 2006)

Clarke, John D., *The Men of HMS Victory at Trafalgar* (Darlington, 1999)

Cohn, Raymond, L., 'Deaths of Slaves in the Middle Passage', *Journal of Economic History*, 45 (1985), pp. 685–92

Cohn, Raymond L., 'Maritime Mortality in the Eighteenth and Nineteenth Centuries: A Survey', *International Journal of Maritime History*, 1 (1989), pp. 159–91

Cohn, Raymond L. and Jensen, Richard A., 'The Determinants of Slave Mortality Rates on the Middle Passage', *Explorations in Economic History*, 19 (1982), pp. 269–82

Cook, Gordon C., *Disease in the Merchant Navy: A History of the Seamen's Hospital Society* (Oxford, 2007)

Cook, H.J., 'Practical Medicine and the British Armed Forces after the "Glorious Revolution"', *Medical History*, 34 (1990), pp. 1–26

Cooke, William, *A Brief Memoir of Sir William Blizard* (London, 1835)

Corfield, P.J., *Power and the Professions in Britain, 1700–1850* (London, 2000)

Cormack, A., *Two Royal Physicians: Sir James Clark, Bart., 1788–1870, Sir John Forbes, 1787–1861* (Banff, 1967)

Crimmin, P.K., 'The Sick and Hurt Board and the Health of Seamen, c. 1700–1806', *Journal for Maritime Research* [www.jmr.nmm.ac.uk] (December 1999)

Crimmin, P.K., 'The Shortage of Surgeons and Surgeons' Mates, c.1740–1806: An Evil of a Serious Nature to the Service', *Transactions of the Naval Dockyards Society*, forthcoming

Crumplin, Michael K., *Men of Steel: Surgery in the Napoleonic Wars* (Shrewsbury, 2007)

Curtin, Philip D., '"The White Man's Grave": Image and Reality, 1750–1850', *Journal of British Studies*, 1 (1961), pp. 94–110

Curtin, Philip D., *The Image of Africa: British Ideas and Action, 1780–1850* (Madison, 1964)

Curtin, Philip D., 'Epidemiology and the Slave Trade', *Political Science Quarterly*, 83 (1968), pp. 190–216

Curtin, Philip D., *The Atlantic Slave Trade: A Census* (Madison, 1969)

Curtin, Philip D., *Death by Migration: Europe's Encounter with the Tropical World in the Nineteenth Century* (Cambridge, 1989)

Dabydeen, David and Samaroo, Brinsley (eds), *Across the Dark Waters: Ethnicity and Indian Identity in the Caribbean* (London, 1996)

Davidoff, L. and Hall, C., *Family Fortunes: Men and Women of the English Middle Classes, 1780–1850* (London, 1987)

Drake, B.K., 'The Liverpool-African Voyage c.1790–1807: Commercial Problems', in Roger Anstey and P.E.H. Hair (eds), *Liverpool, the African Slave Trade, and Abolition* (Liverpool, 1976), pp. 126–56

Duffy, M., 'The Establishment of the Western Squadron as the Linchpin of British

Naval Strategy', in M. Duffy (ed.), *Parameters of British Naval Power, 1650–1850* (Exeter, 1992), pp. 60–81

Dunne, Charles, *The Chirurgical Candidate; Or Reflections on Education Indispensable to Complete Naval, Military and Other Surgeons* (London, 1808)

Eltis, David, 'Mortality and Voyage Length in the Middle Passage: New Evidence from the Nineteenth Century', *Journal of Economic History*, 44 (1984), pp. 301–18

Eltis, David, *The Rise of African Slavery in the Americas* (Cambridge, 2000)

Eltis, David, 'The Volume and Structure of the Atlantic Slave Trade: A Reassessment', *William and Mary Quarterly*, 58 (2001), pp. 17–46

Eltis, David and Engerman, Stanley L., 'Fluctuations in Sex and Age Ratios in the Transatlantic Slave Trade, 1663–1864', *Economic History Review*, 46 (1993), pp. 308–23

Eltis, David and Richardson, David, 'Productivity in the Transatlantic Slave Trade', *Explorations in Economic History*, 32 (1995), pp. 465–84

Eltis, David and Richardson, David, 'Prices of African Slaves Newly Arrived in the Americas, 1673–1865: New Evidence on Long-Run Trends and Regional Differentials', in David Eltis, Frank Lewis and Kenneth Sokoloff (eds), *Slavery in the Development of the Americas: Essays in Honor of Stanley L. Engerman* (Cambridge, 2004), pp. 181–218

Eltis, David, Behrendt, Stephen D., Richardson, David and Klein, Herbert S., *The Transatlantic Slave Trade, 1527–1867: A Database on CD-Rom* (Cambridge, 1999)

Eltis, David, Behrendt, Stephen D., Richardson, David and Florentino, Manolo, *The Transatlantic Slave Trade, 1527–1867: A Revised and On-line Database* [www.slavevoyages.com].

Emmer, P.C., 'Caribbean Plantations and Indentured Labour, 1640–1917: A Constructive or Destructive Deviation from the Free Labour Market', *Itinerario* (1997), pp. 73–89

Ennis, Daniel James, *Enter the Press-Gang: Naval Impressment in Eighteenth-Century British Literature* (London, 2002)

Estes, J. Worth, *Naval Surgeon: Life and Death at Sea in the Age of Sail* (Massachusetts, 1998)

Glete, J., *Navies and Nations: Warships, Navies and State Building in Europe and America, 1500–1800* (Stockholm, 1993)

Goddard, J.C., 'An Insight into the Life of Royal Naval Surgeons during the Napoleonic War, Part 1', *Journal of the Royal Naval Medical Service*, 77 (1991), pp. 205–22

Gradish, S., *The Manning of the British Navy During the Seven Years' War* (London, 1980)

Granville, Augustus B., *Autobiography of A.B. Granville: Being Eighty-eight Years of the Life of a Physician who Practised his Profession in Italy, Greece, Turkey, Spain, Portugal, the West Indies, Russia, Germany, France, and England* (London, 1874)

Guthrie, George James, *Commentaries on the Surgery of the War in Portugal, Spain, France, and the Netherlands, 1808–1815. Sixth edition, with Additions relating to the Crimea* (London, 1855)

Haines, Robin, *Emigration and the Labouring Poor: Australian Recruitment in Britain and Ireland, 1831–1900* (London, 1997)

Haines, Robin, *Doctors at Sea: Emigrant Voyages to Colonial Australia* (London, 2005)

Haines, Robin, *Life and Death in the Age of Sail: The Passage to Australia* (London, 2006)

Haines, Robin and Shlomowitz, Ralph, 'Explaining the Modern Mortality Decline:

What Can We Learn from Sea Voyages?', *Social History of Medicine*, 11 (1998), pp. 15–48

Haines, Robin and Shlomowitz, Ralph, 'Explaining the Decline in Mortality in the Eighteenth Century British Slave Trade', *Economic History Review*, 53 (2000), pp. 262–83

Haines, Robin and Shlomowitz, Ralph, 'Causes of Death of British Emigrants on Voyages to South Australia, 1848–1885', *Social History of Medicine*, 16 (2003), pp. 193–208

Haines, Robin and Shlomowitz, Ralph, 'Causes of Death of British Emigrants on Voyages to South Australia 1848–1885', *Journal of the Society for the Social History of Medicine*, 16 (2003), pp. 193–208

Haines, Robin and Shlomowitz, Ralph, 'Deaths of Babies Born on Government-Assisted Emigrant Voyages to South Australia in the Nineteenth Century', *Health and History*, 6 (2004), pp. 113–24

Haines, Robin, Shlomowitz, Ralph and Brennan, L., 'Maritime Mortality Revisited', *International Journal of Maritime History*, 8 (1996), pp. 133–72

Haines, Robin, McDonald, J. and Shlomowitz, Ralph, 'Mortality and Voyage Length in the Middle Passage Revisited', *Explorations in Economic History*, 38 (2001), pp. 503–33

Haines, Robin, Jeffery, Judith and Slattery, Greg, *Bound for South Australia: Births and Deaths on Government-Assisted Immigrant Ships, 1848–1885*, CD-ROM (Adelaide, 2004)

Harding, R., *Amphibious Warfare in the Eighteenth-Century: The British Expedition to the West Indies 1740–1742* (Suffolk, 1991)

Harrison, Mark, *Public Health in British India: Anglo-Indian Preventive Medicine, 1859–1914* (Cambridge, 1994)

Harrison, Mark, 'Medicine and the Culture of Command: The Case of Malaria Control in the British Army during the Two World Wars', *Medical History*, 40 (1996), pp. 437–52

Haycock, David Boyd, 'Exterminated by the Bloody Flux: Dysentery in Eighteenth-Century Naval and Military Medical Accounts', *Journal of Maritime Research* [www.jmr.nmm.ac.uk] (January 2002)

Headrick, D.R., *The Tools of Empire: Technology and European Imperialism in the Nineteenth Century* (Oxford and New York, 1981)

Hill, J.R., *The Prizes of War: The Naval Prize System in the Napoleonic Wars* (Stroud, 1998)

Hooper, R., *Examinations in Anatomy, Physiology, Practice of Physic, Surgery, Materia Medica, Chemistry, and Pharmacy, for the use of Students, who are about to Pass the College of Surgeons, or the Medical or Transport Board* (New York, 1815)

Howell, Raymond, *The Royal Navy and the Slave Trade* (London, 1987)

Hughes, R.E., 'James Lind and the Cure of Scurvy: An Experimental Approach', *Medical History*, 19 (1975), pp. 342–51

Inkster, Ian, 'Marginal Men: Aspects of the Social Role of the Medical Community in Sheffield, 1790–1850', in D. Richards and J. Woodward (eds), *Health Care and Popular Medicine in Nineteenth Century England* (London, 1977)

Ives, Edward, *A Voyage from England to India: In the year MDCCLIV: And an Historical Narrative of the Operations of the Squadron and Army in India* (London, 1773)

Jackson, R.V., 'Sickness and Health on Australia's Female Convict Ships, 1821–1840', *International Journal of Maritime History*, 18 (2006), pp. 65–84

Johnson, Robert, *Sir John Richardson: Arctic Explorer, Natural Historian, Naval Surgeon* (London, 1976)

Kaufman, Matthew H., *The Regius Chair of Military Surgery in the University of Edinburgh, 1806–1855* (Amsterdam and New York, 2003)

Keevil, J.J., *Medicine and the Navy, 1200–1900. Vol. 1: 1200–1649* (Edinburgh and London, 1957)

Keevil, J.J., *Medicine and the Navy, 1200–1900. Vol. 2: 1649–1714* (Edinburgh and London, 1958)

Khan, Munshi Rahman, *Autobiography of an Indian Indentured Labourer*, trans. Kathinka Sinha-Kerkhoff, Ellen Bal and Alok Deo Singh (Delhi, 2005)

King-Hall, L. (ed.), *Sea Saga: Being the Naval Diaries of Four Generations of the King-Hall Family* (London, 1935)

Klein, Herbert S., *The Middle Passage* (Princeton, 1978)

Klein, Herbert S., *The Atlantic Slave Trade* (Cambridge, 2002)

Klein, Herbert S. and Engerman, Stanley L., 'Slave Mortality on British Ships 1791–1797', in Roger Anstey and P.E.H. Hair (eds), *Liverpool, the African Slave Trade and Abolition* (Liverpool, 1976), pp. 113–26

Klein, Herbert S. and Engerman, Stanley L., 'Long-term Trends in African Mortality in the Transatlantic Slave Trade', in David Eltis and David Richardson (eds), *Routes to Slavery: Direction, Ethnicity and Mortality in the Transatlantic Slave Trade* (London, 1997), pp. 36–48

Klein, Herbert S., Engerman, Stanley L., Haines, Robin and Shlomowitz, Ralph, 'Transoceanic Mortality: The Slave Trade in Comparative Perspective', *William and Mary Quarterly*, 58 (2001), pp. 93–117

Knight, R.J.B., 'Politics and Trust in Victualling the Navy, 1793–1815', *Mariner's Mirror*, 94 (2008), pp. 133–49

Lane, Joan, 'The Role of Apprenticeship in Eighteenth-Century Medical Education', in W.F. Bynum and Roy Porter (eds), *William Hunter and the Eighteenth-Century Medical World* (Cambridge, 1985), pp. 57–104

Lawrence, Christopher, 'Disciplining Diseases: Scurvy, the Navy and Imperial Expansion, 1750–1825', in David Miller and Peter Reill (eds), *Visions of Empire: Voyages, Botany, and Representations of Nature* (Cambridge, 1996), pp. 80–106

Lawrence, S.C., *Charitable Knowledge: Hospital Pupils and Practitioners in Eighteenth-Century London* (Cambridge, 1996)

Leveen, E.P., *British Slave Trade Suppression Policies* (New York, 1977)

Lewis, Michael, *The Navy in Transition: A Social History, 1814–1864* (London, 1965)

Lincoln, Margarette, 'The Medical Profession and Representation of the Navy, 1750–1815', in Geoffrey L. Hudson (ed.), *British Military and Naval Medicine, 1600–1830* (Amsterdam, New York, 2007), pp. 201–26

Lind, James, *A Treatise of the Scurvy … and Cure, of that Disease* (Edinburgh, 1753)

Lind, James, *An Essay on the Most Effectual Means of Preserving the Health of Seamen in the Royal Navy* (3rd edn, London, 1774)

Lloyd, C. and Coulter, J.S., *Medicine and the Navy, 1200–1900. Vol. III, 1714–1815* (Edinburgh and London, 1961)

Lloyd, C. and Coulter, J.S., *Medicine and the Navy, 1200–1900. Vol. IV, 1815–1900* (Edinburgh and London, 1963)

Lloyd, Christopher, *The Navy and the Slave Trade* (London, 1949)

Lloyd, Christopher (ed.), *The Health of Seamen: Selections from the Works of Dr James Lind, Sir Gilbert Blane and Dr Thomas Trotter* (London, 1965)

Loudon, Irvine, *Medical Care and the General Practitioner, 1750–1850* (Oxford, 1986)

Lovejoy, Paul E. and Richardson, David, 'Competing Markets for Male and Female Slaves: Slave Prices in the Interior of West Africa, 1780–1850', *International Journal of African Historical Studies*, 28 (1995), pp. 261–93

Lovejoy, Paul E. and Richardson, David, '"This Horrid Hole": Royal Authority, Commerce and Credit at Bonny, 1690–1840', *Journal of African History*, 45 (2004), pp. 363–92

Maehle, A.-H., *Drugs on Trial: Experimental Pharmacology and Therapeutic Innovation in the Eighteenth Century* (Amsterdam, 1999)

Manen, N. van, 'Preventive Medicine in the Dutch Slave Trade, 1747–1797', *International Journal of Maritime History*, 18 (2006), pp. 129–85

Martin, Bernard and Spurrell, Mark (eds), *The Journal of a Slave Trader (John Newton) 1750–1754* (London, 1962)

Maxwell-Stewart, Hamish, 'The Rise and Fall of John Longworth: Work and Punishment in Early Port Arthur', *Tasmanian Historical Studies*, 6 (1999)

Maxwell-Stewart, Hamish, *Closing Hell's Gates: The Death of a Convict Station* (Sydney, 2008)

McBride, W., '"Normal" Medical Science and British Treatment of the Sea Scurvy, 1753–75', *Journal of the History of Medicine and Allied Sciences*, 46 (1991), pp. 160–3

McDonald, J. and Shlomowitz, R., 'Mortality on Convict Voyages to Australia, 1788–1868', *Social Science History*, 13 (1989), pp. 285–313

McIlraith, J., *The Life of Sir John Richardson … Inspector of Naval Hospitals and Fleets, &c.* (London, 1868)

McLean, David, *Public Health and Politics in the Age of Reform: Cholera, the State and the Royal Navy in Victorian Britain* (London, 2006)

McWilliam, James O., *Report on the Fever at Boa Vista* (London, 1847)

McWilliam, James O., *An Exposition of the Case of the Assistant Surgeons of the Royal Navy* (London, 1849)

Middleton, Richard, 'Pitt, Anson and the Admiralty, 1756–61', *History*, 55 (1970), pp. 189–98

Middleton, Richard, 'Naval Administration in the Age of Pitt and Anson, 1755–1763', in J. Black and P. Woodfine (eds), *The British Navy and the Use of Naval Power in the Eighteenth Century* (Leicester, 1988), pp. 109–27

Middleton, Richard, 'British Naval Strategy, 1755–1762: The Western Squadron', *Mariner's Mirror*, 75 (1989), pp. 349–67

Miller, Joseph C., 'Mortality in the Atlantic Slave Trade: Statistical Evidence on Causality', *Journal of Interdisciplinary History*, 11 (1980), pp. 385–434

Morriss, Roger, *Naval Power and British Culture, 1760–1850: Public Trust and Government Ideology* (Aldershot, 2004)

M'William, James O., *Medical History of the Expedition to the Niger during the Years 1841–2, comprising an Account of the Fever which led to its abrupt Termination* (London, 1843)

Northrup, David, *Indentured Labor in the Age of Imperialism, 1834–1922* (Cambridge, 1995)

Pelling, Margaret, *Cholera, Fever and English Medicine, 1825–1865* (Oxford, 1978)

Peterson, J.M., 'Gentlemen and Medical Men: The Problem of Professional Recruitment', *Bulletin of the History of Medicine*, 29 (1985), pp. 138–68

Porter, Roy, 'The Patient's View: Doing Medical History from Below', *Theory and Society*, 14 (1985), pp. 175–98

Postma, Johannes M., *The Dutch in the Atlantic Slave Trade, 1600–1815* (Cambridge 1990)

Pullen, H.F., *The Shannon and the Chesapeake* (Toronto, 1970)

Rasor, E.L., *Reform in the Royal Navy: A Social History of the Lower Deck 1850 to 1880* (Hamden, Conn., 1976)

Rediker, Marcus, *The Slave Ship: A Human History* (London, 2007)

Richardson, David, 'Slave Exports from West and West-Central Africa, 1700–1810: New Estimates of Volume and Distribution', *Journal of African History*, 30 (1989), pp. 1–22

Richardson, David, 'Prices of Slaves in West and West-Central Africa: Toward an Annual Series, 1698–1807', *Bulletin of Economic Research*, 43 (1991), pp. 21–46

Richardson, David, 'Shipboard Revolts, African Authority, and the Atlantic Slave Trade', *William and Mary Quarterly*, 58 (2001), pp. 69–92

Riley, James C., 'Mortality in Long-Distance Voyages in the Eighteenth Century', *Journal of Economic History*, 41 (1981), pp. 651–6

Risse, Guenter, *Hospital Life in Enlightenment Scotland: Care and Teaching at the Royal Infirmary of Edinburgh* (Cambridge, 1986)

Risse, Guenter, 'Britannia Rules the Seas: The Health of Seamen, Edinburgh, 1791–1800', *Journal of the History of Medicine and Allied Sciences*, 43 (1988), pp. 426–46

Rodger, N.A.M., 'Le scorbut dans la Royal Navy pendant la guerre de Sept Ans, 1756–1763', in A. Lottin, J.-C. Hocquet and S. Lebecq (eds), *Les hommes et la mer dans l'Europe du nord-ouest de l'antiquité à nos jours* (*Revue du Nord*, extra number, 1986), pp. 455–62

Rodger, N.A.M., *The Wooden World: An Anatomy of the Georgian Navy* (London, 1988)

Rodger, N.A.M., 'Medicine and Science in the British Navy of the Eighteenth Century', in C. Buchet (ed.), *L'Homme, la santé et la mer* (Paris, 1997), pp. 333–44

Rodger, N.A.M., *The Command of the Ocean: A Naval History of Britain, 1649–1815*, 2nd edn (London, 2005)

Rosner, Lisa, *Medical Education in the Age of Improvement: Edinburgh Students and Apprentices 1760–1828* (Edinburgh, 1991)

Ryan, A.N., 'The Royal Navy and the Blockade of Brest, 1689–1805: Theory and Practice', in M. Acerra, J. Merino and J. Meyer (eds), *Les Marines de guerre européennes, XVII–XVIIIe siècles* (Paris, 1985)

Sheridan, Richard B., 'The Guinea Surgeons on the Middle Passage: The Provision of Medical Service in the British Slave Trade', *International Journal of African Historical Studies*, 14 (1981), pp. 601–25

Shlomowitz, Ralph, 'Mortality and the Pacific Labour Trade', *Journal of Pacific History*, 22 (1987), pp. 34–55

Shlomowitz, Ralph, 'Epidemiology and the Pacific Labor Trade', *Journal of Interdisciplinary History*, 19 (1989), pp. 585–610

Shlomowitz, Ralph, 'Mortality and Voyages of Liberated Africans to the West Indies, 1841–1867', *Slavery and Abolition*, 11 (1990), pp. 30–41

Shlomowitz, Ralph, *Mortality and Migration in the Modern World* (Vermont, 1996)

Shlomowitz, Ralph and Brennan, L., 'Mortality and Migrant Labour en route to Assam, 1863–1924', *Indian Economic and Social History Review*, 27 (1990), pp. 313–30

Shlomowitz, Ralph and Brennan, L., 'Mortality and Indian Labour in Malaya, 1877–1913', *Indian Economic and Social History Review*, 29 (1992), pp. 57–75

Shlomowitz, Ralph and Brennan, L., 'Epidemiology and Indian Labour Migration at Home and Abroad', *Journal of World History*, 5 (1994), pp. 47–67

Shlomowitz, Ralph and McDonald, J., 'Mortality of Indian Labour on Ocean Voyages, 1843–1917', *Studies in History*, 6 (1990), pp. 35–65

Staniforth, M., 'Diet, Disease and Death at Sea on the Voyage to Australia, 1837–1839', *International Journal of Maritime History*, 8 (1996), pp. 119–56

Steckel, Richard H. and Jensen, Richard A., 'New Evidence on the Causes of Slave and Crew Mortality in the Atlantic Slave Trade', *Journal of Economic History*, 46 (1986), pp. 57–77

Stevenson, C., *Medicine and Magnificence: British Hospital and Asylum Architecture, 1660–1815* (London, 2000)

Swinton, Jane, *Journal of a Voyage with Coolie Emigrants, from Calcutta to Trinidad* (London, 1859)

Syrett, D., 'The Methodology of British Amphibious Operations during the Seven Years and American Wars', *Mariner's Mirror*, 58 (1972), pp. 269–80

Thomas, Hugh, *The Slave Trade: The History of the Atlantic Slave Trade, 1440–1870* (London, 1997)

Thursfield, H.G. (ed.), *Five Naval Journals, 1789–1817* (London, 1951)

Tinker, Hugh, *A New System of Slavery: The Export of Indian Labour Overseas, 1830–1920* (London, 1974)

Tröhler, U., *'To Improve the Evidence of Medicine': The Eighteenth-Century British Origins of a Critical Approach* (Edinburgh, 2000)

Trotter, Thomas, *Observations on the Scurvy: With a Review of the Opinions Lately Advanced on that Disease, and a New Theory Defended* (2nd edn, London, 1792)

Trotter, Thomas, *A Practicable Plan for Manning the Royal Navy, and Preserving our Maritime Ascendency, without Impressment: Addressed to Admiral Lord Viscount Exmouth, K.G.B.* (Newcastle, 1819)

Turnbull, William B., *The Naval Surgeon: Comprising the Entire Duties of Professional Men at Sea. To which are Subjoined, a System of Naval Surgery, and a Compendious Pharmacopoeia* (London, 1806)

Watt, James, 'Some Forgotten Contributions of Naval Surgeons', *Journal of the Royal Society of Medicine*, 78 (1985), pp. 758–62

Watt, James, 'Nelsonian Medicine in Context', *Journal of the Royal Naval Medical Service*, 86 (2000), pp. 64–71

Watt, James, 'The Health of Seamen in Anti-Slavery Squadrons', *Mariner's Mirror*, 88 (2002), pp. 69–78

Watt, James, 'Surgery at Trafalgar', *Mariner's Mirror*, 91 (2005), pp. 266–83

Worboys, Michael, 'The Emergence of Tropical Medicine: A Study in the Establishment of a Scientific Speciality', in G. Lemaine *et al.* (eds), *Perspectives on the Emergence of Scientific Disciplines* (The Hague, 1977), pp. 76–98

Index